Evidence Synthesis
for Decision Making in Healthcare

Statistics in Practice

Series Advisors

Human and Biological Sciences
Stephen Senn
CRP-Santé, Luxembourg

Earth and Environmental Sciences
Marian Scott
University of Glasgow, UK

Industry, Commerce and Finance
Wolfgang Jank
University of Maryland, USA

Statistics in Practice is an important international series of texts which provide detailed coverage of statistical concepts, methods and worked case studies in specific fields of investigation and study.

With sound motivation and many worked practical examples, the books show in down-to-earth terms how to select and use an appropriate range of statistical techniques in a particular practical field within each title's special topic area.

The books provide statistical support for professionals and research workers across a range of employment fields and research environments. Subject areas covered include medicine and pharmaceutics; industry, finance and commerce; public services; the earth and environmental sciences, and so on.

The books also provide support to students studying statistical courses applied to the above areas. The demand for graduates to be equipped for the work environment has led to such courses becoming increasingly prevalent at universities and colleges.

It is our aim to present judiciously chosen and well-written workbooks to meet everyday practical needs. Feedback of views from readers will be most valuable to monitor the success of this aim.

A complete list of titles in this series can be found at
www.wiley.com/go/statisticsinpractice

Evidence Synthesis for Decision Making in Healthcare

Nicky J. Welton
School of Social and Community Medicine
University of Bristol, UK

Alexander J. Sutton
Nicola J. Cooper
Keith R. Abrams
Department of Health Sciences
University of Leicester, UK

A.E. Ades
School of Social and Community Medicine
University of Bristol, UK

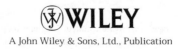
A John Wiley & Sons, Ltd., Publication

This edition first published 2012
© 2012 John Wiley & Sons, Ltd

Registered office
John Wiley & Sons Ltd., The Atrium, Southern Gate, Chichester, West Sussex, PO19 8SQ,
United Kingdom

For details of our global editorial offices, for customer services and for information about how to apply
for permission to reuse the copyright material in this book please see our website at www.wiley.com.

Library of Congress Cataloging-in-Publication Data

Evidence synthesis for decision making in healthcare / Nicky J. Welton . . . [et al.].
     p. ; cm.
  Includes bibliographical references and index.
  ISBN 978-0-470-06109-1 (cloth)
  I. Welton, Nicky J.
  [DNLM: 1. Decision Support Techniques. 2. Statistics as Topic. 3. Evidence-Based
Medicine–economics. 4. Models, Statistical. WB 102.5]

  362.1068′4–dc23

                                                                2011051684

A catalogue record for this book is available from the British Library.

ISBN: 978-0-470-06109-1

Typeset in 10/12pt Times by Laserwords Private Limited, Chennai, India.
Printed and bound in Singapore by Markono Print Media Pte Ltd.

Contents

Preface

This book is intended to be used in a wide variety of ways. The book will serve as an introduction to evidence synthesis, leading from relatively simple to intermediate level examples. Everything is set within a Bayesian framework, and within a decision-making context, and for those unfamiliar with either of these fields this book should provide a useful introduction. At the same time, the book can be simply taken as a treatise on evidence synthesis.

The book provides a practical guide on how to carry out meta-analyses, indirect comparisons and mixed treatment comparisons in a decision-making context. Through a series of illustrative examples, it also outlines a general approach to synthesis which can be applied to a very wide range of evidence structures, including multiple outcomes, epidemiological models, and the role of observational studies of treatment efficacy. The methods are designed to be fully compatible with National Institute of Health and Clinical Excellence (NICE) methods guidance in the sense that, if built into a decision model, they deliver a probabilistic decision analysis. NICE methods guidance is relatively nonprescriptive; it is also regularly reviewed and in a process of continuous development. We cannot therefore say that certain forms of analysis are 'approved' for use in NICE submissions. However, we can say that the kinds of analysis suggested will be understood by those who are tasked with making evidence-based recommendations about new health technologies as valid ways of statistically combining available evidence.

Statisticians, even those who are experienced in meta-analysis, will find that unfamiliar questions will be asked about how to statistically combine evidence on different parameters that are related through an underlying model. This will lead to further questions about the consistency of evidence. These are related to, but differ from, questions of model fit and influence that might arise in, say, a regression analysis.

It is those with a background in health economics or decision modelling who are likely to find the greatest challenges to their established modus operandi. This is because we have turned a large portion of the decision model into an essentially statistical exercise. Models will *not* be just 'populated' with values from the literature. Instead, we will require demonstrations that models actually *fit* the data. External validation will be turned into a relatively formal question of evidence consistency. Finally, because the methods faithfully convert uncertainty in evidence into uncertainty in the decision, it becomes worthwhile to pay closer attention to the assessment of uncertainty. This demands greater emphasis on criteria for evidence inclusion and exclusion than is often seen in decision models, and sensitivity of results to data.

We also intend the book to provide a practical introduction to Bayesian thinking and to WinBUGS, albeit in a somewhat restricted context, and readers should emerge with a reasonable working understanding of Bayesian hierarchical models. A great advantage of WinBUGS is that its entire syntax can be inferred from even the simplest example. In theory, a reader armed with a single WinBUGS program, together with the lists of functions and distributions in the online manual 'knows' the software in its entirety. This contrasts with certain procedure-based statistical packages which may never be fully mastered in a lifetime! Readers interested in Bayesian data analysis more broadly, of course, will need to study a far wider range of examples in order to be able to use WinBUGS to its full extent.

The intended audience for the book, is, therefore, mixed – just like the participants who have attended the course (of the same name) on which this book is based: decision modellers, health economists, and statisticians who are involved in producing assessments of new interventions for governmental bodies, insurance companies or manufacturers; and academics, students and employees of governments or pharmaceutical companies. Based on experience with the course, we believe the book will also be of interest to people in senior or management roles, who may not wish to learn 'how to' skills for WinBUGS, but who have a responsibility to manage the production of technical assessments, who need to know what these new methods can and cannot accomplish. Similarly, those with an interest in the production of systematic reviews will also find much that is both new and highly relevant to their work.

There are some 'prerequisites' in terms of the statistical knowledge or mathematical skills. We assume a basic understanding of methods such as logistic regression and the concepts of interaction and confounding. Readers who plan to use the book to help learn WinBUGS are strongly encouraged to download the software, and work through the online tutorial and the BLOCKER example before taking on other examples.

This book includes an accompanying website. Please visit www.wiley.com/go/decision_making_healthcare

1

Introduction

This book is at heart about a fusion of ideas from medical statistics, clinical epidemiology, decision analysis, and health economics. These are distinct academic disciplines, each with its own history and perspectives. Recently, though, developments within these separate fields, together with political changes across the developed world in attitudes to funding public services, have conspired to bring particular strands of thought from each of these disciplines together in a fruitful and compelling way. Before describing the contents of the book, we shall therefore start with a look at these wider developments. This contextual background has two purposes. It will give readers from each discipline an essential introduction to the others, but it will also explain why this book has come about.

1.1 The rise of health economics

The last 20 years has witnessed an enormous change in how new medical technology is deployed. Previously, clinicians were free to treat their patients in whatever way seemed best. The perceived efficacy or treatments, taking account of course the risk of adverse side effects, was the dominant factor. In countries with a centralised state-funded health service there were clearly budget constraints, which could be realised through limits on the numbers of hospitals, doctors or nurses. But the idea that health care itself should be *rationed* would not only have been regarded as politically infeasible, but was rejected by the medical professions as a threat to 'clinical freedom'.

Clinical freedom, placing no limit on the costs of health care, is an open invitation to pharmaceutical and medical device manufacturers to enter the market place with a stream of genuinely new products and 'me-too' products. Eventually, both nationalised and insurance-based health systems have had to find ways of curtailing

Evidence Synthesis for Decision Making in Healthcare, First Edition. Nicky J. Welton,
Alexander J. Sutton, Nicola J. Cooper, Keith R. Abrams and A.E. Ades.
© 2012 John Wiley & Sons, Ltd. Published 2012 by John Wiley & Sons, Ltd.

clinical freedom by considering not only the clinical efficacy of new procedures, but also their economic implications. The numbers of economic evaluations has mushroomed accordingly, and in many countries including the UK, Netherlands, France and Germany, the introduction of new clinical treatments as well as new screening programmes is routinely accompanied by some form of economic analysis.

Economic analyses have been subdivided into *cost-benefit, cost-effectiveness* and *cost-utility analyses*. All compare the costs of an intervention with the 'outcomes'. Cost-benefit considers benefits as seen by the recipients of the intervention, and as they would be evaluated in cash terms. Cost-effectiveness studies compare costs and 'effects' measured for example as the number of patients cured, or the average weight-loss measured in kilograms. Cost utility is similar, but the 'effects' are measured in Quality Adjusted Life Years (QALYs) or Disability Adjusted Life Years (DALYs). The output of all these forms of analysis tends to be a ratio measure of the additional costs of the intervention divided by the additional benefits, effects, or utilities. In cost-effectiveness analysis this is called the Incremental Cost-Effectiveness Ratio (ICER).

There is one particular form of economic analysis, net benefit analysis [1, 2], that has had a major influence on the field. Its advent has opened the way for many of the developments described in this book, but it also reveals a great deal about how public attitudes have changed. Net Benefit analysis unifies the three approaches by translating the utilities into their money 'values' using an exchange rate λ, which is simply the money value attributed to the unit of health gain. If U is the lifetime utility of some intervention and C its lifetime cost, the Net Benefit is: $U\lambda - C$. If we now agree to always use QALYs to represent the measure U, Net Benefit immediately becomes a very powerful decision-making tool:

- First, health planners can, in principle, evaluate any intervention on the same level playing field: dialysis for end-stage renal disease, herceptin for breast cancer, group counselling for smoking cessation, or newborn screening for sickle cell disease.

- Secondly, planners can choose rationally between alternative treatment strategies for the same condition by selecting the one with the highest net benefit, S^*:

$$NB(s) = U(s)\lambda - C(s)$$
$$S^* = ArgMax_s(NB(s))$$

(1.1)

Here, the function $ArgMax_s$ picks out the strategy s which yields the highest Net Benefit.

- Finally there is its mathematical convenience. We avoid the difficulties associated with ratios of costs and benefits/effects/utilities (for example, how does one interpret a negative ICER?), and instead can deal with a single quantity, Net Benefit, on a well-understood scale. This will become particularly useful when we consider uncertainty (Section 1.2).

Under this regime, health economic evaluation becomes a *modelling* exercise. Based on the evidence available, a model of the disease process under each of the interventions of interest, s, is constructed in order to arrive at values of $U(s)$ and $C(s)$. We are left, in effect, with a *decision analysis* and we will shortly turn to see how the methods routinely used in *operations research* can be used to carry this out.

However, the legitimacy of this entire exercise (and indeed much of this book!) rests on whether defensible values of λ and U can be arrived at. We would be misleading readers who are unfamiliar with health economics if we were anything but frank about the foundations that this book rests on. We shall summarise the situation briefly.

To set λ a decision maker must answer a question that sounds very simple, but which is in fact profoundly difficult: how much am I willing to pay to gain one QALY for a single patient? One way to justify a range of figures is to consider a wide selection of noncontroversial, accepted interventions, and to look at the QALY gain, net of costs, that they appear to confer. Exercises of this sort [3] offer a benchmark range of figures against which proposed new interventions can be assessed. For many years, officials at the Department of Health (London, UK) have considered that interventions that gain one QALY at a cost of £10 000 would be 'a bargain', while those that cost over £30 000 would be 'too expensive', but these figures were never made officially public. However, it is public knowledge that the National Institute for Health and Clinical Excellence (NICE) in the UK, uses a range of $\lambda = £20\,000 - 30\,000$ as a benchmark to decide whether new technologies should be adopted by the National Health Service. The fact that this is openly known illustrates that, even if the British public are not yet aware that their health is being valued this way, at least British policy makers have owned up to what they are doing. Ten years ago, if these ideas were presented to a British audience there would still be angry challenges from clinicians. Now, the reality of health care rationing in this form is unlikely to raise any complaints. At the same time, it is only fair to acknowledge that the entire basis for decision making that this assumes is far from being accepted by all health economists. To some extent the opposition is based on philosophical considerations underpinning health economic theory [4]. The controversy is also fuelled by the considerable doubts about how QALYs are measured [5]. It is important to recognise that patients, clinicians, decision analysts, decision makers are, quite rightly, openly sceptical about whether existing measures and methods really allow us to put treatments for Alzheimer's disease on the same basis as cancer drugs, or whether cancer treatment can be in any way equated to newborn screening. But, in spite of these doubts, decisions still have to be made, and if they cannot be made on a perfect basis, they must be made on the best basis that current methods will permit. The attempt to create the 'level playing field' may not have succeeded in flattening all the dips and lumps in the grass – it may never do so. However, the commitment to the aspiration may be more important than the success – or even the feasibility – of its execution.

1.2   Decision making under uncertainty

1.2.1   Deterministic models

Once the concept of Net Benefit is accepted, decision modelling *in principle* becomes an essentially mechanical exercise. (Only in principle, as the question of where the parameter values come from – a major focus of this book – is far from simple.) The Net Benefit of each alternative strategy is calculated and the decision maker simply chooses the strategy with the highest net benefit. The nature of the task can be made plain by a *decision tree*. The example in Figure 1.1 shows a *choice node* between two strategies for managing a particular condition. The choice node is depicted as a small square. Each strategy corresponds to a treatment. Standard Treatment 1 has a probability p_1 of success, new Treatment 2 has probability p_2. These probabilities would hopefully be based on evidence from Randomised Controlled Trials (RCTs) (see Section 1.3). To complete the tree we need only add the (lifetime) costs C_1, C_2 and QALYs attaching to treatment success U^+ and treatment failure U^-.

Note the assumption that the QALYs attaching to each strategy are based solely on the proportion of patients experiencing 'success', not on the treatment itself. This assumption is not required.

$$NB_1 = \lambda[p_1 U^+ + (1 - p_1)U^-] - C_1$$
$$NB_2 = \lambda[p_2 U^+ + (1 - p_2)U^-] - C_2$$

(1.2)

Economic evaluation (Section 1.1) is concerned with a comparative analysis of the available options. The critical measure is therefore the Incremental Net Benefit (INB). This leads to an important simplification:

$$INB = NB_2 - NB_1$$
$$= \lambda[(p_2 - p_1)(U^+ - U^-)] - (C_2 - C_1)$$

(1.3)

$$= \lambda \Delta_p \Delta_U - \Delta_C$$

The INB of new Treatment 2 compared with standard Treatment 1 can be expressed in terms of the *difference* Δ_p in the probabilities of successful treatment, the QALY *difference* Δ_U between the success and failure outcomes, and the cost difference Δ_C. The ambitious data collection project required to identify the absolute lifetime costs and lifetime QALYs under each treatment is reduced to the far simpler – though still difficult – task of finding differences between the treatments. The epidemiologist is therefore still in familiar territory. All the parameters can be informed by controlled, i.e. comparative, studies. Δ_p in particular can be informed by an RCT. The decision now depends on whether INB is positive (NB_2 is greater than NB_1, choose new Treatment 2) or not (choose standard Treatment 1).

It is worth noting that the results of the economic evaluation will depend on the treatment difference on the absolute probability scale. This contrasts with the ratio measures – Odds Ratio, Risk Ratio or Hazard Ratio – that are typically reported

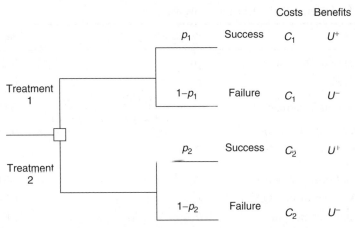

Figure 1.1   A simple decision tree with two treatment options, a binary (success/failure) outcome, and costs C for each treatment and utilities U for each outcome.

in RCTs, and the Log Odds Ratios (LORs), Log Risk Ratios and Log Hazard Ratios commonly used in meta-analysis (see Section 1.3). The decision analyst is therefore likely to need to map from the ratio quantities familiar from clinical epidemiology into the absolute quantities required for economic analysis. For example, one will need to transform information on a LOR δ into information on p_2 at a specified p_1:

$$\delta = \frac{\text{logit}(p_2)}{\text{logit}(p_1)}$$

$$p_2 = \frac{\exp(\text{logit}(p_1) + \delta)}{1 + \exp(\text{logit}(p_1) + \delta)} \qquad (1.4)$$

$$\Delta_p = \frac{\exp(\text{logit}(p_1) + \delta)}{1 + \exp(\text{logit}(p_1) + \delta)} - p_1$$

Finally, then, substituting this expression for Δ_p back into Equation (1.3), INB emerges as a function of $p_1, \delta, \Delta_U, \Delta_C$. Given values for these inputs, we can derive values for p_2, and then for Δ_p, and finally for *INB*. This is illustrated in Table 1.1. Given the inputs provided, the INB of Treatment 2 compared with Treatment 1 is £4795. This is above zero, so Treatment 2 emerges as the optimal strategy.

Figure 1.1 represents a particularly simple situation. In applications, the decision trees downstream and upstream of the treatment can become far more extensive. Frequently they may include a Markov model of disease progression (Chapter 10). These consist of a series of states representing different stages of illness. Probability or rate parameters describe the expected numbers of transitions from one state to another in a given time period.

Table 1.1   Deterministic decision analysis.

Parameter	Symbol	Value
Pr(success) on Treatment 1	p_1	0.25
Log Odds Ratio	δ	0.8
Pr(success) on Treatment 2	$p_2 = \dfrac{\exp(\text{logit}(p_1) + \delta)}{1 + \exp(\text{logit}(p_1) + \delta)}$	0.425897
Difference in Pr(success)	$\Delta_p = p_2 - p_1$	0.175897
QALY gain for successful outcome	Δ_U	2
Incremental cost Treatment 2	Δ_C	£4000
Monetary value of one QALY	λ	£25 000
Incremental Net Benefit	$INB = \lambda\Delta_p\Delta_U - \Delta_C$	£4794.838

1.2.2   Probabilistic decision modelling

The previous section laid out what has been called a *deterministic* decision model. It takes no account of uncertainty in the parameter values. Of course, the analyst is free to vary the input parameters to see whether this will reverse the sign of the INB and thus change the decision. Perhaps the confidence intervals on the original published parameter estimates, $p_1, \delta, \Delta_U, \Delta_C$, would be used to guide the choice of input parameters in a *deterministic sensitivity analysis*. There are a number of difficulties with the deterministic approach to analysing uncertainty [6]. First, there are usually far too many parameters for one to try out all the combinations. Secondly, the decision maker would usually like to know, in view of the uncertainty in the input parameters, whether a decision based on INB is secure. A deterministic procedure does not actually deliver a clear, interpretable metric. Finally, once we admit uncertainty in parameters, a deterministic procedure may not even guarantee to deliver the correct decision, as we will see below.

To take account of parameter uncertainty, each parameter is characterised by a probability distribution. For example, the probability of success on standard treatment p_1 might be characterised as a Beta distribution (see Appendix 2), which is the natural choice for probabilities. If it is based on a particular study where 10 successful outcomes were observed in 40 patients, a Beta(10,30) distribution would be appropriate. Typically, information on p_2 is introduced indirectly, via the LOR δ, as shown in Equation (1.4), δ would be assigned a normal distribution with a mean and variance taken from the meta-analysis. Table 1.2 sets out all the parameters needed to define INB, together with their probability distributions.

Because INB is a function of these parameters, it now also has a probability distribution. It can be shown that, under conditions of uncertainty, the optimal decision is based on the *expected net benefit*. The expectation, of course, is over the parameters $p_1, \delta, \Delta_U, \Delta_C$; in other words, we must average the INB over all the values of the input parameters. Writing INB as a function of parameters, the decision will be based on the expectation:

$$E[INB(p_1, \delta, \Delta_U, \Delta_C)] \tag{1.5}$$

The simplest way to carry out this integration is via Monte Carlo simulation. Values are drawn from the distributions of each of the input parameters, and INB is evaluated for each set of input parameter values. This is done thousands of times, creating in numerical form a *distribution* of INB (Figure 1.2). The analyst can then compute the mean of all these samples, to be used as an estimate of expected INB (Equation (1.5)), and can also examine the variance and centiles.

Monte Carlo simulation has formed the basis for probabilistic decision analysis [7, 8] for many years, as it has for modelling in general throughout the physical, biological and social sciences. It is important to note, however, that besides providing us with an analysis of *uncertainty*, probabilistic analysis has the further advantage that it gives a correct computation of expected INB under uncertainty, namely Equation (1.5). A deterministic analysis is almost invariably based on the mean values of the input parameters.

$$INB(E[p_1], E[\delta], E[\Delta_U], \Delta_C) \tag{1.6}$$

But the mean of a function of parameters (Equation (1.5)) is not necessarily equal to the same function applied to the parameter means (Equation (1.6)). This 'short-cut' computation of the mean of a function of parameters is correct under certain special circumstances: the function must be *linear* in all parameters (or multi-linear), and the parameters must not be correlated. In this particular example these conditions are not met. INB is linear in p_1 and Δ_U, but it is *not* linear in δ, as in evident from Equation (1.4). In this example the expected INB from the probabilistic analysis is £4871, nearly 2% higher than the deterministic analysis – not a huge amount, but enough to illustrate the point.

We may also compute a probability that the optimal decision based on the evidence inputs is the correct decision: this is simply the area to the right of the point of neutrality, $INB=0$. In our example, this probability is 0.64. There is a 36% chance therefore that the optimal decision is the wrong decision. This statement may sound nonsensical to some: if so, imagine that if all uncertainty was eliminated, the

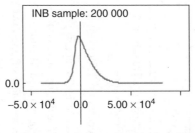

Figure 1.2   Distribution of Incremental Net Benefit, based on 200 000 samples from a Monte Carlo simulation.

Table 1.2 Probabilistic decision analysis, based on 100 000 Monte Carlo simulations. We distinguish between the true mean of the input distribution and the estimate based on the simulation.

Parameter	Symbol	Distribution	Mean	Estimated mean (95% CI) from simulation
Pr(success) on Treatment 1	p_1	Beta(10,30)	0.25	0.2501 (0.13, 0.39)
Log Odds Ratio	δ	Normal(0.8,0.7²)	0.8	0.8002 (−0.5766, 2.171)
Pr(success) on Treatment 2	$p_2 = \dfrac{\exp(\text{logit}(p_1) + \delta)}{1 + \exp(\text{logit}(p_1) + \delta)}$			0.4278 (0.1308, 0.7710)
Difference in Pr(success)	$\Delta_p = p_2 - p_1$			0.1776 (−0.08876, 0.4836)
QALY gain for successful outcome	Δ_U	Normal(2,0.5)	2	0.1998 (0.6171, 3.378)
Incremental cost Treatment 2	Δ_C	Constant	£4000	
Monetary value of one QALY	λ	Constant	£25000	
Incremental Net Benefit	$INB = \lambda \Delta_p \Delta_U - \Delta_C$			4871 (−8442, 25120)

variance of INB would be zero, and the probability of making a 'wrong' decision would be zero. Deterministic sensitivity analysis tends to be used to answer the question 'what if this (these) parameter(s) took this (these) value(s)?', but it fails to pay much attention to how likely the various scenarios are. The probabilistic approach allows us to take the extent of parameter uncertainty much more seriously. The uncertainty in the input parameters is *propagated* faithfully through the model, to be faithfully reflected in the uncertainty in the decision.

1.3 Evidence-based medicine

Evidence-Based Medicine (EBM) has taken the form of a 'movement'. While it would seem to be almost a truism that clinical practice should be based on 'evidence', the EBM movement has grown up alongside the ideas of *systematic review*. The essential insight is that any review of the literature on, for example, the effect of Treatment 2 compared with Treatment 1, must have a defined *protocol*, with a clear rationale for inclusion and exclusion of studies. The aim is to prevent arbitrary selection of studies and put the process of deriving a summary estimate of the treatment effect on an objective and repeatable basis. At the same time, careful and thorough searching of literature would strengthen the summary estimate, reducing uncertainty [9].

The EBM movement has also been concerned with grading the quality of evidence. Direct RCT evidence on clinical end-points is graded as superior to evidence from observational studies, or evidence of surrogate end-points, or indirect evidence of various kinds. A 'hierarchy of evidence' has been established [10]. Further quality assessment is undertaken within each the category of studies: for example, studies of disease prevalence, or studies of diagnostic tests, are also graded on their own specific quality criteria. In general, evidence of the highest grade available is used.

EBM has been a response to the massive increase in the sheer volume of evidence. Its insistence that every systematic review must have a clear *method* governing study inclusion and exclusion, translates directly into the purposes of this book. Putting it into our terms, there must be a clear method underlying the selection of evidence to inform every model parameter. There can be no arbitrary selection or exclusion of evidence. But, having said what we would share with EBM, we must also be explicit about where we differ.

First, the position taken in this book tends to be more inclusive about evidence. We would generally argue that evidence of different sorts should be 'synthesised', that is statistically combined within a single coherent model. Methods for carrying out this kind of synthesis are discussed in Chapters 7–10. While certain studies or types of evidence may be definitely or potentially biased, we would see it as wrong to treat them as totally irrelevant. Our preference would therefore be to include them, but to explicitly account for and adjust biases (see Chapter 11). However, the broader question of what evidence to include or exclude deserves much greater discussion than we can give it in this book.

Secondly, we would probably go further in the analysis of study-specific bias than is typical in a Cochrane review. The desire to make systematic reviews repeatable and objective is worthy, but it has given rise to the unrealistic belief that the review process and the construction of the summary measure can be mechanised to the extent that any computer-literate person can do it. Our view is that no economic analysis can be undertaken without considerable input from individuals with clinical and epidemiological expertise in the relevant areas. The subjective element cannot be eliminated. Indeed, there is no reason to eliminate it: instead – and in fact very much in line with EBM core procedures – the analysis of study-specific bias, and the elicitation of expert opinion could be put on a far more systematic basis [11].

A third, related, point of difference has to do with the concept of 'summary measure'. In Cochrane reviews, the summary measure tends to be seen as a 'summary of the literature', and meta-analysis is simply seen as a process that produces it. Our view is, again, a little different because 'summary of the literature' does not exactly capture what an economic assessment requires. The decision maker has a specific target population and a specific protocol in mind. What the decision analyst therefore requires is an estimate of, for example, the treatment effect in this particular group with this specific protocol. Very possibly, there may be no evidence that addresses this precise question, but there may be quite a lot of evidence from possibly imperfect studies using *similar* protocols in *similar* patients. The evidence synthesis task is then to take account of both internal biases, and the possibility that the target parameter may differ from the parameters estimated in the studies available. Input from knowledgeable experts and clinicians is obviously essential. At the same time of course, meta-analysis is not just a procedure that is applied to a bunch of studies to derive a summary: it is a set of statistical models. Statisticians have a large toolbox for evaluating models, and we will be opening this box regularly in Chapters 6 and 8–10. This introduces a statistical element to decision modelling that most decision modellers will be unfamiliar with.

Finally, EBM has spawned evidence-based decision making and evidence-based policy. In the UK, even government ministers make frequent reference to the 'evidence base' in their response to each public health emergency that confronts them. At first sight this seems wholly laudable. However, closer examination reveals a belief that one can go directly from 'evidence' to decision. Our view would be that the role of evidence is to inform a *model*. Even when the evidence appears to arise from studies that seem to replicate exactly the decision question at hand, there is still an implicit model that relates the historical evidence to what would be expected to happen following a decision to be made in the future. In fact the expression 'evidence-based modelling' would not be out of place in the title of this book.

1.4   Bayesian statistics

The first defining feature of the Bayesian approach is the focus on parameter uncertainty, or more generally how we can draw inferences about uncertain parameters given the data, rather than what we can say about the likelihood of the data at specific values of the parameters. It is evident from the discussion of decision making under uncertainty (Section 1.2) that the exercise this book is embarked on is necessarily going to be a Bayesian exercise, and this has been widely recognised [12, 13].

However, the way the example in Section 1.2 was presented is somewhat ambiguous regarding the second major defining feature of Bayesian data analysis, the updating of prior distributions with data to form posterior distributions (see Chapter 2). The approach adopted in Section 1.2, which corresponds to what is done in the vast majority of probabilistic decision models, makes no explicit mention of prior distributions being updated to form posteriors. What has happened is this: the evidence on each parameter has been summarised and characterised as a distribution. This is followed by 'forward' Monte Carlo simulation from what could be considered 'informative priors' (see Sections 3.5 and 8.1).

There is nothing inherently wrong with this, except that we are forced to treat each parameter as an independent item. This severely limits the way evidence can be used, and eventually would even limit *which* evidence can be used. A full use of Bayesian methodology, providing us with posterior distributions, will allow us to be much more flexible in our use of data. In particular, we will be able to combine evidence on parameters, such as in Table 1.1, with indirect evidence, and with evidence on complex functions of the parameters (Chapter 8–10). The decision context actually *requires* a Bayesian posterior analysis just because this is the only way to make sure that all available evidence will be included.

Until recently, Bayesian analysis, except in particularly simple circumstances, was accessible only to those with considerable mathematical and computing skills. The situation has dramatically changed with the recent the arrival of flexible Markov Chain Monte Carlo (MCMC) software in the form of WinBUGS [14]. Models that previously would have presented intractable difficulties can be estimated conveniently by users with relatively little mathematical knowledge. Even so, we must warn readers that Bayesian estimation with WinBUGS requires a degree of care and thought that goes beyond the use of standard frequentist software. In the decision-making context of this book, however, MCMC methods have the very obvious attraction of being simulation based. MCMC therefore allows us to replace simulation from unrelated prior distributions by simulation from a joint posterior parameter distribution. Immediately, we can now integrate the statistical estimation step with the calculation of net benefit in a single, one-step process (Chapter 7). Furthermore rather than propagate evidence uncertainty 'forward' from parameter distributions, we propagate it 'back' from data, onto parameters, then forward through the decision model.

1.5 NICE

In England and Wales the National Institute for Health and Clinical Excellence (NICE), has the responsibility to decide whether new interventions will be reimbursed by the National Health Service. NICE is one of many similar bodies worldwide though it was regarded by the World Health Organisation as pre-eminent in 2003. The role of NICE is to ensure that new products and procedures are properly appraised before being introduced. The purpose is both to limit expenditure, but, equally importantly to stop what had come to be called the 'postcode lottery', by which the treatments that patients received simply depended on which hospital they attended.

NICE's procedures emphasise transparency. Because its decisions are scrutinised by manufacturers, clinicians' professional organisations, and the Department of Health – as well as being open to public inspection – transparency of method is essential to maintain credibility and to create a process in which stakeholders who may on occasions have fundamentally different objectives can nevertheless participate and reach a degree of consensus. Once the specific decision question is set, specifying the patient group, the new technology and the comparator technologies, manufacturers are invited to make submissions which include analyses of the efficacy and cost-effectiveness of the products in question. Or, if multiple new technologies are to be compared, a Technical Assessment Report is produced by one of the academic units contracted to undertake this kind of work. This includes an independent assessment of efficacy and cost-effectiveness, as well as a review of previous cost-effectiveness analyses and of the manufacturers' submission.

NICE methods guidelines [15] bring together all the key elements described above: economic analyses are generally based on net benefit analysis; probabilistic decision analysis is the expected primary analysis, and clear reasons must be advanced if submissions depart from this; submissions adhere to the general principles of 'hierarchy of evidence', with explicit protocols for the literature search and study inclusion or exclusion. Many submissions include Bayesian evidence synthesis with simulation from a posterior distribution in WinBUGS.

1.6   Structure of the book

Each chapter includes running worked examples, and ends with suggestions for further reading, and exercises. The further reading suggestions are carefully selected to lead readers into slightly more complex syntheses, as well as to provide a broader exposure to the important issues which must be addressed in cost-effectiveness modelling, but which we cannot cover in this book. The full WinBUGS code for all the examples and exercises, as well as solutions, are available from the publisher's website www.wiley.com/go/decision_making_healthcare. Sections with more advanced material, and more difficult exercises, are asterisked.

Chapter 2 introduces Bayesian reasoning and explains why it is suited to decision modelling. It also provides an introduction into the practical use of the WinBUGS software. Chapter 3 introduces deterministic and stochastic decision models and how cost-effectiveness acceptability curves can be constructed. Chapter 4 describes a Bayesian approach to fixed and then random effects meta-analysis for pairs of treatments, which is then extended to meta-regression and the use of baseline as a covariate in Chapter 5. Chapter 6 asks how users can evaluate meta-analysis models, and what issues to consider when choosing between Fixed and Random Effects models. Chapter 7 shows how the synthesis methods developed this far can be embedded within cost-effectiveness analyses.

Chapters 8 and 9 take two different evidence structures in turn, epidemiological models, then mixed and indirect treatment comparisons, and introduce multi-parameter evidence synthesis techniques. These all involve simultaneous estimation using 'direct' evidence on model parameters *and* 'indirect' evidence on functions of model parameters. Chapter 10 introduces WinBUGS programming for Markov models of disease progression. Chapter 11 takes on the challenge represented by data that is relevant, but potentially biased – such as observational studies of treatment efficacy. Chapter 12 briefly describes Expected Value of Information analysis, and gives some guidance on how this can be computed in the presence of the complex correlations between parameters that are induced by multi-parameter evidence synthesis.

The book includes a listing of all abbreviations used (Appendix 1), and a guide to common distributions (Appendix 2).

1.7   Summary key points

Developments in several distinct fields have coalesced to create an environment for the development of the methods described in this book.

• In health economics Net Benefit analysis has put health gains and costs on the same basis, and creating an environment where Bayesian Expected Value decision making can be carried out.

• Probabilistic decision modelling became the preferred way to evaluate cost-effectiveness analyses, as it faithfully maps parameter uncertainty into decision uncertainty, and correctly delivers Expected Net Benefit.

• EBM insists on a protocol for inclusion and exclusion of evidence in reviews and summary measures, and has acted to generally raise awareness of issues around the quality of evidence, and thus the uncertainty in estimates derived from it.

• Simultaneously, the development of Bayesian MCMC methods has made Bayesian data analysis routinely accessible, and dovetails exactly with the growing popularity of probabilistic cost-effectiveness models.

1.8   Further reading

Statisticians seeking a more rounded idea of health economics could consult Hunink *et al.* [16] or Briggs *et al.* [17] could be used as a good introduction to medical decision modelling.

Health economists and decision modellers interested in Bayesian statistics and its implications are recommended Spiegelhalter *et al.* [18]. Standard textbooks on Bayesian methods are: Berry [19], O'Hagan and Luce [20] and Lee [21].

The philosophy behind the Evidence-Based Movement is well captured in a series of papers 'Users Guide to the Medical Literature' [10, 22–27]. The dominant force in EBM methodology is the Cochrane Collaboration handbook [28]. For some recent literature that raises more open questions about evidence inclusion, Cooper *et al.* [29] can be consulted. A completely different approach to grading studies, which is fully compatible with the approach taken in this book, can be found in Turner *et al.* [11].

In line with its policy of complete transparency, all NICE guidelines and guidance, as well as the vast majority of the submitted evidence, can be found on the NICE website. Readers may find the methods guidelines of particular interest [15].

References

1. Claxton K., Posnett J. An economic approach to clinical trial design and research priority-setting. *Health Economics* 1996;**5**:513–524.

2. Stinnett A., Mullahy J. Net health benefits: a new framework for the analysis of uncertainty in cost-effectiveness analyses. *Medical Decision Making* 1998;**18**: S68–S80.

3. Laupacis A., Feeny D., Detsky A.S., Tugwell P.X. How attractive does a new technology have to be to warrant adoption and utilization? Tentative guidelines for using clinical and economic evaulations. *Canadian Medical Association Journal* 1992;**146**: 473–481.

4. Coast J. Is economic evaluation in touch with society's health values ? *British Medical Journal* 2004;**329**: 1236.

5. Dolan P., Cookson R. A qualitative study of the extent to which health gain matters when choosing between groups of patients. *Health Policy* 2000;**51**:19–30.

6. Ades A.E., Claxton K., Sculpher M. Evidence synthesis, parameter correlation and probabilistic sensitivity analysis. *Health Economics* 2005;**14**:373–381.

7. Doubilet P., Begg C.B., Weinstein M.C., Braun P., McNeill B.J. Probabilistic sensitivity analysis using Monte Carlo simulation: a practical approach. *Medical Decision Making* 1985;**5**:157–177.

8. Critchfield G.C., Willard K.E. Probabilistic analysis of decision trees using Monte Carlo simulation. *Medical Decision Making* 1986;**6**:85–92.

9. Mulrow C.D. Rationale for systematic reviews. In: Chalmer I., Altman D.G., eds. *Systematic Reviews*. London: BMJ Publishing Group, 1995;1–8.

10. McAlister F., Laupacis A., Wells G.A., Sackett D.L. Users' guides to the medical literature. XIX Applying clinical trial results. B. Guidelines for determining whether a drug is exerting (more than) a class effect. *Journal of the American Medical Association* 1999;**282**:1371–1377.

11. Turner R.M., Spiegelhalter D.J., Smith G.C.S., Thompson S.G. Bias modelling in evidence synthesis. *Journal of the Royal Statistical Society, Series A* 2009;**172**:21–47.

12. Felli J.C., Hazen G. A Bayesian approach to sensitivity analysis. *Health Economics* 1999;**8**:263–268.

13. Briggs A.H. A Bayesian approach to stochastic cost-effectiveness analysis. *Health Economics* 1999;**8**:257–261.

14. Lunn D.J., Thomas A., Best N., Spiegelhalter D. WinBUGS – a Bayesian modelling framework: concepts, structure, and extensibility. *Statistics and Computing* 2000;**10**: 325–337.

15. National Institute for health and Clinical Excellence. *Guide to the Methods of Technology Appraisal*. London: NICE, 2008.

16. Hunink M., Glasziou P., Siegel J., *et al. Decision Making in Health and Medicine: Integrating Evidence and Values*. Cambridge: Cambridge University Press, 2001.

17. Briggs A., Sculpher M., Claxton K. *Decision Modelling for Health Economic Evaluation*. Oxford: Oxford University Press, 2006.

18. Spiegelhalter D.J., Abrams K.R., Myles J. *Bayesian Approaches to Clinical Trials and Health-Care Evaluation*. New York: John Wiley & Sons, Ltd, 2004.

19. Berry D.A. *Statistics: A Bayesian Perspective*. London: Duxbury, 1996.

20. O'Hagan A., Luce B. *A Primer on Bayesian Statistics in Health Economics and Outcome Research*. www.bayesian-initiative.com: Bayesian Initiative in Health Economics and Outcomes Research, MedTap Intl, 2003.

21. Lee P.M. *Bayesian Statistics: An Introduction*. London: Arnold, 1997.

22. Drummond M.F., Richardson W.S., O'Brien B.J., Levine M., Heyland D. Users' guides to the medical literature. XIII. How to use an article on economic analysis of clinical practice. A. Are the results of the study valid? Evidence-Based Medicine Working Group. *Journal of the American Medical Association* 1997;**277**:1552–1557.

23. Guyatt G.H., Sinclair J., Cook D.J., Glasziou P. Users' guides to the medical literature. XVI. How to use a treatment recommendation. *Journal of the American Medical Association* 1999;**281**:1836–1843.

24. Guyatt G.H., Sackett D.L., Cook D.J. Users' guides to the medical literature. II. How to use an article about therapy or prevention. A. Are the results of the study valid? Evidence-Based Medicine Working Group. *Journal of the American Medical Association* 1993;**270**:2598–2601.

25. Guyatt G.H., Haynes R.B., Jaeschke R.Z., *et al.* Users' guides to the medical literature: XXV. Evidence-based medicine: principles for applying the users' guides to patient care. *Journal of the American Medical Association* 2000;**284**:1290–1296.

26. Oxman A.D., Cook D.J., Guyatt G.H. Users' guides to the medical literature. VI. How to use an overview. Evidence-Based Medicine Working Group. *Journal of the American Medical Association* 1994;**272**:1367–1371.

27. Oxman A.D., SACKETT D.L., Guyatt G.H. Users' guides to the medical literature. I. How to get started. The Evidence-Based Medicine Working Group. *Journal of the American Medical Association* 1993;**270**:2093–2095.

28. Higgins J.P.T., Green S. *Cochrane Handbook for Systematic Reviews of Interventions Version 5.0.0 [updated February 2008]*. Chichester: The Cochrane Collaboration, John Wiley & Sons, Ltd, 2008.

29. Cooper N.J., Sutton A.J., Abrams K.R., Turner D., Wailoo A. Comprehensive decision analytical modelling in economic evaluation: a Bayesian approach. *Health Economics* 2003;**13**:203–226.

2

Bayesian methods and WinBUGS

2.1 Introduction to Bayesian methods

2.1.1 What is a Bayesian approach?

There are two distinct approaches to statistical inference, the Frequentist (or Classical) approach and the Bayesian approach. The two approaches have much in common, but differ in their interpretation of probability and hence in their view of uncertainty regarding parameters. In a Frequentist approach parameters are viewed as fixed quantities that can be estimated by data with uncertainty in these estimates arising from sampling error. In the Bayesian approach, parameters are viewed as random variables with probability distributions that reflect the beliefs about the parameters resulting from all the available evidence. The approach requires an initial belief about the parameter (that comes from external sources to the data), which is then updated to reflect the evidence provided by the data. In a healthcare context Spiegelhalter *et al.* [1] define a Bayesian approach to be:

> The explicit quantitative use of external evidence in the design, monitoring, analysis, and interpretation of a health-care evaluation.

External evidence may come from subjective sources such as elicited expert opinion, objective sources such as a meta-analysis of previous trials evaluating the healthcare technology, or may simply be a very wide distribution over the feasible range of a parameter to represent the lack of evidence available. As the Bayesian

Evidence Synthesis for Decision Making in Healthcare, First Edition. Nicky J. Welton,
Alexander J. Sutton, Nicola J. Cooper, Keith R. Abrams and A.E. Ades.
© 2012 John Wiley & Sons, Ltd. Published 2012 by John Wiley & Sons, Ltd.

approach requires an initial distribution to represent belief about the parameter in advance of collecting data, it can be used to help design a study to collect evidence on the parameter (for example to inform sample size calculations – see Chapter 12). The technique of updating the belief (probability distribution) given new data lends itself to trial monitoring to perform interim analyses to make decisions to stop or continue with a trial (adaptive trial designs). The data obtained from the trial can be combined with the external evidence to form a new belief about the parameter given the data. The resulting probability distribution can be interpreted using probability statements, such as 'the probability that the mean treatment effect is negative is 0.01' in contrast to the interpretation of frequentist p-values which rely on a repeated sampling statement.

The main attractions of taking a Bayesian approach are that it is:

- *Flexible*. Since the 1980s the development of Markov Chain Monte Carlo (MCMC) simulation has meant that one computational approach can be used for most models making it relatively straightforward to fit very complex models that would be difficult using a Frequentist approach.

- *Efficient*. It uses all available evidence relevant to the parameter(s) of interest.

- *Useful*. The interpretation of parameters as random variables means that it is straightforward to make predictions for future populations or studies that can be used as inputs to decision making, planning of new research and public policy.

- *Ethical*. Its use of all available evidence fully exploits the experience of past patients, and its use in the design of future studies only randomises the patients necessary given previous evidence.

Note that the statistical models themselves are the same for both approaches (so for example a logistic regression would be used in both approaches where there is binary outcome data) – it is only the method of parameter estimation and computation that differs.

2.1.2   Likelihood

Statistical inference is concerned with learning about the underlying distribution (*population*) of the quantities (*parameters*) of interest using observations (*data*). We will denote parameters by θ and the observed data by y. For example, θ could be the mean relative treatment effect (Log Odds Ratio (LOR) of mortality) of beta-blockers compared with placebo, and y could be the observed LORs of mortality observed with standard error se in a set of trials of beta-blockers vs placebo. The distribution of the data y given a particular value of the parameter θ (written $f(y \mid \theta)$ and read 'distribution of y given θ') can be interpreted as telling us how likely the observed data are for a given value of θ. This distribution may take any feasible shape, but it is usually assumed that the distribution takes a standard shape (parametric form), for example Binomial for binary data and Normal for continuous data (see Appendix 2 for common probability distributions). Such assumed distributional forms are known as statistical models. Suppose for example that $f(y \mid \theta)$ has a Normal distribution with population mean θ:

$$f(y \mid \theta) \sim \text{Normal}(\theta, se^2)$$

If we observe $y = -1$ with standard error $se = 0.2$, then it would be very unlikely that the observed data were generated from a model with $\theta = 0$, in fact $f(y \mid \theta = 0) = 0.07$. It is more likely that it was generated from a model with $\theta = -0.5$ where $f(y \mid \theta = -0.5) = 0.48$, and more likely still that it was generated from a model with $\theta = -1$ where $f(y \mid \theta = -1) = 0.89$. For this reason $f(y \mid \theta)$ is known as the likelihood function, often written $L(y \mid \theta)$ or $L(\theta)$. With more than one data point, the likelihood function is the product of the individual likelihoods for each data point (this assumes that each data point is independent of the others given the model).

The Frequentist approach to statistical inference estimates the parameter θ as the (fixed) value that is best supported by the observed data, i.e. that which has the highest likelihood. The value of θ that maximises the likelihood function is known as the Maximum Likelihood Estimate (MLE), and much of Frequentist statistics is concerned with writing down the likelihood function and finding computational methods to find the parameter values that maximise it.

The likelihood function is central to the Bayesian approach to statistical inference too, because it summarises all the information that the data y can tell us about parameters θ. However, the Bayesian approach considers the parameters to be random variables with a probability distribution, and combines the information from the data about the parameters with information from external sources.

2.1.3 Bayes' theorem and Bayesian updating

Scientific enquiry is about updating our *prior beliefs* regarding an event or situation *in the light of new evidence* to provide an assessment of our *current state of knowledge*. The Bayesian approach follows this logic by starting with a probability distribution, $f(\theta)$, that describes our prior belief about the parameters θ arising from external sources. $f(\theta)$ is known as the *prior distribution*. The information provided by the new evidence is the *likelihood function*, $f(y \mid \theta)$. The prior distribution is then updated in light of the evidence provided by the data to give a new updated belief about the data, $f(\theta \mid y)$, known as the *posterior distribution*. The updating process uses Bayes' theorem.

Bayes' theorem was published in 1763 after it was found posthumously amongst the papers of the Rev. Thomas Bayes. Bayes' theorem is a mathematical relationship that holds between marginal and conditional probability densities of any two random variables. In itself Bayes' theorem is a statement of fact and is used uncontroversially in many applications, for example in diagnostic testing to find the probability of having a disease conditional on giving a positive test result.

In the context of Bayesian updating with parameters θ and data y the joint probability density $f(y, \theta)$ can be written as a product of the conditional probability density $f(y \mid \theta)$ and the marginal probability density $f(\theta)$:

$$f(y, \theta) = f(y \mid \theta) f(\theta) \qquad (2.1)$$

The same relationship holds if we instead condition on y instead of θ, giving:

$$f(y, \theta) = f(\theta \mid y) f(y) \qquad (2.2)$$

Equating Equations (2.1) and (2.2) gives Bayes' theorem:

$$f(\theta \mid y) = \frac{f(y \mid \theta) f(\theta)}{f(y)} \qquad (2.3)$$

The denominator $f(y)$ does not depend on the parameters θ and is therefore just a constant that ensures that $f(\theta \mid y)$ integrates to 1. So we can write Equation (2.3) as:

$$f(\theta \mid y) \propto f(y \mid \theta) f(\theta) \qquad (2.4)$$

or, in words, the posterior distribution is proportional to the likelihood multiplied by the prior:

$$\text{posterior} \propto \text{likelihood} \times \text{prior} \qquad (2.5)$$

Figure 2.1 illustrates the process of Bayesian updating, showing the posterior that results from the prior and likelihood for two examples. In Figure 2.1(a) the prior distribution is very flat representing only weak prior evidence compared with the information provided by the data. We might expect this to be the case when there is no external evidence. The posterior distribution always lies between the prior and the likelihood, but in this case since the prior evidence is weak it is dominated by the likelihood and lies close to it. Inference would be very similar from both the Bayesian and Frequentist approaches in this case. In Figure 2.1(b) the prior evidence is very strong compared with the evidence provided by the data. We might expect this to be the case when there is substantial external evidence, such as a meta-analysis of previous trials of the same health technology as that evaluated in a new trial providing the current data. The posterior must lie between the prior and the likelihood, but in this case it is dominated by the prior. Inference would be very different from Bayesian and Frequentist approaches in this case.

Writing the posterior distribution down in closed form is often not possible because of difficulties in calculating the denominator in Equation (2.3):

$$f(y) = \int f(y \mid \theta) f(\theta) d\theta \qquad (2.6)$$

although there are some special cases. In particular there are certain pairs of distributions, known as conjugates, for the prior and the likelihood that combine to

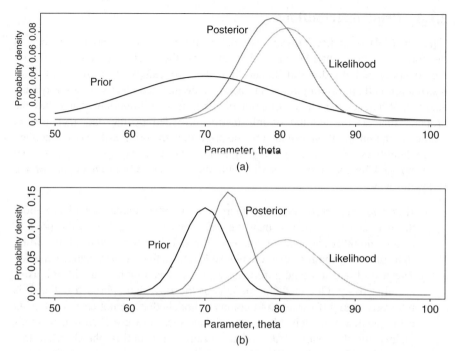

Figure 2.1   Illustration of the posterior probability densities that arise from two examples of prior distribution and likelihood function, where (a) the likelihood dominates the prior and (b) the prior dominates the likelihood.

give a posterior distribution that is in the same family as the prior. For example, if the data have a Binomial likelihood and there is a Beta prior distribution then the posterior also has a Beta distribution. Specifically, if r is the number of observed events and $(n - r)$ the number of nonevents, and a Beta(a, b) prior is used, the posterior is a Beta$(a + r, b + (n - r))$ distribution.

Where it is not possible to write the posterior distribution down in closed form numerical methods are required to find the integral in Equation (2.6). Until the 1980s the main approaches were asymptotic approximations, such as Laplace approximations, and numerical integration techniques, such as quadrature. These approaches are technical and cannot be easily applied to more complex models. More recently, MCMC simulation methods (see Section 2.1.8) have been developed, which can be performed easily in standard software (e.g. WinBUGS [2] or JAGS (http://mcmc-jags.sourceforge.net/)) and can cope with more complex models. The development of MCMC simulation has meant that instead of a Bayesian approach being technically more difficult than a Frequentist approach, it is now easier – especially for complex models. This has lead to an explosion in the number of applications that take a Bayesian approach. We assume in the rest of this book that an MCMC simulation approach is taken for parameter estimation.

2.1.4   Prior distributions

Equation (2.4) is in itself uncontroversial, it is the use of external evidence in the form of a prior distribution, rather than just the likelihood function, that is controversial and divides statisticians into the two camps. The choice of prior distribution is therefore important and needs to be justified clearly in any Bayesian analysis. Whatever the choice of prior distribution it is important that it has the property that, as the amount of information provided by the data increases in relation to the information provided by the prior, then the prior will be overwhelmed by the likelihood. This will hold as long as the prior does not exclude values that are supported by the data. Prior distributions are usually chosen in one of the following ways:

- *Vague/noninformative priors*. If there were no other available evidence about the parameters of interest than the data, then one would wish the prior to contain no information about the parameters. This can be achieved by putting 'flat' prior distributions over the plausible ranges that the parameters can take. The use of vague or noninformative priors is common to avoid criticisms of subjectivity. One of the attractions of the Bayesian approach is that it is relatively straightforward to fit complex models that are not easy to fit using a Frequentist approach. Many statisticians therefore use Bayesian methods mainly for this reason rather than because of a philosophical belief that external evidence should be incorporated as a prior. Vague/noninformative priors are therefore used to obtain inference close to that which would be obtained by frequentist methods.

- *Reference priors*. Some priors are chosen to have specific desirable properties. The most common is the Jeffreys' prior, which has the property that it is invariant to re-parameteristion.

- *Sceptical/enthusiastic*. This is a form of sensitivity analysis where an extreme prior distribution is used centred on a null effect, but with a pre-specified probability of a positive (or negative) effect. For example Higgins and Spiegelhalter [3] used a sceptical prior centred on 0 that represented a 5% chance that magnesium would reduce the odds of mortality by more that 25%. One can then ask what data would be needed to persuade a sceptic that the treatment is effective (or an enthusiast that it is not effective).

- *Subjective*. Prior information can be elicited from individual experts or groups of experts. Many criticisms of Bayesian methods are based on a worry about the use of subjective opinions as priors. As a result subjective priors are not commonly used, although they have an important role to play in cases where there are no data available or where the available data are weak and bounds need to be placed on the feasible range that the parameters can take. The use of informative priors allows one to transparently include expert opinion in a decision-making process.

- *Previous evidence/studies*. Prior information may represent a meta-analysis of previous trials of the health technology of interest. If may also represent other previous information from less rigorous studies such as observational studies or trials with methodological flaws. Priors based on less rigorous studies can be adjusted or down-weighted for potential biases (see Chapter 11).

2.1.5   Summarising the posterior distribution

While a Frequentist approach produces a point estimate (the MLE) of the parameter together with a confidence interval, a Bayesian approach produces a probability distribution for the parameter. The posterior distribution can then be summarised in a variety of ways. Note that typically the posterior distribution will have been computed using MCMC simulation, and thus it will not be possible to write it in parametric form. All of the summaries below will therefore be approximations obtained from the simulated parameter values.

The marginal posterior distributions can be displayed graphically using kernel density estimation [4]. Point estimates can be obtained, most commonly by using the posterior mean or posterior median, although the posterior mode is also a useful summary because its interpretation as the most likely value for the parameter equates most closely to the Frequentist MLE (but is difficult to calculate from MCMC output). The posterior standard deviation is also useful for symmetrical posterior distributions.

Bayesian credible intervals (written CrI to distinguish them from Frequentist confidence intervals) give a range of values for the parameter where there is a certain posterior probability that the parameter lies in this range, for example 95% credible intervals have a probability of 0.95 that the parameter lies in the range. Note the natural interpretation of the credible interval which is different to the interpretation of a Frequentist confidence interval (but is how many misinterpret confidence intervals). Credible intervals are not unique, but usually found as the interval that has equal tail probability (2.5% for a 95% CrI) on each side. For skew distributions the Highest Posterior Density (HPD) interval, which is the smallest interval that has 95% posterior probability, is a sensible alternative [5].

Direct probability statements can be made easily, for example the posterior probability that the parameter exceeds 0, $\Pr(\theta > 0)$. Again these statements have a natural interpretation that is different to the interpretation of a Frequentist p-value (but is how many misinterpret p-values).

Posterior distributions for functions of parameters can also easily be obtained. For example if θ is a LOR we may also want to report summaries for the absolute probability of an event on treatment, α, in a population that has a 10% probability of an event without the treatment. Then the log-odds of the event on treatment is equal to the log-odds of the event without treatment plus the LOR, θ:

$$\log\left(\frac{\alpha}{1-\alpha}\right) = \log\left(\frac{0.1}{0.9}\right) + \theta$$

which gives:

$$\alpha = \frac{0.11 * e^{\theta}}{1 + 0.11 * e^{\theta}}.$$

Using MCMC simulation it is straightforward to calculate α for each simulated value of θ, and then find posterior summaries for α in the same way as for θ.

2.1.6   Prediction

The Bayesian approach is well suited to problems of prediction through the use of the *predictive distribution*. Suppose we want to make a prediction for a new random event x that depends on the parameter θ. Commonly used examples are a prediction for a new observation with the same likelihood or a prediction for a new study in a meta-analysis. If $f(x \mid \theta)$ is the probability distribution of x given θ, then the posterior prediction for x given observed data y is found by averaging over the posterior distribution $f(\theta \mid y)$:

$$f(x \mid y) = \int f(x \mid \theta) f(\theta \mid y) d\theta \qquad (2.7)$$

Again it is straightforward to form the posterior predictive distribution using MCMC simulation by drawing from the distribution $f(x \mid \theta)$ for each simulated value of θ.

Posterior prediction is useful in the monitoring of trials, where it is used to predict the eventual trial result based on the data collected so far and obtain the predictive probability of eventually demonstrating a difference. It is also useful in predicting the results of a new study population that is 'similar to' the studies in a meta-analysis for use in decision models [6].

Equation (2.7) can also be adapted to make predictions from the prior rather than the posterior distribution for θ, known as prior prediction:

$$f(x) = \int f(x \mid \theta) f(\theta) d\theta \qquad (2.8)$$

Prior prediction is useful in the design of trials, where it is used to predict the probability that a trial will demonstrate a difference.

2.1.7   More realistic and complex models

Evaluations of healthcare interventions rarely concern a single summary statistic. For example analyses of multiple endpoints, multiple subsets of patients, multiple treatment group contrasts, and meta-analyses of multiple studies. So far we have focused on the case where there is a single parameter θ, but Bayes' theorem applies equally to multiparameter models with a vector of parameters $\boldsymbol{\theta}$. The main difference is that the posterior distribution is now a *joint distribution* across all of the parameters, $f(\theta_1, \theta_2, \ldots, \theta_m \mid y)$. Inference for each parameter is usually obtained by averaging over all of the other parameters, which gives the posterior marginal distributions:

$$f(\theta_1 \mid y) = \int_{\theta_2,\ldots,\theta_m} f(\theta_1,\ldots,\theta_m \mid y)d\theta_2 \ldots d\theta_m \qquad (2.9)$$

Posterior summaries can then be reported from these marginal distributions.

An important example of multi-parameter models is where the parameters $\theta_1, \theta_2, \ldots, \theta_m$ represent a measure taken on m units, for example a meta-analysis of LORs from m studies. There are three possible assumptions (models) that can be assumed: (i) all of the θ_j are identical (Fixed Effect model); (ii) the θ_j are unrelated and analysed separately; and (iii) the θ_j are 'similar' (exchangeable) and can be considered to come from a population of effects (hierarchical or random effects model). These models are described in more detail in Chapter 4.

2.1.8   MCMC and Gibbs sampling

MCMC simulation works by drawing values for each parameter repeatedly in such a way that eventually the samples come from the posterior distribution. Suppose that we have several parameters, $\theta_1, \theta_2, \ldots, \theta_m$. We begin at an initial guess for the value of these parameters $\theta_1(1), \theta_2(1), \ldots, \theta_m(1)$, and at each subsequent iteration we sample new values based on the values of the previous iteration. The property that current values depend on the past only through the previous value is known as the Markov property (hence *Markov Chain* in MCMC). There are several sampling methods available to do this, but one of the simplest and that which is used in the WinBUGS software is the Gibbs sampler (a special case of the Metropolis–Hastings algorithm). Suppose that after t iterations the values of the parameters are $\theta_1(t), \theta_2(t), \ldots, \theta_m(t)$. Gibbs sampling works by taking each parameter in turn and drawing a value from its posterior distribution *conditional* on the values of all the remaining parameters being fixed at their current value, which for the first parameter is $f(\theta_1(t + 1) \mid \theta_2(t), \theta_3(t), \ldots, \theta_m(t))$ and so on. These distributions are known as the *full conditional distributions* and are often much easier to sample from than the joint distribution – not least because they are univariate distributions.

Initially our samples may not represent the target distribution particularly well, but it can be shown that in general the simulated values will eventually settle down to the joint posterior distribution that we are interested in. The chain of simulated values is said to *converge* to the posterior distribution. The simulations prior to convergence are known as the 'burn-in' sample and are discarded. Once convergence has occurred, a large number of further iterations of the Markov Chain are run to obtain a sample from the joint posterior distribution. If the number of samples is large enough, then summary measures calculated from this sample, for example the mean, will provide a good estimate of summary measures from the posterior marginal distributions. This approach to obtaining parameter estimates is known as Monte Carlo simulation (hence *Monte Carlo* in MCMC).

The most commonly used software to perform MCMC simulation is WinBUGS (http://www.mrc-bsu.cam.ac.uk/bugs/), but note that there are others, for example JAGS (Just Another Gibbs Sampler; http://www-fis.iarc.fr/~martyn/software/jags/). All of the examples in this book were performed using WinBUGS and we provide codes for all of the examples in the text and online.

2.2   Introduction to WinBUGS

2.2.1   The BUGS language

WinBUGS uses the BUGS (Bayesian Inference Using Gibbs Sampling) language to generate samples from the posterior distribution. It is freely available from: http://www.mrc-bsu.cam.ac.uk/bugs/. At the time of writing WinBUGS1.4.3 is a stable version of the package and unlikely to be developed further. Future developments are the focus of the OpenBUGS project, which also provides the open source code (see http://www.openbugs.info).

The BUGS language has a similar syntax to R and S-plus, and WinBUGS files are saved as compound documents that have an .odc file extension. WinBUGS requires five key elements: specification of the likelihood, a description of the statistical model linking parameters to the likelihood, specification of prior distributions for the parameters, the data, and initial values for the sampler. Further statements to calculate functions of parameters can also be included. We introduce the BUGS language through an example.

Example 2.1   Beta-blockers vs placebo for myocardial infarction (MI).

We illustrate how to perform MCMC in WinBUGS using a pairwise meta-analysis of 22 trials of beta-blockers *vs* placebo for patients following myocardial infarction [7]. This is the Blocker example in the WinBUGS *Help_Examples Vol I* file. The data are displayed in Table 2.1 where for each study j the LOR, Y_j, and its variance (standard error squared), V_j, are reported. We focus in this chapter on the coding and running of the WinBUGS program. The random effects meta-analysis model used is described in detail in Chapter 4.

Components of a WinBUGS .odc file

In WinBUGS use either *File>New* or *File>Open* to create a new document or open an existing one. The model, data, and initial values for each chain are each loaded separately, and can either be contained in the same file or in different files. Every WinBUGS model is described by statements within the curly brackets of a model statement. The data and initial values are loaded in list and/or column

Table 2.1   Log odds ratio, Y_j, and its variance (standard error squared), V_j, reported in 22 trials of beta-blockers *vs* placebo for patients following a myocardial infarction.

Trial, j	Y_j	V_j	Trial, j	Y_j	V_j
1	0.028171	0.723016	12	−0.03891	0.052652
2	−0.741	0.233435	13	−0.59325	0.180767
3	−0.54062	0.318729	14	0.281546	0.042208
4	−0.24613	0.019095	15	− 0.32133	0.088631
5	0.069453	0.078768	16	−0.13535	0.06808
6	−0.58416	0.456588	17	0.140606	0.132623
7	−0.51239	0.019234	18	0.32205	0.305416
8	−0.07862	0.041612	19	0.444381	0.513586
9	−0.42417	0.075061	20	−0.21751	0.067518
10	−0.33482	0.013705	21	−0.59108	0.066155
11	−0.2134	0.037975	22	−0.6081	0.07419

format (described below). Any text on a line that follows a '#' are comments and not read as code. An *.odc* file containing all of these elements therefore can take the following structure:

```
#Model
model{
   <likelihood specification>
   <statistical model statements>
   <prior specification>
   <functions of parameters>
}

#Data
   <List or column format>

#Initial values
   <List or column format for chain 1>
   <List or column format for chain 2>
   <etc.>
```

Note that several different lists and sets of columns can be loaded to fully specify the data and initial values. Also, if preferred, the model, data and initial values can be specified in separate *.odc* documents. The order of the statements in the model is not important as long as statements depending on indexes (e.g. study number) belong within loops over that index.

Specification of the likelihood

The observed LORs have a Normal likelihood with mean LOR δ_j:

$$Y_j \sim \text{Normal}(\delta_j, V_j) \tag{2.10}$$

WinBUGS specifies the Normal distribution in terms of its precision, $P_j = 1/V_j$. The WinBUGS code to specify the likelihood is:

```
for (j in 1:Nstud){           #Loop over the Nstud=22 studies
  P[j]<- V[j]                  #Precision = 1/Variance
  Y[j]~dnorm(delta[j],P[j])    #Normal likelihood for data Y[j]
}
```

The syntax

```
for (j in 1:Nstud){
...
}
```

means that the statements inside the curly brackets are carried out for $j = 1$, $j = 2$, up to $j = Nstud$, where *Nstud* is the number of studies (22 in this example). The square brackets indicate vector elements, so P[j] is the jth element of the precision vector (i.e. the precision for study j). The '<-' syntax represents a logical operation, where the calculation on the right-hand side is carried out and the result assigned to the variable on the left-hand side (like '=' in many other programming languages). Here the precisions are set equal to the reciprocal of the variances. The '~' syntax is used to indicate distributions for random variables and can be read as 'is distributed as' – in this case the observed LORs have a Normal distribution (dnorm) for the likelihood. Note the same syntax is used for distributions for likelihoods, priors, the statistical model, and straight simulation. The meaning should be clear from the code. Here the variable on the left-hand side is data, so it must be a likelihood statement.

Description of the statistical model

The study-specific mean LORs δ_j are assumed to come from a common Normal random effects distribution:

$$\delta_j \sim \text{Normal}(d, \tau^2) \tag{2.11}$$

where d is the overall mean LOR and τ^2 the between-studies variance of the study-specific LORs. Equation (2.11) shows the relationship between the parameters that have priors (d and τ^2) and the parameters that feed into the likelihood (δ_j). The statistical model is described by adding the following statement within the loop over j:

```
delta[j]~dnorm(d,prec)        #Random Effects model
```

and the following statement outside the loop over j to calculate the between studies precision *prec* from the variance τ^2:

```
prec<- 1/(tau*tau)            #precision = 1/ tau-squared
```

Specification of the prior distributions

We put a very flat Normal prior on the overall mean LOR, d, and a very wide Uniform prior on the between-studies standard deviation for the LORs, τ:

$$d \sim \text{Normal}(0, 10^6) \quad \tau \sim \text{Uniform}(0, 10) \qquad (2.12)$$

The following code added outside the loop over j specifies these priors (noting that the Normal distribution is specified in terms of its precision which is the reciprocal of the variance, $1/10^6 = 10^{-6}$).

```
d~dnorm(0,1.0e-6)            #Flat Normal prior for d
tau~dunif(0,10)              #Wide Uniform prior for tau
```

Functions of parameters

At each iteration of the MCMC simulation functions of parameters can be calculated. The resulting chain of values is a sample from the posterior distribution for the function of parameters. For example, if we wish to make inference on the overall mean Odds Ratio, the following line of code can be added to the model:

```
OR<-exp(d)                   #odds ratio = exp(log-odds ratio)
```

Bayesian p-values can be calculated by taking advantage of the step function in WinBUGS. step(e) returns a 1 if $e \geq 0$ and a 0 otherwise producing a chain of 0's and 1's. The posterior mean of this chain is the probability that $e \geq 0$ (i.e. the proportion of 1's). For example, we may wish to find the probability that the overall mean Odds Ratio is 1 or more, $OR \geq 1$. We can achieve this by adding the following line to the model:

```
prob.OR1<-step(OR-1)         #posterior mean = p(OR>=1)
```

Monitoring prob.OR1 and finding its posterior mean gives the probability that $OR \geq 1$. Equivalently, we can write this in terms of the LOR because $p(OR \geq 1) = p(d \geq 0)$, so the following code would produce the same results:

```
prob.OR1<-step(d)            #posterior mean = p(OR>=1)
```

Data

The data can be entered in list format, which is convenient if exporting data from R or S-plus:

```
list(Nstud=22, Y=c(0.028, -.741, ..., -.6081),
     V=c(.723016, .233435, ..., .07419))
```

Constant values (e.g. Nstud) must be entered in list format, but vectors can be entered as columns which can be more convenient if exporting data from a spreadsheet such as Excel. The above data could therefore also have been entered as:

```
list(Nstud=22)

Y[]     V[]
0.028   .723016
-.741   .233435
.

.
-.6081  .07419
END
```

The values for Y[ ] and V[ ] can be cut-and-paste from a spreadsheet into the *.odc* file, but when pasting you must use ***Edit>Paste Special>Plain Text***. There must be a carriage return following the END statement.

Arrays can be entered in either list using the structure statement (see Chapter 10 for an example) or in column format where the header row indicates which column is entered, so for example the matrix

$$x = \begin{pmatrix} 1 & 2 & 3 & 4 \\ 5 & 6 & 7 & 8 \\ 9 & 10 & 11 & 12 \end{pmatrix}$$

can be entered in with the following code:

```
x[1,]   x[2,]   x[3,]   x[4,]
1       2       3       4
5       6       7       8
9       10      11      12
END
```

Initial values

Initial values need to be specified for each MCMC chain that is run. It is advisable to run at least (and preferably more than) two chains so that convergence can be assessed (see Section 2.2.4) using very different initial values. Results obtained prior to convergence will be incorrect. Initial values are required for all stochastic variables (nodes), i.e. all nodes that are on a left-hand side of a '~' sign but are not specified as data. In our example initial values are required for δ, d and τ. WinBUGS can generate initial values, but often produces unusually big or small values that can lead to numerical errors. It is generally better for the user to specify the initial values to ensure that they are reasonably sensible, although for some higher level hierarchical variables where the lower level variables are given sensible initial values by the user, it is fine to let WinBUGS generate the initial values. Initial values can be specified in either list or column format, as for data. In the beta-blocker example we used:

list(delta=c(0,0,0,0,0, 0,0,0,0,0, 0,0,0,0,0, 0,0,0,0,0, 0,0),d=0,tau=1)

For a second chain quite different initial values should be used, for example:

list(delta=c(10,10,10,10,10, 10,10,10,10,10, 10,10,10,10,10, 10,10,10,10,10, 10,10),d= −10,tau=8)

We have used equal values for each element of δ, but that is not necessary and in fact different values can sometimes help avoid numerical errors with the sampler. Because δ is from a hierarchical model depending on d and τ, if sensible values are specified for d and τ, it is probably fine to use WinBUGS to generate initial values for δ. Some types of variable are particularly sensitive to the choice of initial value, such as variables that are constrained to lie within certain limits (e.g. probabilities, standard deviations) and rate parameter. Many numerical 'Trap' errors generated by WinBUGS, which prevent the sampler from updating, can often be solved by choosing different, more sensible, initial values.

If WinBUGS has been used to generate initial values you can view them using *Model>Save State*.

2.2.2   Graphical representation

The types of model that can be fitted in WinBUGS can be illustrated in a Directed Acyclic Graph (DAG) [8]. The graphs consist of Nodes, Plates and Edges:

- Nodes represent all the data, variables and constants in the model. They are rectangles for constants, and ellipses for all other node types (stochastic or logical).

- Plates illustrate indexes, for example a plate would cover all variables indexed by study j, and indicate which statements need to be within a loop over j. Any global parameters relevant to all studies lie outside the plate for j.

- Edges join up nodes and indicate the direction of the relationship between them. Single lines indicate a stochastic relationship, and double lines represent a logical relationship.

A DAG is Acyclic, meaning that there is no circularity in the graph (it is not possible to follow edges to get back to where you started), and Directed, so that arrows display the directions of relationships between variables. Arrows go from parent nodes to children nodes. Each node is independent of all other nodes conditional on its parents, and it is this property of DAGs that is exploited by the MCMC samplers used in WinBUGS. Writing the model as a DAG can help when writing a

WinBUGS program, and in fact if you draw a DAG in WinBUGS, it can generate the code for you (see **Help_Doodle help**). Note that WinBUGS does not always do this in the most efficient way (in particular it writes out a loop for each statement rather than grouping statements into a single loop), so for complicated models it is recommended that you write your own code – not least because it can be easier to debug.

Example 2.1 revisited   Beta-blockers vs placebo for MI.

The DAG for the random effects meta-analysis model for the beta-blockers example (Equations (2.10)–(2.12)) is shown in Figure 2.2.

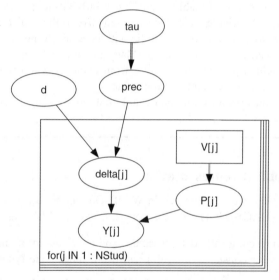

Figure 2.2   Directed Acyclic Graph for the Random Effects model for the beta-blockers example (Equations (2.10–2.12)).

Nodes d, prec, and tau lie outside the plate (loop) over j because they do not depend on study j. Nodes d and prec are 'parents' of node delta[j] because the distribution for delta[j] depends on d and prec (Equation 2.11).

2.2.3   Running WinBUGS

Once the model, data and initial values have been coded in an *.odc* (or text) file the mode needs to be loaded into WinBUGS using the model specification tool (**Model_Specification** ...):

- Highlight the word 'model' at the top of the program, then click **check model**.

- For data in list format, highlight the word 'list' and for column data highlight the first variable name, and then click on **load data**. Repeat this for each set of data.

- Enter the number of chains that you wish to run, then click on **compile**.

- Highlight the word 'list' at the beginning of the initial values, and then click on **load inits**. Repeat for each chain.

- If you have not initialised everything, then you can get WinBUGS to generate the remaining initial values by clicking on **gen inits**. Note that these may not always be sensible, so it is best in general to provide your own initial values.

Once the model has been successfully specified, MCMC samples can be generated using the **Model_Update** tool:

- First set sample monitors for all nodes that results are required for using the **Inference_Samples** tool. Type variable name then click **set** for each node.

- In the **updates** box type in the number of simulations that you want to run, then click **update**. Note that nothing will be saved unless sample monitors have been set.

2.2.4   Assessing convergence in WinBUGS

At first the MCMC sampler will not be sampling from the joint posterior distribution of interest, but under most situations will eventually settle down to the right distribution. The burn-in simulations before convergence should be discarded, but it is not always easy to tell how many simulations are needed for convergence to occur.

With a single chain one can look at history plots (**Inference_Samples_history**) of the simulated values for each node to see when they 'settle down' but this is difficult to judge by eye. If there is any obvious structure in the plot it is an indication of slow convergence. MCMC chains are correlated due to the Markov Chain that generates the samples, measured by the autocorrelation statistics that show the correlation between sampled values for specified numbers of iterations apart (known as the lag). For example, correlations between sampled values 2 iterations apart would be at lag 2. The autocorrelation should drop off with increasing lag, and if it does not do so it indicates slow convergence. This can be diagnosed by inspecting autocorrelation plots (**Inference_Samples_auto-cor**) that plot the autocorrelation for different lags, although this does not in itself help identify when convergence has occurred.

Most convergence checking methods rely on running multiple chains, and compare the simulated values from the different chains to identify when they become 'similar'. History plots with the different chains superimposed (in different colours) can be useful to quickly see if the chains are very different, although less easy to see if they are the same distribution. Comparing posterior summaries for each chain

(*Inference_Sample_stats*) for different burn-in periods until the burn-in period is sufficiently big that the chains give the same results (to within an acceptable accuracy). Note the number of samples after burn-in should be sufficiently large too. There are various diagnostic statistics that have been proposed and can be run using the CODA and BOA packages (available at www.mrc-bsu.cam.ac.uk/bugs). See Cowles and Carlin [9] for a comparison of the methods. The diagnostic that is provided within WinBUGS is the Brooks–Gelman–Rubin diagnostic [10, 11] (*Inference_Samples_bgr diag*). This produces a plot with three coloured lines: the green line is the width of an 80% credible interval from the simulations pooled from all of the chains (a measure of between-chain variability), the blue line is the average width of the 80% credible intervals for each chain separately (a measure of within-chain variability), and the red line is the ratio of the between- and within-chain measures. Convergence is deemed to have occurred when the red line settles down to close to 1 and the blue and green lines converge together to stability. Note the *bgr diag* tool cannot be used with binary nodes, for example if you have included a node/parameter to calculate the posterior probability that a parameter/node exceeds a specific value.

Example 2.1 revisited   Beta-blockers vs placebo for MI.

History plots from a single chain with 30 000 updates are shown in Figure 2.3 for parameters d and τ. There are a few points in the chain where the sampler gets 'stuck' where consecutive sampled values are close together. There seem to be more spikes in the history plot for τ, suggesting that this parameter is slower to converge, which is typically the case for variance parameters relative to mean parameters. However, it is difficult just looking at these plots to assess whether and when convergence occurs.

The autocorrelation plots (Figure 2.4) also show that convergence is expected to be slower for τ compared with d because the autocorrelation drops off much more slowly with lag time with still a reasonably high correlation between simulated values 40 iterations apart.

The Brooks–Gelman–Rubin diagnostic (*bgr diag*) plots based on 30 000 iterations show that convergence seems satisfactory – the bottom two lines have settled together to stability and the top line has converged to 1 (Figure 2.5). Discarding the first 30 000 iterations as 'burn-in' and then running a further 30 000 iterations, we obtain the following summary statistics for the 2 chains (entering in 'chains 1 to 1' for chain 1, etc.), which give posterior means and standard deviations the same to two decimal places:

```
#Chain 1
node  mean      sd       MC error  2.5%      median    97.5%     start    sample
d     −0.2488   0.0641   0.001408  −0.3713   −0.2503   −0.1172   30 001   30 000
tau    0.1289   0.08272  0.003112   0.00463   0.1216    0.3115   30 001   30 000
```

```
#Chain 2
node  mean     sd       MC error   2.5%      median    97.5%    start   sample
d     -0.2457  0.06622  0.001599  -0.3727   -0.2462   -0.1141   30001   30000
tau    0.1336  0.08045  0.003094   0.00775   0.1257    0.311    30001   30000
```

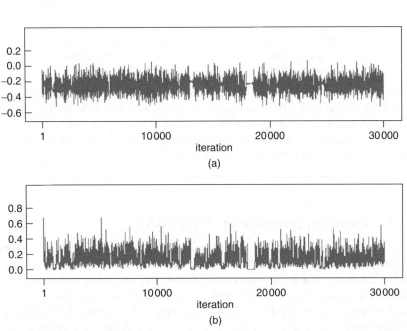

Figure 2.3   History plots from a single chain of the MCMC sampler. Plots are shown for (a) the overall mean LOR, d, and (b) the between studies standard deviation, τ for the beta-blockers example.

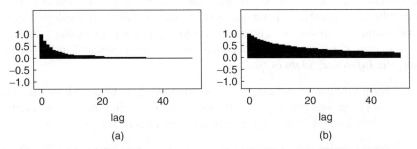

Figure 2.4   Autocorrelation plots plotted against lag times for a single chain of the MCMC sampler. Plots are shown for (a) the overall mean LOR, d, and (b) the between studies standard deviation, τ for the beta-blockers example.

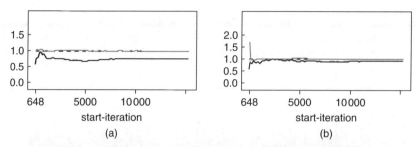

*Figure 2.5   Brooks-Gelman-Rubin diagnostic (**bgr diag**) plots for (a) the overall mean LOR, ḋ, and (b) the between studies standard deviation, τ for the beta-blockers example, based on 2 chains with 30 000 updates. Bottom lines: between- and within-chain variability (blue and green in WinBUGS). Top line: the ratio of between- and within-chain variability (red in WinBUGS).*

2.2.5   Statistical inference in WinBUGS

Once convergence is satisfactory, further updates can be run to obtain summary statistics from the posterior distribution. A large enough sample must be run for reliable inference, but how large should this be? A reliable approach is to keep running further iterations until the posterior summaries become stable. A rule of thumb proposed in the WinBUGS help pages (***Help_User manual_Tutorial***) is to compare the Monte Carlo error for each parameter (***MCerror***) with the posterior standard deviation for that parameter. The ***MCerror*** can be interpreted as the standard error of the posterior mean, but adjusted for the autocorrelation in the posterior samples on which the posterior mean is based. The rule of thumb is for the simulation to be run until the ***MCerror*** for each parameter of interest is less than 5% of the posterior standard deviation. Another rule of thumb that gives similar results is to run the same number of iterations again as were required for convergence, and report summary statistics for all chains pooled together on this further sample.

Summary statistics from the marginal posterior distributions can be obtained using the ***Inference_Samples*** tool.

- For each node of interest, type it in the ***node*** box, then click on ***set***. Then run further updates. Type * in the ***node*** box to monitor all set nodes, or type a node name to obtain summaries for individual nodes.

- Set the chains that summaries are required for, e.g. 'chains 1 to 2' will give results pooled for chains 1 and 2.

- Make sure that the burn-in iterations are discarded by setting ***beg*** equal to the first iteration after burn-in, e.g. 30 001 in the beta-blocker example.

– *stats* displays the posterior mean, standard deviation, median, 95% credible limits, and *MCerror*.

– *density* displays the estimated marginal posterior density for each node.

The *Inference_Compare* tool can be used to obtain plots of summaries from the marginal posterior distributions. For example, caterpillar plots plot the posterior mean plus 95% credible interval for each element of a vector specified in node. Note that *beg* needs to be specified on this tool as for *Inference_Samples*.

Example 2.1 revisited   Beta-blockers vs placebo for MI.

Posterior summaries from 30 000 iterations from 2 chains (giving a sample of 60 000 in total) after a burn-in of 30 000 (beg = 30 001) for nodes d, OR, tau, prob.OR1 are:

node	mean	sd	MC error	2.5%	median	97.5%	start	sample
OR	0.7826	0.05128	8.347E-4	0.6893	0.78	0.8912	30001	60000
d	−0.2473	0.06519	0.001069	−0.3721	−0.2484	−0.115	30001	60000
prob.OR	15.833E-4	0.02415	1.267E-4	0.0	0.0	0.0	30001	60000
tau	0.1313	0.08163	0.002198	0.0059	0.124	0.311	30001	60000

The posterior mean for the mean LOR is −0.2473 with 95% credible interval (−0.3721, −0.1152) and the posterior mean on the odds-ratio scale is 0.7826 with 95% credible interval (0.6893, 0.8912). The posterior median between study standard deviation is 0.1237 with 95% credible interval (0.005906, 0.3113) – note that this interval is different from the Uniform(0,10) prior, so is not being limited by the prior. The posterior probability that $OR \geq 1$ is 5.833E-4 = 0.0005833. This suggests strong evidence that beta-blockers have a protective effect against mortality following MI. The density plots in Figure 2.6 show the marginal posterior distributions graphically.

Figure 2.7 shows a caterpillar plot which displays the estimated posterior mean and 95% credible interval for the 22 study-specific mean LORs, δ_j (elements 1:22). Note these are model estimates and not the raw observed values commonly displayed in a forest plot (see Chapter 4 for details). Posterior summaries for the overall mean LOR, d, is displayed at the bottom of the graph in element 26. This was achieved by adding in the following line of code to the model:

```
delta[26]<-d              #element 26 of delta = d for caterpillar plot
```

Note this trick is necessary because only a single vector can be plotted at once in a caterpillar plot.

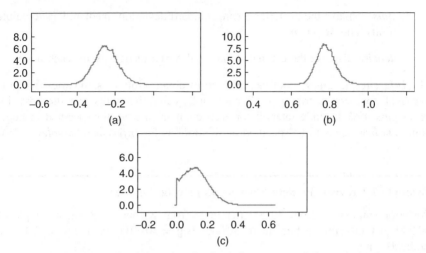

Figure 2.6 *Density plots showing the kernel-estimate of the marginal posterior distributions from the simulated chains. Plots are shown for (a) the overall mean LOR,* d, *(b) the overall mean Odds Ratio and (c) the between studies standard deviation,* τ, *for the beta-blockers example, based on 2 chains with 30 000 updates following a burn-in of 30 000.*

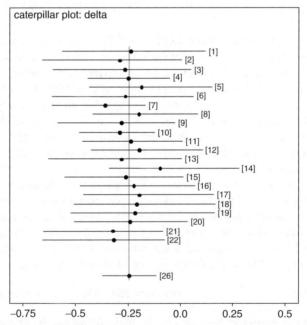

Figure 2.7 *Caterpillar plot showing posterior mean and 95% credible intervals for the study-specific mean LORs (elements 1:22) and for the overall mean LOR,* d *(element 26).*

2.2.6   Practical aspects of using WinBUGS

Error (Trap) messages are displayed at the bottom of the screen and can also be seen in the log (*Info_Open Log*). However, the error messages are often unhelpful! The WinBUGS user manual (*Help_User manual*) is very useful – in particular see the section on *Tips and Troubleshooting*. Also, searching through past messages or sending a new query to the BUGS discussion list (details at www.mrc-bsu. cam.uk/bugs) can usually find a solution. Using sensible initial values can avoid many problems of WinBUGS producing Trap messages.

The WinBUGS user manual (*Help_User manual*) is the best place for help with the BUGS language. In particular, help with the syntax for the different distributions can be found by clicking *Model Specification_The bugs language: stochastic nodes_Distributions* and help with the syntax for logical function can be found by clicking *Model Specification_logical nodes*.

The examples volumes I and II (*Help_...*) cover a wide range of models, and a good strategy is to find a similar model and then modify it.

If many programs are to be run, then using the point-and-click menus can get very repetitive. Instead, WinBUGS can be run in 'batch mode' from script files, which can help automate the running of models. Details can be found in the user manual (*Help_User manual_Batch-mode: Scripts*). Script files have led to it being possible to call WinBUGS from other packages (Excel/R/SAS/Stata/Matlab – links are provided at www.mrc-bsu.cam.ac.uk/bugs), which can be useful if WinBUGS is to be called repeatedly within simulations, and also for preparing data and post-processing WinBUGS samples.

Finally, note that MCMC simulation is a numerical method and results should always be checked to see if they are sensible and robust to choice of burn-in period and further samples for inference. Sensitivity to choice of prior distributions should also be considered, especially when there are variance parameters or when a large number of particularly vague prior distributions have been used.

2.3   Advantages and disadvantages of a Bayesian approach

The key criticism of a Bayesian approach is that the use of prior distributions introduces an element of subjectivity, and even when 'vague' prior distributions are used there are some parameters (in particular variance parameters) where there is no obvious candidate and results can be sensitive to the form of distribution chosen. Historically there has been a reluctance to use Bayesian methods due to a fear of acceptance, but this is changing with most journals now accepting Bayesian analyses and also regulatory and reimbursement bodies such as the National Institute of Health and Clinical Excellence (NICE) [12] in the UK and the Food and Drug Administration (FDA) [13] in the US. Computational difficulties have in the past been a barrier to the use of Bayesian methods. The advent of MCMC has made the Bayesian approach much more accessible, however some see

MCMC as a black box that is difficult to understand. The lack of tests of statistical significance is another criticism of the approach, although Bayesian p-values can be calculated.

On the plus side it is easy to fit very complex models – although this could be a considered a disadvantage if complexity is achieved at the expense of intuitive understanding. The simulation environment provided by MCMC methods makes it easy to estimate credible intervals, complex functions of parameters, make predictions about future quantities, and make direct probability statements. As such it is ideal for integrating meta-analyses and more general types of evidence synthesis into decision models (see Chapter 7 and other examples throughout this book). However, it is crucial that all of the evidence and prior distributions used be clear, explicit and transparent so that they can be challenged and subject to critique.

2.4   Summary key points

- A Bayesian approach views parameters as random variables with probability distributions whereas a Frequentist approach views parameters as fixed quantities that are estimated with sampling error.

- External evidence (represented by prior distributions) is combined with observed data (represented by the likelihood function), using Bayes' theorem to form a posterior distribution representing the updated belief about the parameters.

- Prior distributions can be vague/noninformative, be chosen to have specific properties, be based on previous evidence, be elicited from experts, or represent the views of an enthusiast or a sceptic in a sensitivity analysis.

- MCMC simulation is the main method for computation of the posterior distribution, which can be performed in WinBUGS, OpenBUGS and JAGS amongst other software.

- MCMC is a numerical simulation procedure and needs to be used with care. In particular, convergence should be assessed and sufficiently large samples taken on which to base inference.

- The marginal posterior distributions can be summarised graphically using kernel density estimation, and summary statistics such as the posterior mean, standard deviation, median, credible intervals, and direct probability statements.

- The simulation environment makes it straightforward to fit complex models and make predictions for new observations or new studies.

- All assumptions made should be clear, explicit and transparent, so that they can be subject to critique.

2.5   Further reading

There are many introductory texts on Bayesian statistics, and here we list just a few. Berry, Gelman *et al.*, Gilks *et al.* and Lee [5, 14–16] are general texts, whereas Spiegelhalter *et al.* [1] is specific to clinical trials and healthcare evaluation and O'Hagan and Luce [17] is specific to health economics and outcomes research. Congdon [18, 19] covers a very wide range of examples and also provide the WinBUGS code used to fit them. WinBUGS links and resources can be found at www.mrc-bsu.cam.ac.uk/bugs/.

2.6   Exercises

2.1 Using the model in *BLOCKER.odc*, cut and paste the data for the 22 trials (in terms of the LOR and variance for each) from *BLOCKER.xls* into WinBUGS. Go through the steps of checking the model, loading the data and compiling it. Update your model for 10 000 iterations (the 'burn-in'), monitor d and tau using the *Sample Monitor Tool*, and update for a further 10000 iterations. Use the *Sample Monitor Tool* to obtain summaries and graphical displays of the posterior distributions. Try rerunning your model for fewer or more iterations in both the 'burn-in' and the sample – do you get different results?

2.2 Modify the model in *BLOCKER.odc* so that you can obtain the posterior distribution for the Odds Ratio (OR) and the posterior probability that the OR is greater than or equal to 1. Remember that step(x) returns 1 when $x \geq 0$.

2.3 Try running your model using multiple chains and assess whether there is evidence of convergence using the Brooks–Gelman–Rubin diagnostic plots (use the *bgr diag* button on the *Sample Monitor Tool*) – remember that you will have to specify a set of starting values for *each* chain, and that these should be very different in order to assess convergence properly.

2.4 In WinBUGS run *BLOCKER binomial.odc* which models directly the binomial data for the 22 trials – compare your results with those from models 1–3 above which use the LOR. In particular, monitor delta (the LOR) and use the *Compare Tool* to obtain a 'caterpillar plot' of both the individual and pooled LORs. Remember you will have to store the pooled LOR (d) in a previously unused element of delta, say delta[26], in order that both the individual and pooled LORs appear on the same plot – you also have to add sufficient NAs to the vector of starting values for delta, where NA represents a missing observation. Modify the code and rerun the model so that you can obtain the posterior distributions for the OR in each study and the pooled OR, and produce a 'caterpillar plot' on an OR scale.

References

1. Spiegelhalter D.J., Abrams K.R., Myles J. *Bayesian Approaches to Clinical Trials and Health-Care Evaluation*. New York: John Wiley & Sons, Ltd, 2004.

2. Lunn D.J., Thomas A., Best N., Spiegelhalter D. WinBUGS – a Bayesian modelling framework: concepts, structure, and extensibility. *Statistics and Computing* 2000; **10**:325–337.

3. Higgins J.P.T., Spiegelhalter D.J. Being sceptical about meta-analyses: a Bayesian perspective on magnesium trials in myocardial infarction. *International Journal of Epidemiology* 2002;**31**:96–104.

4. Silverman B.W. *Density Estimation*. London: Chapman and Hall, 1986.

5. Gelman A., Carlin J.B., Stern H.S., Rubin D.B. *Bayesian Data Analysis*. London: Chapman & Hall, 2004.

6. Ades A.E., Lu G., Higgins J.P.T. The interpretation of random effects meta-analysis in decision models. *Medical Decision Making* 2005;**25**:646–654.

7. Carlin J.B. Meta-analysis for 2 × 2 tables: a Bayesian approach. *Statistics in Medicine* 1992;**11**:141–158.

8. Spiegelhalter D.J. Bayesian graphical modelling: a case-study in monitoring health outcomes. *Journal of the Royal Statistical Society, Series C* 1998;**47**:115–133.

9. Cowles M.K., Carlin B.P. Markov Chain Monte Carlo convergence diagnostics: a comparative review. *Journal of the American Statistical Association* 1996;**91**:883–904.

10. Brooks S.P., Gelman A. Alternative methods for monitoring convergence of iterative simulations. *Journal of Computational and Graphical Statistics* 1998;**7**:434–455.

11. Gelman A., Rubin D.B. Inferences from iterative simulation using multiple sequences. *Statistical Science* 1992;**7**:457–472.

12. National Institute of Health and Clinical Excellence. *Guide to the Methods of Technology Appraisal*. 2008. http://www.nice.org.uk/media/B52/A7/TAMethodsGuideUpdated June2008.pdf.

13. Food and Drug Administration. *Challenge and Opportunity on the Critical Path to New Medical Products*. 2004. http://www.fda.gov/downloads/ScienceResearch/ SpecialTopics/CriticalPathInitiative/CriticalPathOpportunitiesReports/ucm113411.pdf.

14. Berry D.A. *Statistics: A Bayesian Perspective*. London: Duxbury, 1996.

15. Gilks W.R., Richardson S., Spiegelhalter D.J. *Markov Chain Monte Carlo in Practice*. London: Chapman & Hall/CRC, 1996.

16. Lee P.M. *Bayesian Statistics: An Introduction*. London: Arnold, 1997.

17. O'Hagan A., Luce B. *A Primer on Bayesian Statistics in Health Economics and Outcome Research*. www.bayesian-initiative.com. Bayesian Initiative in Health Economics and Outcomes Research, MedTap Intl, 2003.

18. Congdon P. *Bayesian Statistical Modelling*. Chichester: John Wiley & Sons, Ltd, 2001.

19. Congdon P. *Applied Bayesian Modelling*. Chichester: John Wiley & Sons, Ltd, 2003.

3

Introduction to decision models

3.1 Introduction

It is rare for an individual study to provide all the evidence required to evaluate the cost- effectiveness of competing interventions; and even if one did, it would be exceptional if this were the only study which provided evidence for this assessment. While it is not uncommon for individual trials to collect economic data and estimate cost-effectiveness, such evaluations often have limitations in terms of comparisons considered, time horizons, and generalisability of the results beyond the healthcare system where the trial was conducted. Further, synthesis of such cost-effectiveness estimates across multiple studies is problematic due to fundamental differences between studies such as different costings for different countries (although some examples of this type of analysis do exist [1]).

Due to this, reliance is often placed on decision-analytical models for economic evaluations of healthcare interventions. These have the objective of providing information to allow scarce healthcare resources to be allocated efficiently [2, 3]. For example, organisations worldwide, such as the National Institute for Health and Clinical Excellence (NICE) in the UK and the Canadian Agency for Drugs and Technology in Health (CADTH), are increasingly being required to utilise economic decision models when making decisions regarding which healthcare interventions and programmes to fund from the limited resources available to healthcare systems. Such models have a range of uses [4], not least to produce cost or cost-effectiveness results of interest not obtainable from trial data directly. Aspects of economic evaluation which decision modelling techniques can address include: (i) the synthesis of data from a variety of sources; (ii) the temporal extrapolation of outcome

Evidence Synthesis for Decision Making in Healthcare, First Edition. Nicky J. Welton,
Alexander J. Sutton, Nicola J. Cooper, Keith R. Abrams and A.E. Ades.
© 2012 John Wiley & Sons, Ltd. Published 2012 by John Wiley & Sons, Ltd.

data beyond the endpoints of relevant trials; (iii) making comparisons between treatments for which no 'head-to-head' trial evidence exist; (iv) investigation of how cost-effectiveness of clinical strategies/interventions changes as values of key parameters are varied (often not observable in primary (RCT) data analysis); (v) the linking of intermediate endpoints to ultimate measures of health gain (e.g. QALYs); and (vi) the incorporation of country specific data relating to disease history and management [5, 6].

The aim of this chapter is to introduce decision analytical models including: (i) consideration of the types of data required to populate such models; and (ii) the different approaches that can be taken to specify and evaluate such models. In respect of the latter, one of the challenges of such evaluations is to make appropriate allowance for all uncertainties – an issue we believe the Bayesian MCMC approach we adopt throughout is well suited to address. While much of this book considers methods for evidence synthesis, and emphasis is placed throughout on using all relevant evidence in economic evaluations, in this introductory chapter, exactly one source of evidence is assumed to exist for each model parameter (and these parameter estimates are assumed to be independent). This is done to allow the motivating principles of decision modelling to be explained ahead of methods for combining multiple sources of evidence on the relevant decision model parameters. The use of meta-analyses and more complex synthesis models to populate decision models are considered in Chapters 7 and 9, respectively.

3.2   Decision tree models

Decision models provide an explicit quantitative and systematic approach to decision making. Decision trees, such as the one depicted in Figure 3.1 for the use of prophylactic antibiotics to prevent wound infection following Caesarean section, provide a simple way to structure problems of decision making under uncertainty [7] whilst describing the major factors involved.

A decision tree depicts a branching system in which each branch represents an event that may take place in the future (i.e. time flows from left to right) and branches from a decision or choice node (□) represent the options, and branches from a chance node (○) represent the possible outcomes assigned a probability of occurrence (p). In this example, the decision node (and hence the decision being

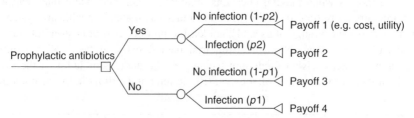

Figure 3.1   Example decision model: implications of using prophylactic antibiotics to prevent wound infection following Caesarean section.

evaluated) is whether or not to give prophylactic antibiotics and following this, patients can either get an infection or not (the chance nodes). It is important that all outcomes are represented and payoffs are assigned for each pathway through the model. Economists are usually interested in both the resource use and health outcomes associated with healthcare interventions, thus payoffs are expressed in terms of costs and utilities. How such parameters are estimated is initially considered in Section 3.3 and is the primary motivation for much of the remainder of this book. The decision tree is evaluated by 'rolling back' the tree to calculate the expected payoffs (see Section 3.4). It should not be forgotten that the usefulness of the results obtained from such models depends on the source and quality of the estimates input into the model [7]. That is, the results are only as reliable as the model's poorest data input, though, the extent to which this has a qualitative effect will depend on whether 'poor' evidence is used for parameters that strongly influence the model results [i.e. key driver(s) in the model].

3.3 Model parameters

For health technology assessments, decision models usually evaluate both the clinical and cost-effectiveness of interventions/strategies. Therefore, to parameterise the model, data are required on clinical effectiveness, disease progression rates, resource use, costs and patient outcomes (often with utility scales).

In this section, consideration is given to the outcome measures which are commonly encountered for informing parameters in decision models. These are discussed below under the four broad headings of effects of interventions, quantities relating to the clinical epidemiology of the underlying medical condition, utilities, and costs. These groupings cover the majority of the parameter types encountered when constructing decision models. Although meta-analysis is not addressed in depth until Chapter 4, a note on meta-analysis specific to the different types of outcomes is provided below.

3.3.1 Effects of interventions

It will be necessary to estimate the clinical effects of the competing alternative interventions in the decision model. The effects of a treatment may be characterised in terms of both benefit and harm outcomes. It is common to estimate the effect of interventions from comparative studies with two or more groups; very often using a randomised controlled trial (RCT) design due to the benefits randomisation offers in balancing confounding factors between groups and minimising bias [8]. In this section the examples presented use RCT data but the principles apply to nonrandomised studies also, although, obviously, concerns regarding the validity of estimates from nonrandomised data exist. Ways of combining randomised and non-randomised evidence whilst acknowledging potential biases in the latter are given consideration in Chapter 11. How such comparative estimates of effect are used to estimate parameters in a decision model is the topic of Chapter 7, however, it is important to stress here that although, ultimately, absolute effects of treatments will usually be required for modelling, data should be meta-analysed on comparative scales to maintain randomisation.

Most commonly RCTs have two intervention arms and traditionally meta-analysis has been used to estimate comparative effects between pairs of interventions using such paired data. This is the format of the data considered in this chapter. Clearly, when the decision question involves more than two interventions it will be necessary to consider either multiple pairwise meta-analyses, or often, more desirably, more complex synthesis models allowing the simultaneous synthesis of RCTs comparing different combinations of the treatments of interest. It may also be desirable to extend the evidence base to include RCTs making comparisons with interventions which are not of direct relevance to the decision question. These extensions to meta-analysis methods are covered in detail in Chapter 9, but for now we restrict our attention to the scenario where a single pairwise comparison is of interest.

We also restrict ourselves to consideration of independent, parallel group studies in which intervention is allocated at the individual patient level. Alternative designs are used, such as cross-over clinical trials [9] and cluster allocated studies [10]. While result data from such alternative designs are readily included in a synthesis, alternative formulae are required to estimate effect sizes and their variances due to the design features of these studies. The necessary details to allow inclusion of such studies are available elsewhere [11].

Binary, continuous, and ordinal outcomes, and outcomes which do not fall neatly into one of these three categorisations, are considered in turn below.

3.3.1.1   Binary outcomes

The most commonly used type of outcome measure are those which measure the presence or absence of an event, e.g. cured or not, alive or dead, etc. Binary outcome data of the form reported in a single comparative two-arm study are presented in Table 3.1

There are a number of ways such data *could* be summarised and synthesised across multiple studies. Firstly, let us highlight the incorrect approaches. As mentioned above, although decision models require separate parameter estimates for the effect of the different treatments, do not be seduced into estimating these separate parameters from these data. Although probabilities of events on placebo and aspirin *could* be obtained in this way, this would 'break' randomisation and abandon the benefits inherent in such data. Secondly, when synthesising this type of

Table 3.1   Binary outcome data for a two-arm study.

	Failure	Success
Treatment A (Experimental)	*a*	*b*
Treatment B (Control)	*c*	*d*

data, it may also look appealing to aggregate the data across all trials to produce a single summary 2×2 table of the form illustrated in Table 3.1. Again, this is not statistically sound and can lead to erroneous conclusions [12] and should be avoided. What is required is an approach that maintains the comparison of patients within the same study and synthesises these within study comparisons. In order to do this, *comparative* measures of effect are calculated for each study.

Several viable comparable outcome measures exist for such data. These include the commonly used Odds Ratio (OR), Relative Risk (RR) and the Risk Difference (RD). These are defined below using the notation of the 2×2 table in Table 3.1 together with associated variances, which provides a measure of uncertainty due to them being estimated from a finite sample (sampling error).

The OR outcome gives a relative measure of chance of the event of interest in the form of the ratio of the odds of an event in the two groups.

$$OR = \frac{ad}{bc} \tag{3.1}$$

For an undesirable outcome, an OR estimate of less than one, when comparing experimental treatment to the control, would indicate an improvement on the new treatment; while a ratio greater than one would imply the new treatment was less effective than control (the converse is true for desirable outcomes).

For the purposes of combining, it is recommended, to transform the data by taking the natural logarithm of the OR, ln(OR) [13], as this should provide a measure which is approximately normally distributed [14]. An estimate of the variance of the ln(OR) is given by:

$$\text{Var}(\ln(\text{RR})) = \frac{1}{a} + \frac{1}{b} + \frac{1}{c} + \frac{1}{d} \tag{3.2}$$

The RR is defined as the probability of an event in the treatment group divided by the probability of an event in the control group:

$$RR = [a/(a+b)]/[c/(c+d)] \tag{3.3}$$

This is the ratio of the probabilities of the event in the two groups, and as for ORs, for an undesirable outcome, an RR estimate of less than one, when comparing experimental treatment with the control, would indicate an improvement on the new treatment, etc. Again, it is usual to use the natural logarithm scale when combining studies; the variance of the log Relative Risk is given by:

$$\text{var}(\ln(\text{RR})) = \frac{1}{a} - \frac{1}{a+b} + \frac{1}{c} - \frac{1}{c+d} \tag{3.4}$$

The RD is defined by:

$$(RD) = [a/(a+b)] - [c/(c+d)] \tag{3.5}$$

It can be interpreted as the difference between the probabilities of an event occurring in the two groups. For an undesirable outcome, an RD estimate of less than zero, when comparing experimental treatment with the control, would indicate an improvement on the new treatment, etc. The variance of this measure is calculated by:

$$\text{var(RD)} = \frac{p_1(1-p_1)}{n_1} + \frac{p_2(1-p_2)}{n_2} \qquad (3.6)$$

where p_1 and p_2 are the observed rates of occurrence of the given event in the treatment and control groups, respectively. Thus in terms of Table 3.1, $p_1 = a/a + b$ and $p_2 = c/c + d$, $n_1 = a + b$ and $n_2 = c + d$ and the estimate of the RR $= p_1/p_2$.

Note that while the OR and RD scales are symmetric [i.e. the OR for the undesirable outcome (e.g. mortality) is 1/OR for the desirable outcome (e.g. survival)], this is not the case on the RR scale, so different estimates will be obtained depending on whether the outcome events are defined in terms of benefit or harm.

With multiple competing outcome scales available to conduct meta-analysis on, this raises the question: Which one should be used in a given situation? While the reader should be aware that choice of outcome scale for the meta-analysis will influence derived parameter estimates for the decision model (although differences will often be small, this is not always the case), there is no definitive answer to this question. Deeks and Altman [15] observe that there are several factors to take into consideration: consistency of effect across studies, mathematical properties and ease of interpretation. When considering consistency, empirical investigation has shown that the OR and the RR, both relative measures, are equally and more consistent than the absolute measure, the RD. ORs are not as easy to interpret as RRs or RDs (often ORs are incorrectly interpreted as RRs!) but they do allow logistic regression type analyses to be conducted which have desirable statistical properties (see Chapter 4).

In situations where OR or RR is undefined due to zero cells in the 2×2 table (i.e. Table 3.1) it is common practice to add a continuity correction of 0.5 to each cell of the 2×2 table to enable the OR or RR to be calculated. More sophisticated correction factors exist [16] which may be worthwhile pursuing if data are very sparse, as is sometimes encountered when evaluating adverse events, although Bayesian models which model the 2×2 table data directly, and, hence avoid the need for correction factors altogether, are considered in Chapter 4 and present a viable alternative.

3.3.1.2   Continuous outcomes

Not all outcomes are discrete events, some may be continuous (e.g. duration of an illness). In such contexts the Mean Difference (MD) between groups is an appropriate statistic to calculate for each study, assuming each study has measured the outcome on the same continuous scale, i.e.

$$MD = \mu_t - \mu_c \qquad (3.7)$$

where μ_t and μ_c are the mean responses in the (experimental) treatment and control groups, respectively. The variance of this treatment difference is:

$$\text{var}(T) = \sigma^2(1/n_t + 1/n_c) \tag{3.8}$$

where n_t is the sample size of the treatment group, n_c is the sample size of the control group, and σ^2 is the variance, assumed common to both groups. σ^2 needs estimating from the data, and this estimate is denoted s^{*2}. s^* can be defined in different ways, each of which will yield a different estimate. Common and intuitive choices for s^* are s^{t*} and s^{c*} which are the standard deviation of the response in the treatment and control groups, respectively. In Section 9.8 consideration is given on how to model continuous outcomes at the arm level rather than as the difference between arms.

Alternatively, a pooled standard deviation (s^{p*}) combining both s^{t*} and s^{c*} can be constructed. Hedges and Olkin [17] suggest using s^{p*} if it is reasonable to assume equal population variances. The formula they propose for s^{p*} pooled sample is:

$$s^{p*} = \sqrt{\frac{(n_t - 1)(s_t^{t*})^2 + (n_c - 1)(s^{c*})^2}{n_t + n_c - 2}} \tag{3.9}$$

where n_t and n_c are the treatment and control group sample sizes, respectively.

Note that when continuous outcomes are reported on different scales in different studies it is common practice in meta-analysis to calculate a standardised effect size by dividing reported outcomes by their standard deviation [17]. However, since interpretation of standardised effect sizes is limited, it is unlikely such an outcome will have a role in informing a decision model. Therefore, a more sophisticated analysis may be required for synthesis in which the relationships between the different outcomes are modelled [18].

A complicating issue with continuous effect sizes is that sometimes outcomes are reported as medians rather than means. This is sometimes done on clinical interpretation grounds [18], but can also be because the distribution of outcomes are skewed. In the former case, it may be possible to obtain the required mean statistics directly from the original study researchers. Note that the mean is the summary statistic of interest as it allows decision makers to calculate the total cost of adopting a new therapy and the total effect received in return for incurring this cost [19]. Regarding the situation where outcomes are non-normally distributed, the central limit theorem [20] implies that the distribution of the mean statistic *will* be normally distributed if the sample sizes are sufficiently large and hence the assumptions underlying the meta-analysis model are (still) satisfied.

3.3.1.3   Ordinal outcomes

Ordinal outcomes (i.e. ordered categorical response scales) are used occasionally to measure effectiveness in medical research (e.g. disease severity scales) and such data could inform a decision model. The reader is referred elsewhere for an account of analysing this type of outcome data [21].

3.3.1.4   Other outcomes

We outline some other outcomes below. In addition, the analysis of rate data is considered in Section 9.8.

Multiple events   Sometimes it is possible that individuals experience multiple (nonfatal) events in the duration of the study (e.g. multiple infections, or epileptic seizures). Sometimes such data are dichotomised by defining the outcome of interest as being one or more events during the study and thus treated as a binary outcome as described above. Alternatively, if events are frequent, the outcome could be defined as being a number of events during the study and thus can be treated as a continuous outcome in the manner described above. A further possibility is that treatment effects are measured using a rate ratio outcome [22]. The data available and the structure of the decision model (note, chronic or recurring diseases are often modelled using a Markov structure – see Chapter 10) will largely dictate the appropriate approach to analysis.

Survival data   When the outcome of interest is time to event (often time to death, but not necessarily – i.e. time to recovery is sometimes considered), this usually includes individuals who did not experience the event in the duration of the study and hence such censored observations complicate the analysis. Much has been written on how to analyse such data for an individual study [23], with Cox's proportional hazards model becoming a popular approach. Several meta-analysis approaches for survival data exist [14], including the pooling of hazard ratios. Unfortunately, reporting of survival analyses is notoriously patchy which means some manipulation of reported data may be necessary before meta-analysis is possible [24]. Time to event data are commonly used to derive transition probabilities in Markov models which are consider in depth in Chapter 10.

Mixture of scales   The reader should be aware that studies may have used a mixture of different types of outcome scales (i.e. binary, rate, continuous, and ordinal). This presents problems for the meta-analyst. Ultimately it may be necessary to omit results from certain studies, or transform results between outcome scales [21] to enable meta-analysis to be conducted. Alternatively, more advance forms of synthesis which allow synthesis across different outcome measure and definitions may be possible [18].

3.3.2   Quantities relating to the clinical epidemiology of the clinical condition being treated

For decision modelling it will often be necessary to estimate parameters relating to the natural history of the medical condition in question (e.g. the probability a patient will die if treated using standard care). For an intervention to be effective, it will have to modify one or more of these parameters. Depending on the complexity of the disease model, this can vary from estimating a small number of parameters for a simple decision tree, to a much more complicated set of dependent parameters relating to disease progression, often modelled assuming a Markov process (see Chapter 10). Typically, such information will come from (noncomparative) observational data or from the placebo arms of trials.

Standard meta-analysis models (as described in Chapter 4) can be used to estimate single, independent, parameters. Commonly, this will relate to rates or probabilities of certain disease related events. For Markov models it will be necessary to estimate rates/probabilities of transition between different health states via a transition matrix, and methods for estimating such matrices are covered in Chapter 10.

3.3.2.1 Probabilities

Probabilities of events occurring (or equivalently proportions of patients who experience an event) may require estimating to inform a decision model. Due to computational issues with such quantities being bounded between 0 and 1, synthesis is commonly conducted on the natural logarithm odds, ln(Odds), scale, but results can be transformed back to the probability scale as required. The ln(Odds) is defined as follows:

$$\ln(\text{Odds}) = \ln \left(\frac{\text{No. of patients having event}}{\text{No. of patients not having event}} \right) \tag{3.10}$$

The variance of the ln(Odds) is:

$$\text{var}(\ln(\text{Odds})) = \frac{1}{\text{No. of patients having event}} + \frac{1}{\text{No. of patients not having event}} \tag{3.11}$$

ln(Odds) can be transformed onto the probability scale using:

$$\text{Probability} = \frac{e^{\ln(\text{Odds})}}{1 + e^{\ln(\text{Odds})}} \tag{3.12}$$

3.3.2.2 Rates

Estimation of rates of events, which include the notion of time (absent on the probability scale) may be required. For statistical reasons, synthesis is conducted on the log scale

$$\ln(\text{Rate}) = \ln(\text{No. events/time}) \tag{3.13}$$

where time is typically measured in observed person-years. The variance of this rate estimate is:

$$\text{var}(\ln(\text{Rate})) = 1/\text{No. events} \tag{3.14}$$

3.3.2.3 Continuous responses

A continuous response can be summarised by its mean, μ, and corresponding variance, $\frac{s^2}{n-1}$, where s^2 is the estimated standard deviation of the response and

n is the number of observations in the sample. Meta-analysis can be conducted directly using these quantities.

3.3.3 Utilities

Although average utilities for populations, commonly measured on the QALY scale, are commonly estimated through empirical surveys, meta-analysis of such data is rare, although notable exceptions do exist [25] and we support such an approach. Part of the reason for this is that the uncertainty in the outcome measures are often poorly reported restricting the syntheses which can be done. Where variances (or standard errors) of mean utility scores do exist, they can be treated as continuous responses as outlined in the previous section. Where no uncertainty is reported, or obtainable, or utilities have been derived from approaches which do not consider uncertainty (e.g. asking an expert for their best 'guess') a standard meta-analytic approach is not possible.

3.3.4 Resource use and costs

Estimates of resource use and unit costs of certain events will often be required for decision modelling. To estimate costs, resource use data are usually combined with unit cost data. For example, if a procedure takes 2 h at a unit cost of £50 per hour then the total cost will be £100. Resource use data and unit cost data will usually be acquired from empirical studies and therefore estimated with uncertainty. Ideally, this uncertainty needs to be taken into account by expressing each of the parameters as distributions (see Example 3.2). Exceptions where costs may be known with certainty include drug costs, although it would still be advisable to perform sensitivity analysis to explore what would happen if the drug costs change, which they inevitably will over time. Where resource use and unit costs data are estimated, through empirical studies, then it is potentially relevant to meta-analyse the data [1]. However, there are inevitably issues relating to the relevance of estimates of resource use and unit costs in the literature for a given decision context, e.g. studies may be done in different health systems in countries which use different resource allocations and currencies. Distributions of medical costs data are often highly skewed [26] which makes assumptions of normality of mean costs (typically made for meta-analysis – see Chapter 4) questionable if sample sizes are small.

3.4 Deterministic decision tree

When populating a decision tree, data may be entered as point estimates with or without their associated uncertainty (reflecting the fact the data are a quantity estimated with error and not known). If the former approach to parameter specification is taken, the resulting model is often referred to as deterministic (i.e. there is no uncertainty in it). If parameter estimation uncertainty is represented in the model (usually by specifying probabilistic distributions for each parameter) the model is referred to as stochastic. In this section we will consider a deterministic model where a single piece of information is used to inform each of the model parameters. We do this for educational purposes, and generally advocate using stochastic modelling in practice (see Section 3.5). However, if this type of model is used, sensitivity analysis approaches can be used to explore the potential impact of uncertainty on the model conclusions by varying one or more individual input parameters across predetermined ranges and exploring how this affects the analysis results.

For the model presented in Figure 3.1, assuming all the parameters to be fixed, the expected payoffs for the two options can be calculated as follows:

Option 1. Prophylactic antibiotics:

$$E\_Option1 = (1 - p2) \times Payoff1 + p2 \times Payoff2$$

Option 2. No prophylactic antibiotics:

$$E\_Option2 = (1 - p1) \times Payoff3 + p1 \times Payoff4$$

Such calculations are sometimes called 'rolling back' the decision tree and are obtained by multiplying the chance of each outcome branch occurring by the payoff for that branch and summing all branches associated with each decision node. Using a deterministic approach, where each quantity in the equation has a fixed parameter, these expected payoffs could be calculated in a standard spreadsheet, or even on a calculator; and the calculations required are provided in Example 3.1. However, since this is an intermediate step to evaluating a fully stochastic model in WinBUGS (Section 3.5), it is important that the reader also understands how this can be achieved in WinBUGS. All that is required is that the above equations are included in the 'model specification' and then the model inputs (e.g. $p1$ and $p2$) are defined as 'data'. Alternatively, as in the example below, $p2$ could be derived from an effectiveness parameter (e.g. RR) and $p1$, and thus defined as part of the 'model specification'. Having specified the model and input the data, a deterministic model is compiled and data input in the usual way but no 'updates' of the MCMC sampler are required(!). This is because there is no stochastic element to the modelling which needs evaluating. Values for each of the parameters of interest can be obtained from the *Info_Node info ...* menu.

Example 3.1   Prophylactic antibiotics (cephalosporins) to prevent wound infection following Caesarean section: Cost implications – deterministic.

Background

There is evidence to suggest that the incidence of wound infection following Caesarean section can be significantly reduced by a very short prophylactic course of antibiotics at the time of the operation [27]. Women who experience wound infection following a Caesarean section tend to require:

- a longer postnatal hospital stay,

- more intensive nursing care,

- antibiotic therapy, and

- more laboratory tests

than would normally be the case after a Caesarean section.

Decision model

The simple decision model presented in Figure 3.1 is used to evaluate the cost only implications (for simplicity) of introducing prophylactic antibiotics at a local maternity hospital.

Effectiveness data

For this analysis the data on the effectiveness of the prophylactic antibiotic cephalosporin, compared with no prophylactic antibiotic treatment, on wound infections in women undergoing Caesarean delivery is extracted from one RCT [28] (Table 3.2). (In reality, several relevant RCTs have been conducted and this example will be revisited in Chapter 7 using all the available RCT evidence.) For this analysis, effectiveness is summarised as a relative risk (note, for a binary outcome such as the occurrence of wound infections the analysis could be conducted on other scales, such as OR or RD [29]). Obviously, the formulae given below will need modifying appropriately if other scales are used.

$$RR = \frac{a/(a+b)}{c/(c+d)} = \frac{4/(4+129)}{28/(28+108)} = 0.15$$

Model parameters

The remaining model parameter estimates used in the evaluation are listed in Table 3.3. (Note, these have mostly been obtained from a previous economic evaluation.)

Evaluation of economic model

To evaluate the model we first need to estimate the the payoffs (i.e. costs) associated with each pathway through the model (Figure 3.2).

Table 3.2   Results extracted from Bibi *et al.*'s [28] RCT.

	Infection	No infection	Total
Prophylactic antibiotics	4 (*a*)	129 (*b*)	133
Placebo	28 (*c*)	108 (*d*)	136

Table 3.3 Resource use and unit cost data extracted from Mugford *et al.* [30] except cost of administering the antibiotic which was assumed to be £7, the cost of a nurse per procedure.

Parameters		Estimates	Variable name
Length of stay	Wound infection	8.80 days	*loswd*
	No wound infection	6.70 days	*losnwd*
Cost of inpatient stay	Wound infection	£163.03	*cstwd*
per day	No wound infection	£107.26	*cstnwd*
Cost of prophylactic	Cephalosporin per dose	£5.67	*cstPx*
antibiotics	(3 doses required)		
Cost of administering	Per dose	£7.00	*cstadmin*
the antibiotic			
Number of Caesarean	Total	486	*nc1*
sections (local	Developing wound	41	*rc1*
hospital data)	infection without		
	antibiotics		

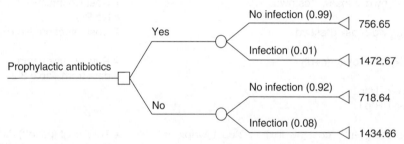

Figure 3.2 Decision tree with estimated parameters: Implications of using prophylactic antibiotics to prevent wound infection following Caesarean section.

Costs

Payoff 1 = (6.7days × £107.26) + 3doses × (£5.67 + £7) = £756.65

Payoff 2 = (8.8days × £163.06) + 3doses × (£5.67 + £7) = £1472.67

Payoff 3 = (6.7days × £107.26) = £718.64

Payoff 4 = (8.8days × £163.06) = £1434.66

Next, we need to estimate *p2*, the probability of developing a wound infection following a Caesarean section with prophylactic antibiotics. This can be calculated from *p1* (i.e. the probability of developing a wound infection following a Caesarean section without prophylactic antibiotics) and *RR*.

$$p2 = \frac{41}{486}(p1) \times 0.15(RR) = 0.01$$

Results

The expected payoffs for the two options are:

Option 1. Prophylactic antibiotics:

$$Costs = ((1 - 0.01) \times £756.65) + (0.01 \times £1472.67) = £765.48$$

Option 2. No prophylactic antibiotics:

$$Costs = ((1 - 0.08) \times £718.64) + (0.08 \times £1434.66) = £779.05$$

Thus, the use of prophylactic antibiotics to prevent infections following Caesarean section is cost saving (difference £13.57).

The WinBUGS code for this model is:

```
model {

cost_nwdpx <-losnwd*cstnwd+dose*(cstPx+cstadmin)    # Cost(No infection/Px)
cost_wdpx<-loswd*cstwd+dose*(cstPx+cstadmin)         # Cost(Infection/Px)
cost_nwd <-losnwd*cstnwd                             # Cost(No Infection/
                                                     # No Px)
cost_wd<-loswd*cstwd                                 # Cost(Infection/ No Px)


RR<-(a/(a+b))/(c/(c+d))                              # Relative risk using
                                                     # data from Table 3.2
p1<-rc1/nc1
p2<-RR*p1

costtrt<-((1-p2) *cost_nwdpx) + p2*cost_wdpx         # Total cost (payoff) Px
costctl<-((1-p1)*cost_nwd) + p1*cost_wd              # Total cost (payoff)
                                                     # No Px


}

list(losnwd=6.7, loswd=8.8, cstnwd=107.26,           # Data
cstwd=163.03, cstdrug=5.67, cstadmin=7, dose=3,
rc1=41, nc1=486, a=4, b=129, c=28, d=108)
```

3.5   Stochastic decision tree

Unlike the deterministic model, that assumes all model parameters to be fixed (i.e. known), a stochastic model incorporates the uncertainty about the true values of the parameters used as inputs in the analysis. This is achieved by specifying each of the model input and payoff parameters as a distribution rather than a point estimate. The distributional form should be determined by the (approximate large-sample) statistical properties of an estimate which will ensure logical bounds are placed on parameters (e.g. probabilities are bounded between 0 and 1 – see Example 3.2). A stochastic model is evaluated by drawing a random sample from each distribution, evaluating the model for these sampled values and repeating the process many times. The resulting (joint) distribution of differences in the outcomes of interest (e.g. costs and effects) between decision options can be used to inform decisions (details of how this can be done are provided in Example 3.2).

This type of analysis is often termed probabilistic sensitivity analysis. However, since in statistics sensitivity analysis refers to analyses which are conducted to assess the robustness of the findings in the primary analysis to the assumptions made, this name is perhaps not ideal, as we consider such a stochastic analysis to be the primary analysis. It is important to note that if the model includes a nonlinear component (e.g. the transformation of ln(RR) to RR) then the estimated mean values of the model outputs will be erroneous from a deterministic analysis (and hence differ from a stochastic model) [31]. Although distributions for parameters are often specified independently, where correlation exists between the estimated parameters this needs to be accounted for through the specification of joint distributions.

A stochastic decision model evaluated within a Bayesian framework allows the decision maker to estimate useful probability statements such as the probability that a new treatment has greater expected payoffs (e.g. more cost-effective) compared with the existing treatment.

Example 3.2   Prophylactic antibiotics (cephalosporins) to prevent wound infection following Caesarean section: Cost implications – stochastic.

Decision model and parameters

The decision model for this example is the same as for Example 3.1 but now the model parameters and payoffs are expressed stochastically; that is, they are defined in terms of distributions (with the exceptions of cost of inpatient stay per day, and cost of prophylactic antibiotics which are assumed known in this instance) – see Table 3.4. Note that the probability of developing a wound infection without antibiotics is expressed as a Beta distribution; that is, using the notation from Table 3.4:

$$pc1 \sim \text{Beta}(alpha, beta)$$

$$\text{where } alpha = rc1 = 41$$

$$beta = (nc1 - rc1) = 445$$

Effectiveness data

As in Example 3.1, the data on the effectiveness of the prophylactic antibiotic cephalosporin, compared with no prophylactic antibiotic treatment, on wound infections in women undergoing Caesarean delivery is extracted from one RCT, namely that of Bibi *et al.* [28]. However, this time the data are specified with

Table 3.4   Resource use and unit cost data extracted from Mugford *et al*. [30] except cost of administering the antibiotic.

Parameters		Estimates	Distribution	Variable name
Length of stay	Wound infection	8.8 days (sd = 3.5)	Normal	*loswd*
	No wound infection	6.7 days (sd = 7.1)	Normal	*losnwd*
Cost of inpatient	Wound infection	£163.03	Fixed	*cstwd*
stay per day	No wound infection	£107.26	Fixed	*cstnwd*
Cost of prophylactic antibiotics	Cephalosporin per dose (3 doses required)	£5.67	Fixed	*cstPx*
Cost of administering the antibiotic	Per dose	£7 (£4 to £10)	Uniform	*cstadmin*
Timeframe	Days	20		
Number of Caesarean sections (local hospital data)	Total	486	Beta	*nc1*
	Developing wound infection without antibiotics	41		*rc1*

uncertainty by defining the natural logarithm of the relative risk to be distributed normally with mean and variance calculated as follows, using the data and notation of Table 3.2:

$$\ln RR \sim \text{Normal}(theta, var)$$

$$\text{where } theta = \ln\left(\frac{a/(a+b)}{c/(c+d)}\right) = \ln\left(\frac{4/133}{28/136}\right) = -1.92$$

$$var = \frac{1}{a} - \frac{1}{(a+b)} + \frac{1}{c} - \frac{1}{(c+d)} = \frac{1}{4} - \frac{1}{133} + \frac{1}{28} - \frac{1}{136} = 0.27$$

Results

The model was evaluated using MCMC methods implemented in WinBUGS. Thirty thousand iterations were performed with the first 10 000 iterations discarded as the burn-in. The expected payoff for the two options, together with their distributions, are presented in Table 3.5.

As for the deterministic model, the use of prophylactic antibiotics to prevent infections following Caesarean section is shown to be cost saving if we focus on the point estimate, −£12.80. However we can now quantify the uncertainty surrounding this estimate and find the result to be less than conclusive since the

95% CrI ranges from −£39.17 to +£11.19. The probability of a cost saving as a result of introducing prophylactic antibiotics is 0.84.

Table 3.5 Expected payoffs from the stochastic model.

	Expected costs	Distributions
Prophylactic antibiotics	£766.40 (695.10 to 837.40)	
No prophylactic antibiotics	£778.80 (710.1 to 846.50)	
Difference	−£12.80 (−39.17 to 11.19)	

The WinBUGS code for this model is:

```
model {

lnRR~dnorm(theta, prec)                              # Distribution for
                                                     # ln(Relative Risk)
theta <- log(a/(a+b))/(c/(c+d))

prec<-1/((1/a) - (1/(a+b)) +(1/c) - (1/(c+d)))
                                                     # Distribution for
                                                     # Prob(Infection/No Px)
p1~dbeta(alpha, beta)
alpha<-rc1
beta<-nc1-rc1
                                                     # Prob(Infection/Px)
```

```
p2<- exp(lnRR)*p1

loswd~dnorm(mnloswd,precwd)                    # Distribution for length of
                                               # stay with infection
precwd<-1/pow(sdloswd/sqrt(numwd),2)

losnwd~dnorm(mnlosnwd,precnwd)                  # Distribution for length of
                                               # stay w/o infection
precnwd<-1/pow(sdlosnwd/sqrt(numnwd),2)

cstadmin~dunif(4,10)                            # Px administration
                                               # costs ~ Uniform
cst.trt<-(1-p2)*((cstPx+cstadmin)*3+(losnwd*cstnwd))   # Total cost (payoff) Px
      +p2*((cstPx+cstadmin)*3+(loswd*cstwd))
cst.ctl<-(1-p1)*(losnwd*cstnwd)+p1*(loswd*cstwd)  # Total cost (payoff) No Px

diff.cost<-cst.trt-cst.ctl                      # Difference in cost
}

list(rc1=41, nc1=486, cstwd=163.03, cstnwd=107.26,    # Data
mnloswd=8.8, sdloswd=3.5, mnlosnwd=6.7,
sdlosnwd=7.1, numwd=41, numnwd=445, cstPx=5.67,
rt=4, nt=133, rc=28. nc=136, a=4, b=129, c=28,
d=108)
```

3.5.1 Presenting the results of stochastic economic decision models

For simplicity, the decision models presented in Examples 3.1 and 3.2 only considered one outcome – cost (difference). However commonly both (differences in) cost and effects are of interest. Traditionally, the results of cost-effectiveness analyses have been reported in terms of an Incremental Cost-Effectiveness Ratio (ICER) defined as the cost per additional unit of effectiveness.

$$ICER = \frac{C_T - C_C}{E_T - E_C} = \frac{\Delta_C}{\Delta_E} < \lambda \qquad (3.15)$$

Where C_C and E_C are the costs and effects in the control group, and C_T and E_T are the costs and effects in the treatment group. Δ_C and Δ_E are the differences in the costs and effects between the treatment and control groups (i.e. incremental costs and incremental effects). If this ICER is less than the maximum amount a decision maker is willing to pay per additional unit of effectiveness (λ) then the new treatment is considered cost-effective compared with the control.

The ICER results can be presented on a cost-effectiveness plane [32]. As depicted in Figure 3.2, the plane is divided into four quadrants depending on the

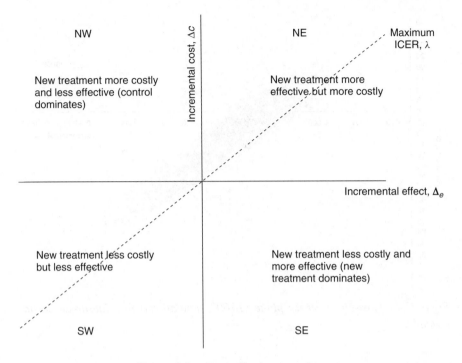

Figure 3.3   Cost-effectiveness plane.

signs of Δ_C and Δ_E. Where the new treatment is less costly and more effective than the alternative then this treatment is said to dominate (i.e. SE quadrant in Figure 3.3). Similarly, the control dominates when the new treatment is more costly and less effective (i.e. NW quadrant). However, in the situation where the new treatment is either more effective but less costly, or, less costly but less effective, then a decision must be made regarding the cost a decision maker is willing to pay per additional health gain (λ). This is depicted on Figure 3.3 as a dashed line where the slope of the line is equal to λ. The points below the dashed line indicate that the new treatment is considered to be cost-effective at the specified threshold, λ. The points above the line indicate that the new treatment is cost-ineffective.

By plotting the simulation results from a probabilistic decision model onto the cost-effectiveness plane, the probability that the new treatment is cost-effective compared with the control can be obtained by simply calculating the proportion of simulations below the dashed line shown in Figure 3.4 for different values of λ.

The amount a decision maker is willing to pay for an additional unit of benefit (λ) may not be disclosed or known exactly. Therefore, the probability that a new treatment is cost-effective is usually calculated for a range of different values of λ and these probabilities are plotted to form a cost-effectiveness acceptability curve (CEAC) [33] (see Figure 3.5).

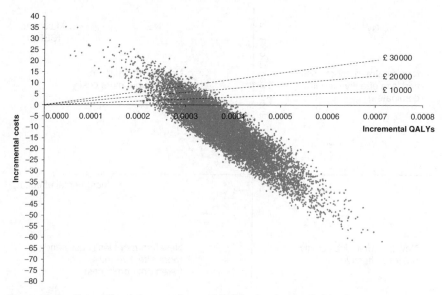

Figure 3.4   Cost-effectiveness plane (10000 simulations) for Caesarean section example.

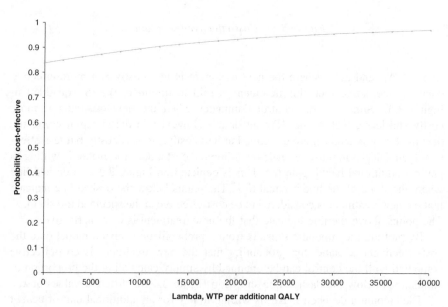

Figure 3.5   Cost-effectiveness acceptability curve for Caesarean section example. WTP, Willingness To Pay.

The interpretation of ICERs is problematic especially when the denominator is negative or zero. Therefore, the Incremental Net Benefit (INB) function [34] has been proposed as an alternative method of presenting cost-effectiveness results. It is defined as:

$$INB = \lambda \Delta_E - \Delta_C > 0 \tag{3.16}$$

INB can be calculated for a range of λ values and plotted together with its credibility intervals (see Figure 3.6(b)). The value at which the INB curve crosses the horizontal axis is the ICER (i.e. Δ_C / Δ_E) [35].

Using the net-benefit framework, the probability that a new treatment is cost-effective compared with the control based on a probabilistic decision model is defined as:

$$p(CE) = \frac{\text{Number of simulations INB} > 0}{\text{Total number of simulations}} \tag{3.17}$$

That is, the number of simulations on the cost-effectiveness plane that fall below the threshold line (i.e. represented by dashed lines in Figures 3.3 and 3.4).

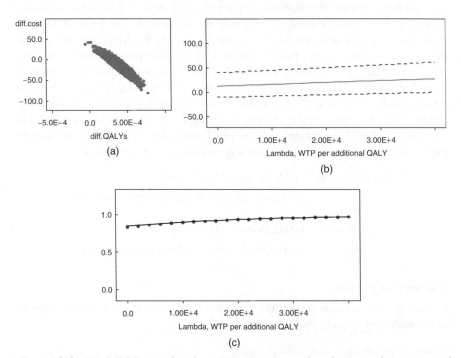

Figure 3.6 WinBUGS graphical output. (a) Joint distribution of incremental QALYs, Δ_E and incremental costs, Δ_C. (b) Expected incremental net benefit and 95% interval for a range of λ. (c) Cost-effectiveness acceptability curve for a range of λ.

INB and the probability that the new treatment is cost-effective compared with the control can be calculated within the WinBUGS program using the following code:

```
for (k in 1:M){
    lambda[k]<-(k-1)*units
    INB[k]<-lambda[k]*delta.effect- delta.cost
    ProbCE[k] <- step(INB[k])}
```

where M represents the number of values of λ to be considered and units the units of λ (e.g. £1000s, £5000s, etc.). delta.cost and delta.effect are the differences in costs and effects, respectively, between the treatment and control groups.

Example 3.3   Prophylactic antibiotics (cephalosporins) to prevent wound infection following Caesarean section: Stochastic economic evaluation.

Decision model and parameters

This example extends the analysis performed in Example 3.2 to a full economic evaluation by including utility values into the analysis in the form of QALYs. Although we would advocate for all data used to inform the decision model parameters to be evidence based, for the purposes of this illustrative example we have simply assumed QALY values associated with a wound infection and without a wound infection following a Caesarean section to be 0.68 (*QALYs.wd*) and 0.88 (*QALYs.nwd*), respectively. Full health is assumed a QALY value of 1.0 (*Fullhealth*). The timeframe for the analysis is assumed to be 20 days (*fllwupdays*). For this analysis, the QALY values are assumed known. The total QALYs for women with wound infection and those without is calculated over 20 days as:

$$totQALYs.wd = ((QALYs.wd/365 \times loswd)$$
$$+ (Fullhealth/365 \times (fllwupdays - loswd))$$

$$totQALYs.nwd = ((QALYs.nwd/365 \times losnwd)$$
$$+ (Fullhealth/365 \times (fllwupdays - losnwd))$$

Economic evaluation

To evaluate the decision model, the costs and QALYs in the two groups need to be calculated by 'rolling back' the tree as follows:

Option 1. Prophylactic antibiotics:

$$cst.trt = (1 - p2) \times ((antibiotic + drugadmin) \times 3 + (losnwd \times inptnwd))$$
$$+ p2 \times ((antibiotic + drugadmin) \times 3 + (loswd \times inptwd))$$

$$QALYs.trt = (1 - p2) \times totQALYs.nwd + p2 \times totQALYs.wd$$

Option 2. No prophylactic antibiotics:

$$cst.ctl = (1 - p1) \times (losnwd \times inptnwd) + p1 \times (loswd \times inptwd)$$

$$QALYs.ctl = (1 - p1) \times totQALYs.nwd + p1 \times totQALYs.wd$$

From these quantities the INB can be calculated and CEACs plotted.

Results

The model was evaluated using MCMC methods implemented in WinBUGS. Thirty thousand iterations were performed with the first 10 000 iterations discarded as the burn-in. The expected payoffs for the two options are presented in Table 3.6.

Table 3.6 Expected payoffs from the stochastic model.

	Expected costs	Expected QALYs
Prophylactic antibiotics	£766.40 (695.10 to 837.40)	0.0525 (0.0523 to 0.0527)
No prophylactic antibiotics	£778.80 (710.10 to 846.50)	0.0521 (0.0519 to 0.0524)
Difference	−£12.79 (−39.50 to 10.57)	0.0004 (0.0002 to 0.0006)

The results from economic evaluation are presented graphically in Figure 3.6. These plots have been created in WinBUGS; however, it is possible to obtain the CODA output from WinBUGS (from the **Inference** menu choose **Samples**, select the required monitored variable and press *coda*) and then copy and paste the output into another software package such as Microsoft Excel® or Stata [36] (Figures 3.4 and 3.5).

The additional WinBUGS code to extend Example 3.2 to the full economic evaluation described above is:

```
totQALYs.wd<- ((QALYwd/365)*loswd) + ((Fullhealth/365)       # QALYs(Infection)
               *(fllwupdays-loswd))

totQALYs.nwd<- ((QALYnwd/365)*losnwd)                         # QALYs(No infection)
               + ((Fullhealth/365)*(fllwupdays-losnwd))

QALYs.trt<-(1-p2)*totQALYs.nwd+p2*totQALYs.wd                 # QALYs(Px)
QALYs.ctl<-(1-p1)*totQALYs.nwd+p1*totQALYs.wd                 # QALYs(No Px)

diff.QALYs<-(QALYs.trt-QALYs.ctl)                             # Difference in QALYs

for (k in 1:M){
        lambda[k]<-(k-1)*2000
        INB[k]<-lambda[k]*delta.QALYs - delta.cost            # Incremental
                                                              # Net Benefit
```

```
ProbCE[k] <- step(INB[k])          # Probability cost
                                   # effective
}
```

```
list(M=21, QALYwd=0.68, QALYnwd=0.88, Fullhealth=1,
fllwupdays=20)                            # Additional data
```

3.6   Sources of evidence

Defining the sources of evidence which should be used to populate a decision model is challenging. This is due in part to issues relating to potential biases in estimates from the different sources of evidence. Consider the typical sources of the evidence required for the different parameters. Although risk of bias for a study will depend on the specifics of that study, as a starting point, it is helpful to consider a potential hierarchy of data sources for the different parameters in an economic decision analysis. Such a hierarchy, as developed by Coyle and Lee [37], and modified by Cooper et al. [38], is presented in Table 3.7. This hierarchy of evidence provides a list of the potential sources for each data component commonly of interest, which in this case are: (i) main clinical effect sizes; (ii) baseline clinical data; (iii) resource use; (iv) costs; and (v) utilities. Sources are ranked on an increasing scale from 1 to 6, with the most appropriate source for each different data component assigned a rank of 1. The last data component within each category (rank 6) is expert opinion, which is often acquired when no other data are available; although it may be used in combination with other sources of data to ensure relevance to the population/decision of interest. Note that for some components there are two levels within a rank to distinguish between evidence from a meta-analysis of trials (denoted by +) and a single trial.

Even with such a hierarchy, producing a definitive answer to the question of which sources of evidence should be used to populate a particular decision model is challenging. For instance, should only evidence from the highest rank obtainable on the hierarchy be used for every parameter? What if the highest rank for some parameters is low on the hierarchy; can allowance be made for this? Further, such a ranking relates to some 'average' study of the type defined and such a hierarchy ignores specific validity issues relating to the specific studies in question.

The authors' belief is that all relevant evidence should be used and synthesised using statistically rigorous methods. However, although potentially relevant, there may be concerns that some evidence is biased. Therefore a, perhaps, utopian vision is to use all relevant evidence, making due allowances for potential biases in the analysis. There are two problems with this. First, methods to assess and adjust for biases are complicated and underdeveloped. Ideally decisions should be based on the validity of each data source (i.e. the likelihood bias exists) with respect to both internal consistency (i.e. comparing what should be happening in the model with what would be expected) and external validity (i.e. validation of the model

Table 3.7 Potential hierarchies of data sources (modified from Coyle and Lee [37].

Rank	Data components
A	**Clinical effect sizes**
1+	Meta-analysis of RCTs with direct comparison between comparator therapies, measuring final outcomes
1	Single RCT with direct comparison between comparator therapies, measuring final outcomes
2+	Meta-analysis of RCTs with direct comparison between comparator therapies, measuring surrogate^a outcomes Meta-analysis of placebo controlled RCTs with similar trial populations, measuring final outcomes for each individual therapy
2	Single RCT with direct comparison between comparator therapies, measuring surrogate^a outcomes Single placebo controlled RCTs with similar trial populations, measuring final outcomes for each individual therapy
3+	Meta-analysis of placebo controlled RCTs with similar trial populations, measuring surrogate^a outcomes
3	Single placebo controlled RCTs with similar trial populations, measuring surrogate^a outcomes for each individual therapy
4	Case control or cohort studies
5	Nonanalytic studies, for example, case reports, case series
6	Expert opinion
B	**Baseline clinical data**
1	Case series or analysis of reliable administrative databases specifically conducted for the study covering patients solely from the jurisdiction of interest
2	Recent case series or analysis of reliable administrative databases covering patients solely from the jurisdiction of interest
3	Recent case series or analysis of reliable administrative databases covering patients solely from another jurisdiction
4	Old case series or analysis of reliable administrative databases. Estimates from RCTs
5	Estimates from previously published economic analyses: unsourced
6	Expert opinion
C	**Resource use**
1	Prospective data collection or analysis of reliable administrative data for specific study
2	Recently published results of prospective data collection or recent analysis of reliable administrative data – same jurisdiction
3	Unsourced data from previous economic evaluations – same jurisdiction
4	Recently published results of prospective data collection or recent analysis of reliable administrative data – different jurisdiction

(*continued overleaf*)

Table 3.7   (*continued*)

Rank	Data components
5	Unsourced data from previous economic evaluation – different jurisdiction
6	Expert opinion
D	**Costs**
1	Cost calculations based on reliable databases or data sources conducted for specific study – same jurisdiction
2	Recently published cost calculations based on reliable databases or data course – same jurisdiction
3	Unsourced data from previous economic evaluation – same jurisdiction
4	Recently published cost calculations based on reliable databases or data sources – different jurisdiction
5	Unsourced data from previous economic evaluation – different jurisdiction
6	Expert opinion
E	**Utilities**
1	Direct utility assessment for the specific study from a sample either:

(a) of the general population
(b) with knowledge of the disease(s) of interest
(c) of patients with the disease(s) of interest

	Indirect utility assessment from specific study from patient sample with disease(s) of interest: using tool validated for the patient population
2	Indirect utility assessment from a patient sample with disease(s) of interest; using a tool not validated for the patient population
3	Direct utility assessment from a previous study from a sample either:

(a) of the general population
(b) with knowledge of the disease(s) of interest
(c) of patients with the disease(s) of interest

	Indirect utility assessment from previous study from patient sample with disease(s) of interest: using tool validated for the patient population
4	Unsourced utility data from previous study – method of elicitation unknown
5	Patient preference values obtained from a visual analogue scale
6	Delphi panels, expert opinion

[a]Surrogate outcomes = an endpoint measured in lieu of some other so-called true endpoint [39] (including survival at end of clinical trial as predictor of lifetime survival).

against other data sets) [40]. Secondly, even if possible, when large quantities of good quality evidence exist, it may be hugely time consuming to find, assess, adjust and include all poorer quality evidence. In such circumstances, the poorer quality evidence will make little material difference to the estimation following its discounting through bias adjustment.

Presently, while evidence synthesis is often carried out to estimate effectiveness from multiple studies – largely based on all relevant systematically identified RCT, we believe it is rare that synthesis is conducted for other decision model parameters. Hence, the 'best' single source of evidence will often be used. This is probably due to issues identified above relating to time constraints and difficulties in adjusting for variable validity (quality). What is currently realistic is probably somewhere between our utopian vision and current practice with many of the issues remaining unresolved.

However, as the ideas presented in the book develop, and issues relating to data on functions of model parameters are explained, the reader will appreciate that, relevancy of evidence should be defined more broadly than afforded in Table 3.1.

Although only at an experimental stage, methods for quality adjusting RCTs in a meta-analysis are evolving (see Chapter 11 for further information), and methods for synthesising estimates of effect from both randomised and observational studies are presented in Chapter 11.

While literature identification methods to identify relevant sources of evidence are beyond the scope of this book, strategies for identifying RCTs are well documented elsewhere. Literature on the noneffectiveness parameters may be trickier to identify [14, 41]. This is due to the fact that often such outcomes will not be a primary outcome of the relevant study and hence indexing on electronic databases will be poor. Recent research by Golder *et al.* [42] investigated the feasibility and efficiency of literature database (e.g. Medline, EMBASE) searching for individual model parameters including baseline event rates, resource use, unit costs, health-related quality of life and outcomes as well as relative clinical effectiveness. Through searching the databases, the authors identified 1237 records of which only 48 contained data relevant to populate their model of interest. The extensiveness of this type of evidence identification process to inform model parameters is undoubtedly labour intensive and limited by financial as well as time constraints of the investigators. A proposed alternative exhaustive searching based on predefined criteria, which is more efficient and pragmatic, is to undertake searches which reflect the complexity of the evidence base used in modelling by adopting an iterative approach to searching. Such approaches to searching include citation searches, 'pearlgrowing' [43] (i.e. using the descriptors/subject indexing of highly relevant articles to conduct new searches to identify other relevant articles) and 'berrypicking' [44] (i.e. using each newly identified piece of information to redefine the initial query resulting in an ever-modifying search strategy). Whilst not exhaustive such approaches are classified as systematic structured identification strategies.

A further issue, which is worth flagging in this introductory chapter, is how to deal with potentially differential effectiveness/cost-effectiveness across different patients. It may be that adoption decisions differ and are dependent on characteristics of patients. This may be due to differential effectiveness or costs (or both) being associated with different patients [45]. Dealing with this issue is challenging since subgrouping data inevitably leads to analyses with diminished power and increased uncertainty. If subgroups of patients are to be looked at individually, then it will often be advantageous to obtain Individual Patient Data (IPD) in order for consistently defined subgroup specific estimates to be obtained.

3.7   Principles of synthesis for decision models (motivation for the rest of the book)

This chapter has outlined the premise for the use of decision models in cost-effectiveness analysis. Both deterministic and stochastic models have been considered and examples of their implementation in WinBUGS provided, where one piece of (independent) evidence per parameter was assumed to exist. While such data are unrealistic of what will be available in practice, this approach forms the basis on which the rest of the book builds. Much of the remainder considers how data should be synthesised where (i) multiple estimates of the same parameter (Chapter 4) and (ii) data relating to functions of the model parameters (Chapters 8 and 10) exist. Consideration of how such synthesis can be integrated into the decision model is provided in Chapter 7. Further, while many decision problems can be represented as decision trees, of the form considered in this chapter, representation of complex trees can often be simplified using Markov models, and these are covered in Chapter 10.

An important aspect of uncertainty in decision modelling which we do not address in this book is uncertainty relating to the structure of the model. While attempts have been made to capture this using sophisticated model parameterisations and techniques which average the result over candidate models [46, 47], we do not address this here.

3.8   Summary key points

- Decision models are routinely used to evaluate the cost-effectiveness of competing interventions.

- It is important that uncertainty in model parameters is accounted for by specifying the model as stochastic.

- Both deterministic and stochastic decision models, assuming one independent piece of evidence per parameter, are presented in this chapter.

- Much of the rest of the book is concerned with estimation of decision model parameters where multiple estimates of parameters are available, and/or evidence is available on functions of the parameters.

3.9 Further reading

Readers are referred to Briggs *et al.* [48] and Petrou and Gray [49] for further reading on decision analytical modelling.

3.10 Exercises

These Exercises concern the following decision model to compare the prophylactic use of neuraminidase inhibitors (NIs) with standard care for influenza:

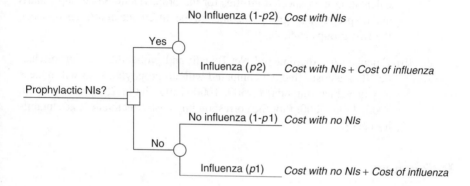

3.1 File ***Model 1 decision model.odc*** contains a decision model where all parameters are specified as known (i.e. with no measure of uncertainty).

   (a) Evaluate the model – **No updates** are required for this model because all parameters are assumed known with no uncertainty. Just check the model specification, load data and compile. Then obtain *values* for costtrt, costctl and diff.cost using the ***node tool*** from the ***info*** menu.

   (b) What are the cost implications of NIs compared with standard care?

3.2 (a) Using the data from a clinical trial given in the table below, calculate the ln(Relative Risk) and its variance. Incorporate these estimates into the model by defining ln(Relative Risk) to have a Normal distribution.

	Flu	No flu	Total
Prophylactic antibiotics	3	268	271
Standard care	19	268	287

    (b) From local hospital data it is observed that under standard care 27 out of 132 patients incur flu (i.e. *p1* in the model). Incorporate these data into the model assuming a beta distribution.

    (c) Evaluate the model obtaining values for p1, RR, costtrt, costctl and diff.cost together with their uncertainty.

3.3 Assume the utility for an individual with influenza is 0.5 and without influenza 0.98.

    (a) Extend the model developed in Exercise 3.2 to include equations for calculating the expected utilities for the prophylactic NIs group (utiltrt) and no prophylaxis group (utilctl), and the difference in utilities between the two groups (diff.util).

    (b) Calculate the Incremental Net Benefit and probability that prophylactic NIs are cost-effective compared with no prophylaxis for willingness to pay values (lambda) 0, 500, 1000, 1500, 2000, 2500, 3000, 3500, 4000, 4500, 5000. Plot the corresponding cost-effectiveness acceptability curve.

References

1. Bower P., Byford S., Barber J., *et al.* Meta-analysis of data on costs from trials of counselling in primary care: using individual patient data to overcome sample size limitations in economic analyses. *British Medical Journal* 2003;**326**:1247–1250.

2. Briggs A., Sculpher M. An introduction to Markov modelling for economic evaluation. *Pharmacoeconomics* 1998;**13**(4):397–409.

3. Hunink M., Glasziou P., Siegel J., *et al.* Constrained resources. In: *Decision Making in Health and Medicine*. Cambridge: Cambridge University Press, 2001;245–304.

4. Brennan A., Akehurst R. Modelling in health economic evaluation: What is its place? What is its value? *Pharmacoeconomics* 2000;**17**(5):445–459.

5. Buxton M.J., Drummond M.F., Van Hout B.A., *et al.*, Modelling in economic evaluation: An unavoidable fact of life. *Health Economics* 1997;**6**:217–227.

6. Briggs A.H. Handling uncertainty in cost-effectiveness models. *Pharmacoeconomics* 2000;**17**(5):479–500.

7. Keeler E. Decision trees and Markov models in cost-effectiveness research. In: Sloan F.A., ed. *Valuing Health Care*. Cambridge: Cambridge University Press, 1996;185–205.

8. Pocock S.J. *Clinical Trials: A Practical Approach*. Chichester: John Wiley & Sons, Ltd, 1983.

9. Senn S. *Cross-over Trials in Clinical Research*. Chichester: John Wiley & Sons, Ltd, 1993.

10. Donner A., Klar N. *Design and Analysis of Cluster Randomization Trials in Health Research*. London: Arnold, 2000.

11. Higgins J.P.T., Green S. *Cochrane Handbook for Systematic Reviews of Interventions Version 5.0.1 [updated February 2008]*. Chichester: The Cochrane Collaboration, John Wiley & Sons, Ltd, 2008.

12. Altman D.G., Deeks J.J. Meta-analysis, Simpson's paradox, and the number needed to treat. *BMC Medical Research Methodology* 2002;**2** (available at: http://www.biomedcentral.com/1471-2288/2/3).

13. Fleiss J.L. The statistical basis of meta-analysis. *Statistical Methods in Medical Research* 1993;**2**:121–145.

14. Sutton A.J., Abrams K.R., Jones D.R., et al. *Methods for Meta-Analysis in Medical Research*. Chichester: John Wiley & Sons, Ltd, 2000.

15. Deeks J.J., Altman D.G. Effect measures for meta-analysis of trials with binary outcomes. In: Egger M., Davey Smith G., Altman D.G., eds. *Systematic Reviews in Health Care. Meta-Analysis in Context*. London: BMJ Publishing Group, 2001.

16. Sweeting M.J., Sutton A.J., Lambert P.C. What to add to nothing? Use and avoidance of continuity corrections in meta-analysis of sparse data. *Statistics in Medicine* 2004;**23**:1351–1375.

17. Hedges L.V., Olkin I. *Statistical Methods for Meta-Analysis*. London: Academic Press, 1985.

18. Welton N.J., Cooper N.J., Ades A.E., et al. Mixed treatment comparison with multiple outcomes reported inconsistently across trials: evaluation of antivirals for treatment of influenza A and B. *Statistics in Medicine* 2008;**27**:5620–5639.

19. Glick H.A., Doshi J.A., Sonnad S.A., et al., Economic evaluation in clinical trials. In: Gray A., Briggs A., eds. *Handbooks in Health Economic Evaluation*. Oxford: Oxford University Press, 2007.

20. Wikipedia. *Central Limit Theorem* (cited December 2008).

21. Whitehead A. *Meta-Analysis of Controlled Clinical Trials*, 1st edn. Chichester: John Wiley & Sons Ltd, 2002.

22. Cooper N.J., Sutton A.J., Lu G., et al. Mixed comparison of stroke prevention treatments in individuals with non-rheumatic atrial fibrillation. *Archives of Internal Medicine* 2006;**166**:1269–1275.

23. Collett D. *Modelling Survival Data in Medical Research*, 2nd edn. New York: Chapman and Hall/CRC, 2003.

24. Parmar M.K.B., Torri V., Stewart L. Extracting summary statistics to perform meta-analyses of the published literature for survival endpoints. *Statistics in Medicine* 1998;**17**:2815–2834.

25. Tengs T.O., Lin T.H. A meta-analysis of quality-of-life estimates for stroke. *PharmacoEconomics* 2003;**21**(3):191–200.

26. Cooper N.J., Sutton A.J., Mugford M., et al. Use of Bayesian Markov Chain Monte Carlo methods to model cost-of-illness data. *Medical Decision Making* 2003;**23**:38–53.

27. Smaill F., Hofmeyr G. Antibiotic prophylaxis for cesarean section. *Cochrane Review* 2001(3).

28. Bibi M., Megdiche H., Ghanem H., *et al.*, L'antibioprophylaxie dans les cesariennes a priori sans 'haut risque infectieux'. *Journal de Gynecologie, Obstetrique et Biologie de la Reproduction (Paris)* 1994;**23**:451–455.

29. Deeks J.J., Altman D.G. Effect measures for meta-analysis of trials with binary outcomes. In: Egger M., Davey Smith G., Altman D.G., eds. *Systematic Reviews in Health Care: Meta-Analysis in Context*. London: BMJ Publishing Group, 2001;313–335.

30. Mugford M., Kingston J., Chalmers I. Reducing the incidence of infection after caesarean section: implications of prophylaxis with antibiotics for hospital resources. *British Medical Journal* 1989;**299**:1003–1006.

31. Ades A.E., Claxton K., Sculpher M., Evidence synthesis, parameter correlation and probablistic sensitivity analysis. *Health Economics* 2006;**15**:373–382.

32. Black W.C. The CE plane: a graphic representation of cost-effectiveness. *Medical Decision Making* 1990;**10**:212–214.

33. van Hout B.A., Malwenn J.A., Gordon G.S., *et al.* Costs, effects and C/E-ratios alongside a clinical trial. *Health Economics* 1994;**3**:309–319.

34. Stinnett A.A., Mullahy J. Net health benefits: a new framework for the analysis of uncertainty in cost-effectiveness analysis. *Medical Decision Making* 1998;**18**(Suppl.): S68–S80.

35. Spiegelhalter D.J., Myles J.P., Jones D.R., *et al.* Methods in health service research: an introduction to Bayesian methods in health technology assessment. *British Medical Journal* 1999;**319**:508–512.

36. StataCorporation, *Stata Statistical Software: Release 10*. College Station, TX: StataCorp LP, 2007.

37. Coyle D., Lee K.M. Evidence-based economic evaluation: how the use of different data sources can impact results. In: Donaldson C., Mugford M., Vale L., eds. *Evidence-Based Health Economics: From Effectiveness to Efficiency in Systematic Review*. London: BMJ Publishing Group, 2002;55–66.

38. Cooper N.J., *et al.* Use of evidence in decision models: an appraisal of health technology assessments in the UK to date. *Journal of Health Services Research and Policy* 2005;**10**(4):245–250.

39. Daniels M.J., Hughesd- M.D. Meta-analysis for the evaluation of the potential surrogate markers. *Statistics in Medicine* 1997;**16**:1965–1982.

40. Philips Z., Ginnelly L., Sculpher M., *et al.* Review of guidelines for good practice in decision-analytic modelling in health technology assessment. *Health Technology Assessment* 2004;**8**(36).

41. CRD. Undertaking systematic reviews of research on effectiveness: CRD's guidance for carrying out or commissioning reviews. In: *Centre for Reviews and Dissemination Report 4*. York: University of York, 2001.

42. Golder S., Glanville J., Ginnelly L. Populating decision-analytic models: The feasibility and efficiency of database searching for individual parameters. *International Journal of Technology Assessment in Health Care* 2005;**21**(3):305–311.

43. Hartley R.J., Keen E.M., Large J.A., *et al. Online Searching: Principles and Practice*. London: Bowker Saur, 1990.

44. Bates M.J. The design of browsing and berrypicking techniques for the online search interface. *Online Review* 1989;**13**:407–424.

45. Sculpher M.J. Subgroups and heterogeneity in cost-effectiveness analysis. *Pharmacoeconomics* 2008;**26**:799–806.

46. Bojke L., Claxton K., Sculpher M., *et al.* Characterising structural uncertainty in decision-analytic models: a review and application of methods. *Value in Health* 2009;**15**(5):739–749.

47. Jackson C.H., Thompson S.G., Sharples L.D. Accounting for uncertainty in health economic decision models by using model averaging. *Journal of the Royal Statistical Society, Series A* 2009;**172**(2):383–404.

48. Briggs A., Sculpher M., Claxton K. *Decision Modelling for Health Economic Evaluation*. Oxford: Oxford University Press, 2006.

49. Petrou S., Gray A. Economic evaluation using decision analytical modelling design, conduct, analysis, and reporting. *British Medical Journal* 2011;**342**:d1766.

4

Meta-analysis using Bayesian methods

4.1 Introduction

Meta-analysis, the statistical synthesis of data from multiple studies [1], has now become an accepted approach and is used extensively to summarise medical research. Although, deservedly, much attention has been given to its use in combining Randomised Controlled Trials (RCTs) evaluating all range of health and medical interventions, it is used to combine all manner of data. For example, meta-analyses of studies evaluating the performance of diagnostic or prognostic factors are not uncommon, nor are meta-analyses estimating the prevalence of a specific disease.

Meta-analysis commonly forms the main statistical component of a systematic review. A systematic review can be defined as a literature review focused on a single question which tries to identify, appraise, select and synthesise all high quality research evidence relevant to that question. Consideration of the nonsynthesis components of a systematic review is beyond the scope of this book, but adoption of such transparent methodology for the identification of the studies to be included in a meta-analysis and the way data are extracted from these studies is a vital component of the analysis and we urge the reader to look elsewhere for guidance on these aspects of a systematic review [2, 3]. Adoption of such an approach for the collation of information ensures that: (i) data are collated systematically; (ii) the estimation process is transparent and reproducible; and (iii) where multiple data sources exist, they can all contribute in a statistically rigorous way.

Although rarely done in practice, there is nothing preventing a systematic review and, where multiple sources of evidence exist, meta-analysis and related

Evidence Synthesis for Decision Making in Healthcare, First Edition. Nicky J. Welton,
Alexander J. Sutton, Nicola J. Cooper, Keith R. Abrams and A.E. Ades.
© 2012 John Wiley & Sons, Ltd. Published 2012 by John Wiley & Sons, Ltd.

synthesis methods (as outlined in much of the remainder of this book) being used to estimate *all* parameters in a decision model. As explained in Chapters 1 and 3, we believe this to be the most rational approach to informing decision models, however we acknowledge for complex models searching and data acquisition could be a time consuming and costly exercise. Further research into evidence identification methods for informing decision models, which are quicker to implement than the typical exhaustive and systematic searches undertaken as part of ('single parameter') systematic reviews, is underway [4]. While meta-analyses of utility and cost data have been undertaken, examples are rare and we focus on measures of effectiveness in this chapter although the principles are broadly applicable.

Much has already been written on methods for meta-analysis, and we have had to be selective in the material covered in this book. We present what, in our experience, we consider to be the most commonly applicable meta-analytic models required to inform decision models. However, variants on such models are readily implemented within the WinBUGS software and may be required for specific contexts. Therefore, emphasis is placed on modelling principles, and many citations are provided to modelling extensions which may be relevant in certain contexts. Fortunately, many of the recent modelling developments in meta-analysis have been implemented in WinBUGS [5], and code is often available from the original papers; we highlight a review considering these in Section 4.7.

The models and principles outlined in this chapter are used and developed extensively throughout the remainder of the book. Indeed, much of the remainder of the book can be viewed as presenting synthesis methods 'beyond' meta-analysis. Although the dividing line between meta-analysis and more advanced synthesis models is undoubtedly blurred, the distinction we make here is that meta-analysis relates to synthesis of multiple pieces of data relating to a single parameter of primary interest. Approaches which combine (i) networks of trial evidence, (ii) matrices of multiple correlated outcomes, (iii) chains of evidence and (iv) data relating to functions of multiple parameters of interest, are covered in subsequent chapters. Further, in this chapter we focus on binary outcomes (although we consider generic models appropriate for other outcomes also). An example of continuous outcomes is covered in Chapter 9 under mixed treatment comparisons. Also, we do not consider the details of how the results of meta-analyses are integrated into the decision model, since this is given in Chapter 7.

Finally, before considering meta-analysis modelling in detail, some consideration of the data that may be available to the analyst is helpful. Meta-analysis is typically conducted using summary data available from study reports, although there are a growing number of instances where meta-analysis has been conducted using the Individual Patient Data (IPD) obtained from the relevant studies [6]. The latter approach has several advantages including; (i) allowing for detailed data checking; (ii) ensuring standardisation of data and the appropriateness of the analysis; (iii) allowing the incorporation of further follow-up data beyond the original publication date of the study; (iv) facilitating the exploration of patient level covariates; and (v) facilitating time-to-event type analyses generally, and, specifically checking whether effects are constant over time. We fully support the use of IPD data for decision modelling generally, and specifically for meta-analysis, but acknowledging that this will often not be possible or feasible due to limited availability and/or time-constraints, so we focus on the use of summary data in this and other chapters. However, we do briefly consider instances when IPD may be particularly valuable in Chapter 5. We welcome the day when internet-based central data repositories make the obtaining of IPD a more routine approach.

Commonly used quantities which require estimation for decision modelling were defined in Section 3.2. In the sections below we consider models to combine multiple estimates of such quantities, using Bayesian meta-analysis methods as implemented in the WinBUGS software. The now standard fixed and random effect approaches to meta-analysis are covered in Sections 4.2 and 4.3, followed by consideration of a specific model for the Odds Ratio (OR) scale. It is hoped that once the material in this chapter has been digested and the exercises attempted, the reader will have confidence in conducting their own meta-analyses using WinBUGS.

4.2   Fixed Effect model

If it is assumed that all effect size estimates to be combined are estimating the same underlying effect, then the estimates can be combined using a Fixed Effect model:

$$Y_i \sim \text{Normal}\left(d, \frac{\sigma_i^2}{n_i}\right) \quad i = 1, \ldots, k \tag{4.1}$$

where Y_i is the effect size in the ith of k studies to be combined, d is the underlying effect size being estimated by the model, and σ_i^2 is the within-study variance for the ith study. In practice, it is usual to assume the σ_i^2 are known, and, hence, the σ_i^2/n_i are replaced by the estimated within-study variances (v_i^2) since this will usually make little practical difference [7].

$$Y_i \sim \text{Normal}(d, v_i^2) \quad i = 1, \ldots, k, \tag{4.2}$$

Such a model assumes that only sampling error is responsible for all variations in the estimated effect sizes across studies. This model includes only one unknown parameter to be estimated from the data: the effect size assumed to be common across studies, d. This parameter requires a prior distribution, if evaluated within a Bayesian framework. If vague prior knowledge is being specified, then a Normal distribution (centred at no effect for comparative outcomes) with a large variance (relative to that of the outcome in question) can be used. For example, for a meta-analysis on the ln(OR) scale (recall, ratio data are log-transformed since this will result in approximately normally distributed outcomes), if the prior distribution

$$d \sim \text{Normal}(0, 10^5) \tag{4.3}$$

was specified, this states a priori we would be 95% certain that the true value of d is between $(0 - 1.96 \times 316)$ and $(0 + 1.96 \times 316)$, where $316 = \sqrt{10^5}$. On an

OR scale that is equivalent to an interval of $(10^{-269}$ to $10^{269})$ which (more than) spans all plausible values for an OR in most medical contexts and is essentially flat (i.e. nonpreferential or noninformative) over the realistic range of interest. This model is essentially 'generic' in the sense that it can be used for any outcome in which effect size and corresponding variance data are available (and many of the common outcomes scales and corresponding formulae were given in Section 3.2); although care should always be taken in specifying a sensible prior distribution for d.

Example 4.1 Fixed effect meta-analysis worked example: Aspirin vs placebo for myocardial infarction (MI).

Table 4.1 provides data for seven RCTs which assessed the effect of aspirin compared with placebo in preventing death from MI [8]. In order to carry out a fixed effect meta-analysis on these data using the model described in the previous section, it is necessary to calculate an effect size and variance for each study. The Log Odds Ratio (LOR) is used here and Equations (3.1) and (3.2) are applied to calculate the necessary quantities.

Table 4.1   Mortality outcome data for seven RCTs evaluating aspirin *vs* placebo for preventing MI.

Study	Aspirin group		Placebo group	
	Total	Survived	Total	Survived
MRC-1	615	566	624	557
CDP	758	714	771	707
MRC-2	832	730	850	724
GASP	317	285	309	271
PARIS	810	725	406	354
AMIS	2267	2021	2257	2038
ISIS-2	8587	7017	8600	6880

For the first study in Table 4.1, MRC-1, the OR is given by: $[(615 - 566) \times 557]/[566 \times (624 - 557)] = 0.718$, which results in a LOR of -0.329. The variance of the LOR is then calculated as:

$$1/(615-566) + 1/566 + (1/624-557) + (1/557) = 0.0389$$

The LORs and variances for all seven studies are presented in Table 4.2. These data can be entered into WinBUGS and synthesised using the code in Figure 4.1, which is a direct translation of Equations (4.2) and (4.3).

This model loops round the seven studies in the meta-analysis (this could be specified directly in the program – i.e. for (i in 1: 7) or, as is done here, specified

Table 4.2   Log Odds Ratios and corresponding variances for the seven RCTs evaluating aspirin *vs* placebo for preventing MI.

Study	Ln(OR)	Var(ln(OR))
MRC-1	−0.3289	0.0389
CDP	−0.3845	0.0412
MRC-2	−0.2196	0.0205
GASP	−0.2222	0.0648
PARIS	−0.2255	0.0352
AMIS	0.1246	0.0096
ISIS-2	−0.1110	0.0015

```
Model {
  for (i in 1:Nstud) {
    P[i] <- 1/V[i]
    Y[i] ~ dnorm(d, P[i]) }
  d ~ dnorm(0, 1.0E-5)
  OR <- exp(d)
}

#Data
list(Y = c(-0.3289, -0.3845, -0.2196, -0.2222, -0.2255, 0.1246, -0.1110), V = c(0.0389,
0.0412, 0.0205, 0.0648, 0.0352, 0.0096, 0.0015), Nstud = 7)

#Initial Values
list(d = 0)
```

Figure 4.1   WinBUGS code for fitting the Fixed Effect model to the seven aspirin RCTs.

as a variable, Nstud, in the data). Recall that WinBUGS deals with precisions (1/variances) which is why the line 'P[i] <- 1/V[i]' is required (alternatively precisions could be specified in the data set and this line could then be omitted). The line 'OR <- exp(d)' back transforms the pooled result back onto the OR scale for ease of interpretation. This code is generic to any outcome (e.g. Relative Risk, Risk Difference, Mean Difference, etc.) which is normally distributed for which effect size and variance data are available (although the aforementioned line 'OR <- exp(d)' can be omitted and care should be taken to ensure the prior distribution placed on d is noninformative (presuming this is intended) for the scale being used).

The code in Figure 4.1 was run in WinBUGS, burning the sampler in for 5000 iterations, followed by a further 10 000 iterations used for estimation. The posterior distribution for the pooled LOR (d) is displayed in Figure 4.2. This corresponds to an OR of 0.90 (95% CrI 0.84 to 0.96) suggesting the odds of death in the aspirin intervention trial arms are lower than in the placebo arms.

For those readers who are familiar with Frequentist approaches to meta-analysis, it may be helpful to note that, when a vague prior distribution is used, the results

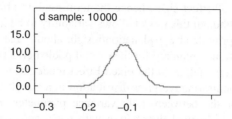

Figure 4.2 Posterior distribution for the pooled LOR.

from WinBUGS will be very similar to Frequentist fixed effect methods of estimation (as commonly used in most statistical software and specific meta-analysis packages). For example, using the inverse variance weighted approach on the data in Table 4.2 results in a pooled OR of 0.90 (95% CI 0.84 to 0.96), i.e. identical to the MCMC estimate to two significant figures.

4.3 Random Effects model

If there is concern that the assumption of the Fixed Effect model is too restrictive to be satisfied by the data, i.e. it is unrealistic to assume all the studies are estimating exactly the same underlying effect size, then a Random Effects model is commonly used which relaxes this strict assumption. Medical studies may vary in a multitude of different ways; for example, patient populations may be different, timings of interventions may vary, etc. In addition, imperfections in the design and conduct of the study may lead to bias. These differences may have an influence on the effect size of interest. If this is so, then this will lead to heterogeneity among the underlying effect sizes each study is estimating. Sometimes the causes of some of the variability are identifiable; when this is the case covariates can be included in the modelling to explicitly model such differences, and approaches to doing this are considered in Chapter 5. However, very often all, or at least a proportion, of the between-study variability will not be explainable. When this is the case, it is common to include a random effect in the model to explicitly allow for variability in effect sizes between studies:

$$Y_i \sim \text{Normal}(\delta_i, v_i^2) \qquad i = 1, \ldots, k$$
$$\delta_i \sim \text{Normal}(d, \tau^2) \qquad i = 1, \ldots, k \tag{4.4}$$

where Y_i and v_i^2 have the same interpretation as in Section 4.2 and δ_i is the unique underlying effect in the ith study. Here, each of the δ_i are assumed to come from a (Normal) distribution with mean d, and variance τ^2, where both of these parameters are estimated from the data. Formally, we say the δ_is are *exchangeable*, which is to say we assume they are different, but, a priori, could not predict the rankings of their magnitudes. Informally, the δ_is can be assumed to be random samples from a distribution of effect sizes, hence the term random effects. It is important to appreciate that although this model allows variability to be incorporated into the model, it does not provide any explanation/insight about what caused it.

A prior distribution is required for the overall pooled effect size d (mean of the distribution of effects), and, as in the Fixed Effect model, $d \sim \text{Normal}(0, 10^5)$ is a good choice if a noninformative prior distribution is required. A prior distribution is also required for the between-study variance parameter, τ^2. Since variances cannot go negative, a Normal distribution with mean zero and large variance is not a viable option. There has been some technical debate over the most suitable choice for a noninformative prior distribution for variance parameters in random effects models. In truth, all candidates are at least slightly informative (so 'vague' is a more appropriate term than completely noninformative) [9]. We are going to specify a uniform distribution on the standard deviation scale, namely:

$$\tau \sim \text{Uniform}(0, 10)$$

As discussed later, a value of 10 for the between study standard deviation is very large on the LOR scale and thus this prior distribution covers all plausible values.

Example 4.2   Random effects meta-analysis worked example: Aspirin vs placebo for MI.

We now reanalyse the seven trials comparing aspirin with placebo for preventing death from MI presented in Example 4.1, this time using a Random Effects model. Note, it is only the model which differs from Example 4.1, exactly the same data, as presented in Table 4.2, are being used. WinBUGS code is presented in Figure 4.3. This code follows Equation (4.4) and subsequent discussion of prior distributions directly (recall WinBUGS works with precisions hence the three lines of code for specifying the prior on τ).

The code in Figure 4.3 was run in WinBUGS, burning the sampler in for 5000 iterations, followed by a further 10 000 iterations used for estimation. The posterior distributions for the mean (d) and variance of the random effect distribution (τ^2) are displayed in Figure 4.4. This corresponds to a mean OR of 1.15 (0.98 to 1.43) and variance 0.02 (0.0002 to 0.21) and this estimate of the OR is similar to that obtained from the fixed effect analysis estimating a single overall mean effect above although the credible interval is wider. The credible interval for d is also slightly wider than when the standard Frequentist approach to random effect meta-analysis is taken (OR = 1.14, 95% CI 1.01 to 1.29) this is because the uncertainty in the between study variance (τ^2) is ignored in the Frequentist computation although little utilised Frequentist methods do exist which do incorporate this [7]. Note that in this example, there is considerable uncertainty in the estimation of the between study variance parameter, this is typical when the number of studies in the meta-analysis is small.

```
Model {
  for (i in 1:Nstud)
  {
  P[i] <- 1/V[i]
  Y[i]    ~ dnorm (delta[i], P[i])
  delta[i] ~ dnorm(d, prec)
  }
  d ~ dnorm(0, 1.0E-5)
  OR <- exp(d)
  tau~dunif(0,10)
  tau.sq<-tau*tau
  prec<-1/(tau.sq)
  }

Data
list(Y = c(-0.3289, -0.3845, -0.2196, -0.2222, -0.2255, 0.1246, -0.1110),
  V = c(0.0389, 0.0412, 0.0205, 0.0648, 0.0352, 0.0096, 0.0015), Nstud = 7)

Initial Values
list(d = 0, tau =1, delta = c(0,0,0,0,0,0,0))
```

Figure 4.3   WinBUGS code for fitting the Random Effects model to the seven aspirin RCTs.

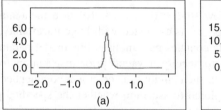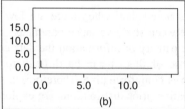

Figure 4.4   Posterior distribution for (a) the mean and (b) the variance of the random effect distribution of treatment effects.

4.3.1   The predictive distribution

It is common to observe the mean of the distribution of effects to be presented at the bottom of a forest plot in the same manner as the fixed effect estimate. However, such a summary ignores the variance of the distribution of effects. For this reason, it has been proposed [10] that a more appropriate summary for a random effect analysis, since it takes into account the between study heterogeneity, is the predictive interval. The predictive distribution can be specified for the underlying effect in a new study and thus acknowledges that individual realisations from the distribution of treatment effects will vary. Algebraically, it is defined as:

$$\delta^{new} \sim \text{Normal}(d, \tau^2) \qquad (4.5)$$

Which can be directly translated into WinBUGS code (back transforming to the OR scale) as:

```
delta.new ~ dnorm(d, prec)
OR.new <- exp(delta.new)
```

Example 4.2 revisited   Random effects meta-analysis worked example: Aspirin vs placebo for MI.

Estimating δ^{new} for the aspirin example results in an estimate of 1.15 (0.75 to 1.88), which has a considerably wider 95% CrI than the mean OR of the distribution as reported above. The issue of which distribution, the mean or the predictive, is most appropriate for use in a decision modelling context has no short answer but relates to the relationship between the populations studied in the trials and the target population of the decision. An in-depth discussion is provided elsewhere [11] and this is considered further in Chapter 7.

4.3.2   Prior specification for τ

It was noted that, when there are few studies (i.e. $<$ ca. 10) in a meta-analysis the between study variance parameter, τ^2, is estimated with large uncertainty, due to the paucity of information the data contains pertaining to this model parameter. Because of this, it can be difficult to specify a vague prior distribution for τ^2 which is noninformative. Therefore, in such circumstances, it is recommended that alternative prior distributions are explored to ascertain whether the specified prior is having an unintentional influence. This issue is discussed in detail elsewhere [9]. One possible alternative prior distribution which could be tried is:

$$\frac{1}{\tau^2} \sim \text{Gamma}(0.001, 0.001) \tag{4.6}$$

A further alternative is to specify a deliberately informative prior distribution for τ^2, which circumvents the problem of specifying vague priors which are unintentionally influential altogether. For example, Higgins and Whitehead [12] consider the construction of informative, empirically based, priors for τ^2 using a distribution for estimates for this parameter from similar meta-analyses. See Chapter 6 for approaches to assessing the goodness of fit of meta-analytic models and choosing between alternative models.

4.3.3   'Exact' Random Effects model for Odds Ratios based on a Binomial likelihood

In the previous sections the model and code presented to conduct meta-analysis could be considered somewhat generic, i.e. it can be used to combine estimates using any outcome scale as long as the effect size and the associated standard error are available from each study.

In this section a specific alternative Random Effects model is presented specifically for use on the OR scale [13]. It is based around using a Binomial likelihood and can be considered as a random effect logistic regression model. This model uses the event data and numbers of individuals in each study arm directly, and this removes the need to calculate LORs and associated standard errors. Further advantages of this approach include: (i) the ability to include studies in which zero/all events are observed in one of the study arms without the need of adding a 'fudge factor' (often too respectfully referred to as a continuity correction factor) to the calculations; (ii) removing the need to assume the LORs from individual studies are normally distributed. Thus, while this model will often give very similar answers to the more generic Random Effects model given above, important differences may be observed, particularly when analysing sparse data as often encountered in investigations of adverse events of interventions [14]. Note that while the random effect version of this approach is considered below, the fixed effect equivalent is given consideration in the Exercises in Section 4.8.

$$
\begin{aligned}
&r_{Ai} \sim \text{Binomial}(p_{Ai}, n_{Ai}) &\quad &r_{Bi} \sim \text{Binomial}(p_{Bi}, n_{Bi}) \\
&\text{logit}(p_{Ai}) = \mu_i &\quad &\text{logit}(p_{Bi}) = \mu_i + \delta_i &\quad (4.7)\\
&\delta_i \sim \text{Normal}(d, \tau^2) &\quad &i = 1, \ldots, k
\end{aligned}
$$

where n_{Ai} and n_{Bi} are the total number of patients in the two arms of the ith study, r_{Ai} and r_{Bi} are the number of events in these two groups, p_{Ai} and p_{Bi} are the probabilities of an event in the two groups. μ_i is the estimate log(odds) of an event in group A, and δ_i, d and τ^2 are as defined in Equation (4.4). In addition to the required prior distributions for d and τ^2, as discussed for Equation (4.4), the μ_is also require a prior distribution, and vague ones can be specified in a similar manner to that specified for d previously, e.g. $\mu_i \sim \text{Normal}(0, 10^5)$.

A variant to Equation (4.7) is to assume the random effects are t rather than normally distributed (and indeed this could be used for the generic model as well) [13]. This may be sensible when the number of studies being combined is small, and it is difficult to assess whether the normality assumption of the random effects has been violated since it provides a more robust estimation procedure (see the **Blocker** example in the WinBUGS examples within the program help menu for how this can be implemented).

Example 4.2 revisited   Random effects meta-analysis worked example: Aspirin vs placebo for MI.

The translation of Equation (4.7) into WinBUGS code, applied to the aspirin trials in Example 4.2, is presented in Figure 4.5.

With a burn in of 5000 iterations followed by 10 000 on which estimation is based, this code produced the following estimates: OR = 0.15 (0.98 to 1.44)

```
Model
    {
        for( i in 1 : Nstud )
        {
                rA[i] ~ dbin(pA[i], nA[i])
            rB[i] ~ dbin(pB[i], nB[i])
            logit(pA[i]) <- mu[i]
            logit(pB[i]) <- mu[i] + delta[i]
            mu[i] ~ dnorm(0.0,1.0E-5)
            delta[i] ~ dnorm(d, prec)
        }
        d ~ dnorm(0.0,1.0E-6)
        tau~dunif(0,10)
        tau.sq<-tau*tau
        prec<-1/(tau.sq)
        OR <- exp(d)
    }

Data
list(rA = c(49,44,102,32,85,246,1570), rB = c(67,64,126,38,52,219,1720),
nA = c(615,758,832,317,810,2267,8587), nB = c(624,771,850,309,406,2257,
8600), Nstud = 7)

Initial Values
list(d = 0, tau = 1, delta = c(0,0,0,0,0,0,0), mu = c(0,0,0,0,0,0,0))
```

Figure 4.5   WinBUGS code for fitting the random effect Binomial likelihood model to the seven aspirin RCTs.

which is very close to the results obtained from using the generic code provided in Figure 4.3.

4.3.4   Shrunken study level estimates

In the account of random effects models above, no consideration was given to the estimation of the δ_is which are the estimates of the treatment effects in each of the i studies. Unlike the Fixed Effect model, the Random Effects model does not assume each study is estimating exactly the same treatment effect, but that treatment effects are related – since they are assumed to be samples from the same random effects distribution. Due to this, the study level estimates 'borrow' information/'strength' from each other, and thus the study level estimates from the Random Effects model are not the same as would be obtained by estimating each study in isolation (the latter being the estimates which are typically drawn on a forest plot). These estimates 'shrink' towards each other and their uncertainty is reduced. Although these shrunken estimates are often only of secondary importance in a meta-analysis, in specific contexts, if the target decision population is more similar that in one of the studies than the others, an argument could be made for considering the shrunken effect size from that study rather than the overall pooled effect in the decision modelling [11].

Example 4.2 revisited   Random effects meta-analysis worked example: Aspirin vs placebo for MI.

The shrunken estimates for the aspirin trials are plotted together with the observed estimates and pooled effect size in Figure 4.6.

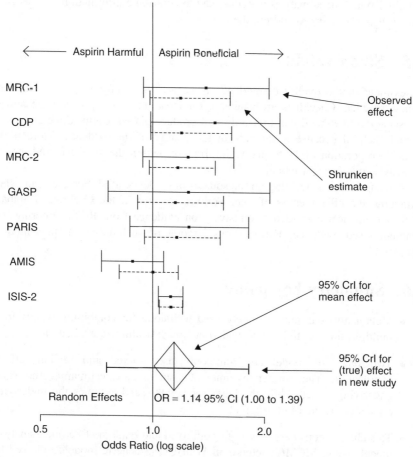

Figure 4.6   Augmented funnel plot showing observed and shrunken study level estimates, mean pooled effect (all with 95% intervals) and 95% prediction interval for the effect in a new study for the aspirin meta-analysis.

4.4   Publication bias

Publication bias is a potential threat to any analysis based on the published literature. Publication bias exists when evidence with significant or favourable results is more likely to be published than that with nonsignificant or unfavourable results. When this occurs, any analysis based on the published literature may be biased. Since a whole book has recently been devoted to publication bias in meta-analysis [15], we do not replicate material here but we do want to make some remarks about publication bias specific to the decision modelling context. First, we support the notion of making an assessment of the likelihood of publication bias where possible. When meta-analysis is being used to contribute information to a decision model, it is necessary to address the bias.

4.5   Study validity

Assessment of the quality of evidence is an accepted stage in good systematic review practice. Checklists are available for most study designs with the aim of assessing the likelihood that the study will produce biased results. Such an assessment is helpful because it can inform the quality of the evidence. More tricky is the incorporation of such quality information within the synthesis and, hence, ultimately, the decision model.

A related issue is deciding on the sources of evidence used. For example, when estimating the effectiveness of interventions, reviews in the Cochrane Database of Systematic Reviews focus exclusively on evidence from RCTs, ignoring any nonrandomised evidence. Further consideration of such issues in presented in Chapter 11.

4.6   Summary key points

- Meta-analysis is now a widely used technique for combining results from multiple similar studies and underpins much healthcare evaluation.

- Two types of model are commonly used – fixed and random effects approaches. The former assumes all studies are estimating the same underlying effect, while the latter relaxes this and assumes the underlying effects are related but different.

- This chapter considers how to fit both fixed and random effect meta-analysis models using MCMC methods in WinBUGS. Generic models followed by those specific to the OR scale are covered. Detailed consideration of prior distributions is also provided.

4.7   Further reading

There is now a vast meta-analysis literature, with several good introductory (predominantly Frequentist based) texts including Borenstein et al. [16]. The Cochrane handbook [3] contains much practical wisdom on conducting meta-analyses of RCTs. A review of recent developments in meta-analysis (many of which were originally implemented in WinBUGS) which cites many relevant papers is also recommended [5].

4.8   Exercises

Model 4.1: Generic Fixed Effect model applied to the cholesterol lowering data set

In this exercise you are going to carry out a fixed effect meta analysis of 34 RCTs to assess the effect of cholesterol lowering interventions on *overall mortality*.
   The data format is:

id	nc	ntg	rc	rt
1	50	50	17	12
2	285	147	70	38
3	156	119	37	40
4	123	129	20	24
..				
..				
33	30	60	0	4
34	311	317	19	12

where **nc** and **nt** are the total number of patients in the control and treatment arms, respectively. **rc** and **rt** are the total number of deaths in the control and treatment arms, respectively. **id** is simply an identification number for each study.
   Open the file: *Cholesterol fixed.odc*
   This file contains the model and data for running the generic Fixed Effect model on the cholesterol study data given above. Since this model uses effect size and variance data these were calculated outside WinBUGS from the binary outcome data. Check you could do this yourself for the first study.

1. Check the model syntax, load both formats of data (i.e. first using 'list' and then by clicking on the arrows to open the 'fold' and load data within the fold by highlighting the variable names), load the initial values given then update the model for 2000 iterations. Monitor d and OR and update a further 5000 iterations.

2. Examine the output of the chains. Dose convergence seem OK by visual inspection (i.e. examine 'history' plots)? Is there any 'autocorrelation'? Generate the statistics for d and OR.

3. Confirm that you could obtain the median and the 2.5% and 97.5% centiles for OR by exponentiating the results for d. Make sure you understand what each of these parameters represents. Interpret the results.

4. Add in a fictitious extra study with log(OR) = 0.2 and var(log(OR)) = 0.1. Run the model and examine how the results have changed.

Model 4.2: Generic Random Effects model applied to the cholesterol lowering data set

Open the file: *Cholesterol random.odc*

This file contains the model and data for running the generic Random Effects model on the cholesterol studies analysed in Model 4.1.

1. As for Model 4.1, load the model, data, compile and load the initial values. You will notice that WinBUGS still needs further initial values not specified in the file. Which of the stochastic nodes does not have an initial value? Add a sensible initial value for this node. Now recompile and run the model.

2. Burn the model in for 2000 iterations. Monitor the parameters of interest (you decide which these are!). And run the sample for a further 5000 iterations.

3. Interpret the output.

Model 4.3: Direct Random Effects OR model applied to the cholesterol lowering data set

Open the file: *Cholesterol random logistic.odc*

This is the version of the Random Effects model explained above (Equation (4.7)) which directly models on the (log) OR scale. It uses essentially the same data as Models 4.1 and 4.2 (without the need to add continuity corrections) but included as raw events and denominators as given above.

1. Load and run the model as for Model 4.2.

2. Compare the results obtained for this model with those for Model 4.2.

3. Derive a predictive distribution for the underlying effect in a new study. (Hint: you will need to add a further line of code and rerun the model.)

4. Obtain the shrunken estimate and 95% credible interval for the first study in the data set. Compare this with the observed effect and 95% interval.

5. Open file: *Cholesterol random logistic 2.odc*. This fits the same model as the previous file but includes code which enables a summary plot to be produced. Load and run the model as before monitoring delta.

6. Go to the *inference* menu and choose the *compare* option. Type delta in the node box and then press the *caterpillar* button. This will produce a plot similar to the forest plot you are used to, but it has important differences. The study specific estimates are the shrunken ones not the observed ones and both the pooled estimate for the mean of the random effects distribution with CrI and predictive interval for the effect in a new study with CrI are plotted. Make sure you understand the importance and difference between these two summaries.

7. *Modify the (random effects) code to fit a fixed effect meta-analysis model using a Binomial likelihood.

8. *It is desirable to be able to make predictions for the observed effect in a future study of a given sample size. This is different from the prediction interval produced above because this is for the underlying effect in a future study not the observed effect which must also incorporate sampling error.

   Modify the file *Cholesterol random logistic 2.odc* to make predictions for future studies with 250, 500, 750 and 1000 persons in each trial arm.
   Hint:

   • Specify the baseline effects (i.e. the log odds of an event on treatment A) as random (the mu[i]s).

   • Create a new vector in the data file containing the trial sizes of interest.

   • Create a node for predicted underlying baseline and treatment effects.

   • Calculated the proportions of events for both arms of a new study:

     logit(pA.pop)<-mu.new

     logit(pB.pop)<-mu.new + d.new.

   • Draw replicate observations (looping over sample size).

   • Calculate the OR and the LOR.

   Comment on the width of the prediction intervals as sample size increases. Is this what you would have expected?

Model 4.4: Direct OR model with built in sensitivity analysis to prior

Open the file: *Cholesterol prior sens.odc*
This file contains code to fit exactly the same model as in Model 4.3. What is novel about this file is that it fits three models simultaneously, each with a different prior distribution placed on the heterogeneity parameter. This gives a more immediate way of visualising influence as we shall see.

1. Load the model, burn it in for a reasonable number of iterations. Monitor OR, update for a few thousand more iterations.

2. Select compare from the influence menu and type in OR, click the caterpillar plot option. This displays a plot of the pooled OR for the three prior distributions. How much has the estimation changed?

3. Repeat the above but produce a plot for the between study variance parameter. Comment.

4. Examine the code so you know what three prior distributions have been specified. If there is time, study the code so you can learn how to set code up to loop around multiple models.

References

1. Sutton A.J., Abrams K.R., Jones D.R., Sheldon T.A., Song F. *Methods for Meta-Analysis in Medical Research*. London: John Wiley & Sons, Ltd, 2000.

2. Deeks J., Glanville J., Sheldon T. Undertaking systematic reviews of research on effectiveness: CRD guidelines for those carrying out or commissioning reviews. Centre for Reviews and Dissemination Report Number 4 (2nd edn). York: York Publishing Services Ltd, 1996.

3. Higgins J.P.T., Green S., eds. *Cochrane Handbook for Systematic Reviews of Interventions 4.2.5 [updated May 2005]*. Chichester: Tne Cochrane Collaboration, John Wiley & Sons, Ltd, 2005.

4. Cooper N.J., Sutton A.J., Ades A., Paisley S., Jones D.R. Use of evidence in economic decision models: practical issues and methodological challenges. *Health Economics* 2007;**16**:1277–1286.

5. Sutton A.J., Higgins J.P.T. Recent developments in meta-analysis. *Statistics in Medicine* 2008;**27**:625–650.

6. Riley R.D., Lambert P.C., Abo-Zaid G. Meta-analysis of individual participant data: rationale, conduct, and reporting. *British Medical Journal* 2010;**340**:c221.

7. Hardy R.J., Thompson S.G. A likelihood approach to meta-analysis with random effects. *Statistics in Medicine* 1996;**15**:619–629.

8. Fleiss J.L. The statistical basis of meta-analysis. *Statistical Methods in Medical Research* 1993;**2**:121–145.

9. Lambert P., Sutton A.J., Burton P., Abrams K.R., Jones D.R. How vague is vague? Assessment in the use of vague prior distributions for variance components. *Statistics in Medicine* 2005;**24**:2401–2428.

10. Spiegelhalter D.J., Abrams K.R., Myles J.P. *Bayesian Approaches to Clinical Trials and Health-Care Evaluation*. Chichester: John Wiley & Sons, Ltd, 2003.

11. Ades A.E., Lu G., Higgins J.P.T. The interpretation of random-effects meta-analysis in decision models. *Medical Decision Making* 2005;**25**:646–654.

12. Higgins J.P.T., Whitehead A. Borrowing strength from external trials in a meta-analysis. *Statistics in Medicine* 1996;**15**:2733–2749.

13. Smith T.C., Spiegelhalter D.J., Thomas A. Bayesian approaches to random-effects meta-analysis: a comparative study. *Statistics in Medicine* 1995;**14**:2685–2699.

14. Sweeting M.J., Sutton A.J., Lambert P.C. What to add to nothing? The use and avoidance of continuity corrections in meta-analysis of sparse data. *Statistics in Medicine* 2004;**23**:1351–1375.

15. Rothstein H.R., Sutton A.J., Borenstein M.E. *Publication Bias in Meta-Analysis – Prevention, Assesment and Adjustments*. Chichester: John Wiley & Sons, Ltd, 2005.

16. Borenstein M., Hedges L.V., Higgins J.P.T., Rothstein H.R. *Introduction to Meta-Analysis*. Chichester: John Wiley & Sons, Ltd, 2009.

5

Exploring between study heterogeneity

5.1 Introduction

In Chapter 4 the possibility that different studies estimate different underlying treatment effects was acknowledged and accounted for through the use of random effects. While such modelling goes some way to accounting for differences between studies, it does not help explain what causes the variation in the first place. This chapter describes ways of extending the meta-analysis models described in Chapter 4 to include study level covariates to create 'meta-regression' analyses.

Before doing this however, it will be constructive to spend a few moments considering the type of covariate information which may be of interest and the broad approaches that can be taken to exploring their impact. Beyond chance, reasons why study results may differ include treatment interactions with: (i) variations in the populations under study or the interventions administered, etc.; or (ii) introduction of different biases due to differences in study design/conduct. Examples of covariates related to differences in populations include ethnic background of patients, or age of patients, etc. Such covariates could truly be study level covariates, i.e. the covariate relates to all patients enrolled in a study. For example, if all individuals were of the same ethnic background in each study then study level covariates could be coded as follows: 0 = European, 1 = Asian, 2 = African, etc. If this were done, then separate subgroup (meta-)analyses could be conducted for each group; and this could be achieved using the models already described in Chapter 4. Alternatively, the ethnicity variable (as coded above) could be included in a (meta-)regression analysis. An advantage of the latter is that the difference between groups with associated uncertainty can be estimated (which is not possible with the former).

Evidence Synthesis for Decision Making in Healthcare, First Edition. Nicky J. Welton,
Alexander J. Sutton, Nicola J. Cooper, Keith R. Abrams and A.E. Ades.
© 2012 John Wiley & Sons, Ltd. Published 2012 by John Wiley & Sons, Ltd.

What if some/all studies included patients of mixed ethnic backgrounds? In this situation, multiple covariate values exist for different patients within the same study. Here, it would be possible to include 'average' patient level values as study level covariates, e.g. percentage of patients of European background could be coded and included in a (meta-)regression analysis. Similarly, for a continuous covariate such as patient age, if studies were conducted on patients in very tight age bands (e.g. children, adults of working age, retired adults) it would be possible to code as study level covariates, but more commonly where studies include patients in multiple age categories, it would be necessary to code as average age within a study and include in a (meta-)regression analysis.

5.2 Random effects meta-regression models

Meta-regression relates the size of the treatment effect to numerical characteristic(s) of the trials included in a meta-analysis. The relationship modelled is like a standard (e.g. least-squares) regression, only the precision of each study's outcome estimate is taken into account (just like in standard meta-analysis models). Either fixed or random effect meta-analysis models can be extended to include covariates, however only the random effects version is pursued here (although the fixed effect version is a straightforward simplification of the model presented). Generally, random effects meta-regression models are preferred since any residual heterogeneity, not explained by the included covariates, is allowed for via the random effect term.

5.2.1 Generic random effect meta-regression model

Thompson and Sharp [1] proposed the following model, which is an extension of Equation (4.4):

$$Y_i \sim \text{Normal}(\delta_i + \beta x_i, V_i) \qquad (5.1)$$

$$\delta_i \sim \text{Normal}(d, \tau^2) \quad i = 1, \ldots, k$$

where β is the regression coefficient for the underlying effect of the covariate, x_i, on the outcome. δ_i is now the treatment effect in the ith study adjusted for the covariate effect (i.e. the treatment effect when the covariate value is 0). Similarly, d is the pooled effect size adjusted for the covariate effect, and all other parameters have the interpretation outlined for Equation (4.4). This model could be extended further to include multiple covariates, or nonlinear terms, etc.

In addition to the prior distributions for d and τ^2, a prior is now also needed for β. Since β is unconstrained and thus can theoretically take any value, a Normal distribution with a large variance can be placed on it (as was done for d previously), for example $\beta \sim \text{Normal}(0, 10^6)$ if a vague prior distribution is required. In the next section we introduce a worked regression example which we analyse using a variant of Equation (5.1) which allows modelling using a Binomial likelihood as introduced in Equation (4.7).

Example 5.1   BCG tuberculosis (TB) vaccine trials.

In a meta-analysis of trials of the BCG vaccine to prevent TB [2] it was proposed that the distance the trial was conducted from the equator would affect the effectiveness of the vaccine. The underlying reason for this was hypothesised as being due to degeneration of the vaccine when stored in hotter and more humid conditions (i.e. near the equator) which would reduce its effectiveness. The outcome data from 13 trials, together with the covariate latitude (measured in degrees from the equator), are presented in Table 5.1. Note that all the trials but one, Trial 9, was conducted in the northern hemisphere as indicated by positive degrees from the equator. For purposes of analysis the absolute degrees are used, so the minus sign in front of the 27 degrees for Trial 9 is removed.

Table 5.1   Outcome data and covariate value for 13 trials of BCG vaccine for the prevention of TB.

Trial	Latitude (degrees from the equator)	Vaccinated		Not vaccinated	
		Disease	No disease	Disease	No disease
1	44	4	119	11	128
2	55	6	300	29	274
3	42	3	228	11	209
4	52	62	13 536	248	12 619
5	13	33	5036	47	5761
6	44	180	1361	372	1079
7	19	8	2537	10	619
8	13	505	87 886	499	87 892
9	−27	29	7470	45	7232
10	42	17	1699	65	1600
11	18	186	50 448	141	27 197
12	33	5	2493	3	2338
13	33	27	16 886	29	17 825

If a random effect meta-analysis is conducted (ignoring the effect of the covariate), then the results in Figure 5.1 are obtained. From this plot it can be seen that there is great variability in the effect sizes from the individual studies, and this is borne out by the relatively large estimate for the between study heterogeneity (τ^2) of 0.39 (95% CrI 0.14 to 1.18). This variability includes both highly effective and harmful treatment effects.

The trial results are presented on a scatter plot against the covariate (distance from the equator) in Figure 5.2. The size of the plotting circles is inversely proportional to the variances of the effect size estimates (i.e. more precise studies have larger circles). It can be seen that there is some evidence that the vaccine is most effective the further from the equator the study is conducted.

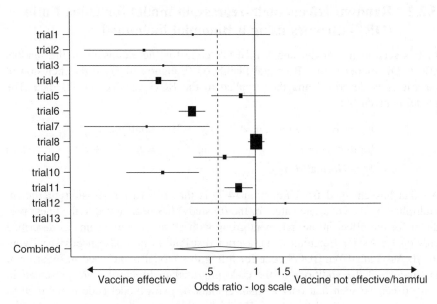

Figure 5.1   Forest plot of BCG vaccine trials.

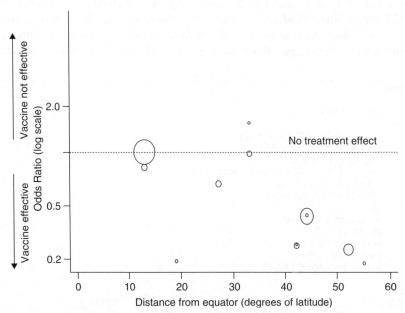

Figure 5.2   Scatter plot of trial effect size estimates versus the distance from the equator the trials were conducted.

5.2.2   Random effects meta-regression model for Odds Ratio (OR) outcomes using a Binomial likelihood

In this section the model and WinBUGS code for the extension of the random effects OR model with a Binomial likelihood (Equation (4.7)) to the inclusion of covariates is described and then applied to the BCG vaccine for TB data. The model is given by:

$$r_{Ai} \sim \text{Binomial}(p_{Ai}, n_{Ai}) \qquad r_{Bi} \sim \text{Binomial}(p_{Bi}, n_{Bi})$$
$$\text{logit}(p_{Ai}) = \mu_i \qquad \text{logit}(p_{Bi}) = \mu_i + \delta_i + \beta x_i \qquad (5.2)$$
$$\delta_i \sim \text{Normal}(d, \tau^2) \qquad i = 1, \ldots, k$$

All that has changed from Equation (4.7) is that βx_i (the regression coefficient multiplied by the covariate value for the ith study) has been added to the linear predictor for the effect in the treatment group with all other components as described previously. As for Equation (5.1), a prior distribution now also needs specifying for β. Associated WinBUGS code for fitting this model is provided in Figure 5.3. In Figure 5.3 the additions to the code provided in Figure 4.5 are presented in bold. It can be seen that only a small amount of extra model code is required to include a covariate in the analysis. Hopefully, this gives some appreciation for the power of WinBUGS for fitting models. A random effect logistic regression model is a nontrivial type of model to fit using Frequentist methods and requires dedicated routines. Since WinBUGS works using a form of simulation where all that is required is a declaration of the model and data, complex models can be fitted and extended with relative ease. While the use of WinBUGS to fit a simple fixed effect

```
Model
{
        for( i in 1 : k )
        {
                rA[i] ~ dbin(pA[i], nA[i])
              rB[i] ~ dbin(pB[i], nB[i])
           logit(pA[i]) <- mu[i]
           logit(pB[i]) <- mu[i] + delta[i] + beta*lat[i]
           mu[i] ~ dnorm(0.0,1.0E-5)
           delta[i] ~ dnorm(d, prec)
        }
        d ~ dnorm(0.0,1.0E-6)
        tau~dunif(0,10)
        tau.sq<-tau*tau
        prec<-1/(tau.sq)
        beta ~ dnorm(0.0,1.0E-6)
}
Data
list(rB = c(4,.........,27),rA = c(11,.........,29),nB = c(123,.........,16913),
        nA = c(139,.........,17854), lat = c(44,.........,33), Nstud = 13)
Initial Values
list(d = 0, tau = 1, delta = c(0,.........,0),     mu = c(0,.........0),beta = 0)
```

Figure 5.3   WinBUGS code for fitting the random effects meta-regression model to the BCG vaccine data.

meta-analysis model may seem like 'overkill', the more complex the modelling becomes, such as the more complex models presented in later chapters, we believe the more appealing the use of WinBUGS becomes, especially when considering the small size of the code files required. A further advantage of WinBUGS is that we believe there is a greater transparency in knowing what model has been fitted, i.e. in WinBUGS code you simply declare the model you wish to fit. In other packages this is not the case, i.e. typically you select a command which allows the fitting of a model within the family you wish to fit, then you specify options to indicate characteristics of the model. There is often no way of verifying that the actual specification of the model fitted is the same as that intended.

Example 5.1 (revisited)   BCG TB vaccine trials.

The WinBUGS code to fit the model in Equation (5.2) to adjust for the covariate latitude in the BCG vaccine for TB example is shown in Figure 5.3. The results of fitting this model to the BCG vaccine are presented graphically in Figure 5.4 via the inclusion of a fitted regression line onto the scatter plot first introduced in Figure 5.2. It can be seen that a strong negative association is estimated (β is estimated to be -0.03 (95% CrI -0.05 to -0.01)), which implies that the Log Odds Ratio (LOR) decreases (linearly) the further away from the equator you are – implying the treatment increases in effectiveness. Hence, this means the

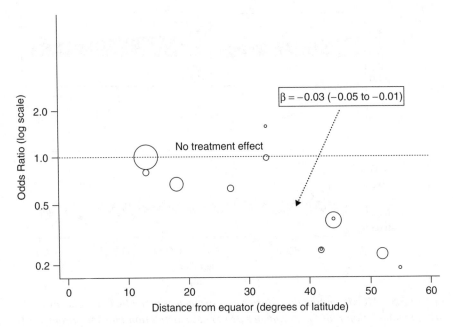

Figure 5.4   Fitted regression line for the BCG vaccine meta-regression.

meta-analysis has not produced a single pooled effectiveness estimate, but implies effectiveness varies with location on the globe.

Note how the fitted regression line is not extrapolated beyond the covariate range of the included studies, as in many contexts extreme caution should be observed if extrapolating. For example, the intercept of the regression line, represented by d (the effect of the vaccine when the covariate value is 0), implies an OR of 1.45, suggesting the vaccine is actually harmful (i.e. it increases the risk of getting TB) but since the closest any of the studies were to the equator is 13 degrees, such a statement would be based on extrapolation. The estimate for the between study heterogeneity, τ^2, is 0.074 (95% CrI 0.001 to 0.67) which is much smaller than was estimated before the inclusion of the covariate, which confirms that much of the between study heterogeneity – but not all – has been explained by the inclusion of the covariate.

5.2.3 Autocorrelation and centring covariates

If you have run the Example 5.1 for yourself, and conscientiously checked some of the Monte Carlo Markov Chain (MCMC) diagnostics available within WinBUGS (as described in Chapter 2), then you may have identified some worrying issues. Figure 5.5 presents the autocorrelation plots for d and β and the history plot for β for 5000 iterations. These indicate that the autocorrelation for both d and β

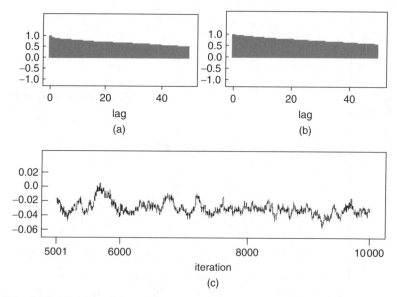

Figure 5.5   MCMC output diagnostics for parameters in the BCG vaccine example: (a) autocorrelation plot for parameter d; (b) autocorrelation plot for parameter β; and (c) history plot for parameter β.

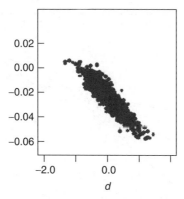

Figure 5.6   Scatter plot of pairs of estimates of the model parameters d and β indicating strong (negative) correlation between them.

are high, and the history plot for appears somewhat less than ideal since the trace 'snakes' slowly around. When such plots are obtained, the possibility of lack of convergence should always be considered. In this instance, as will be explained, the issue here is a poor mixing MCMC chain rather than lack of convergence. In such instances, the MCMC sampler will give valid parameter estimates (as indeed are those presented above), if the model is run for enough iterations, but since successive iterations, even at a lag of 50, are still highly correlated, the sampler is very inefficient. For this relatively simple model, inefficiency will only mean a delay in obtaining estimates of a few minutes, but such inefficiencies could be much more limiting in more complex models so an explanation of what causes the problem together with a solution are presented below.

In Figure 5.6 a scatter plot of pairs of estimates for the model parameters d and β as sampled by WinBUGS are presented. The shape formed by this scatter of points indicates that there is a strong negative association between associated estimates sampled for these parameters (i.e. sampling a high value of β results in a low value of d and vice versa).

It is this correlation between intercept and slope parameter of the regression which is responsible for the poor mixing of the MCMC chains. Figure 5.7(a) illustrates the issue schematically. In this plot, the observed data (represented by stars) are located far away from the origin. If you place a pen along the line of the regression line and move it a little pivoting approximately around the mean covariate value (representing the sampling of different values for the slope parameter at every iteration of the MCMC sampler due to uncertainty in its value), you will notice that the intercept (i.e. where the pen intersects the y-axis) also changes. This change is also predictable – i.e. a steeper slope results in a lower intercept and vice versa. This is what is causing the correlation observed in Figure 5.6 and this dependency restricts the freedom of movement of the MCMC sampler around the distribution of the parameter posterior resulting in the high autocorrelation observed. (Note, for more 'conventional' regression models, WinBUGS avoids this problem since a default setting is to 'block update' all regression parameters simultaneously, which

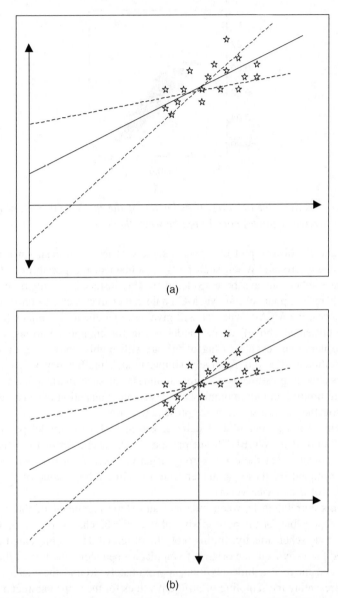

(a)

(b)

Figure 5.7   Illustrative plot of (a) high autocorrelation between intercept and slope parameters (d and β) since a change in one causes a change in the other; and (b) centring the data at the origin removes the dependency of one on the other and hence the problem.

avoids this dependency issue, but not for these meta-regressions.) Fortunately, there
is a relatively simple solution to this problem, which is achieved by centring the
covariates. This means taking the mean covariate value away from each covariate
value, which has the effect of moving the origin of the regression to the mean
covariate value in the centre of the data, as illustrated in Figure 5.7(b). Now if the
pen is placed on the line and 'wiggled' to increase and decrease the slope, since
the pivot point is on the y-axis, the intercept does not move as it did before and
hence the dependency is eliminated.

Centring the covariates can be done outside WinBUGS prior to analysis, or
actually within the analysis code by replacing the line of code:

`logit(pB[i]) <- mu[i] + delta[i] + beta*lat[i]`

with

`logit(pB[i]) <- mu[i] + delta[i] + beta*(lat[i]-mean(lat[]))`

MCMC output diagnostics for this modified code are provided in Figure 5.8.
Figure 5.8(a) indicates the autocorrelation for parameter β is greatly reduced (as it
is for d also – not shown). The scatter plot of β and d in Figure 5.8(b) also shows
a more random scatter with no perceivable correlation. This lack of dependence is
also indicated in the better mixing (more 'spikey') history plot for β presented in
Figure 5.8(c).

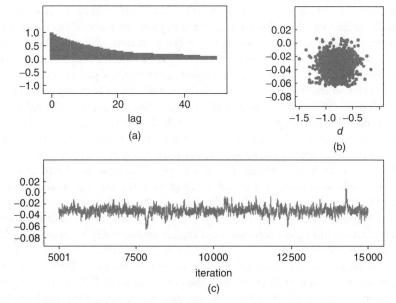

*Figure 5.8   MCMC output diagnostics for parameters in the BCG vaccine example
when the covariate is centred: (a) autocorrelation plot for parameter β; (b) scatter
plot of pairs of estimates of the model parameters d and β; and (c) history plot for
parameter β.*

Once the model is fitted with this new line of code and parameter estimates obtained, it is important to interpret the results correctly and, if necessary, transform the parameters to remove the centring (i.e. the model should produce exactly the same results but the latter is a different parameterisation of the first and the parameters need transforming to give the same interpretation as the uncentred model). As fitted, the interpretation of the parameter d is the treatment effect at the mean covariate value where before it was the effect when the covariate value was 0. To obtain the latter, beta x mean(lat[]) is subtracted from the intercept (d) to remove centring and this can be done within WinBUGS through the creation of a new node, i.e.

```
d.uncent <- d - beta*mean(lat[ ])
```

5.3   Limitations of meta-regression

Exploring how covariates effect treatment effects across studies may seem a very appealing prospect. Indeed the example presented above may reinforce the viewpoint. However, this example is not typical, and in many instances exploration of heterogeneity via covariates will be much less conclusive. The typical numbers of studies in a meta-analysis severely limits the power such analyses have in many contexts [3]. Where analyses are based on aggregate patient level covariates (e.g. % white, average age, etc.), typically, such analyses will have much less power than if the analysis was carried out at the patient (rather than the study) level through the use of Individual Patient Data (IPD) [4]. Further, such analyses are potentially prone to ecologic biases also which implies that associations estimated at the aggregate level may not reflect the underlying relationships at the individual level.

While the use of IPD for meta-analysis is beyond the scope of this book, it is recommended where feasible, and exploring the effect of patient level covariates is a context where IPD will be particularly valuable [5]. The fitting of meta-analysis models to IPD [6–8] in WinBUGS is relatively straightforward, and models to combine IPD and aggregate data, where IPD is not available, are also considered elsewhere [9]. In some contexts, it may be possible to reconstruct the IPD from data available in a trial report. For example, where a binary outcome and a binary patient level covariate are of interest, if the outcome by treatment group 2×2 table were reported for each level of the covariate, this would be sufficient to allow reconstruction of the IPD. Also, it should not be forgotten that meta-regression analyses, whether conducted at the aggregate or the individual level, are observational in nature and causation cannot automatically be assumed between a covariate and outcome.

A further issue in fitting regression models is that often there is concern that the severity of illness interacts with the effectiveness of the intervention. For this reason the effect of 'baseline risk' on outcome is commonly explored through meta-regression. However, a complication with this analysis is that the covariate of interest is actually also part of the outcome definition. A specific model which allows for this is considered in the next section.

5.4 Baseline risk

The influence of baseline risk on treatment effect may be of interest, and a meta-regression analysis may seem a sensible option for exploring such an effect. Heterogeneity in baseline risk among trials is likely to reflect differences in patient characteristics (e.g. age, medical history, co-morbidities, etc.) and thus baseline risk may be considered a proxy, or surrogate, for such underlying factors; data for which may not be available to the analyst

However, if we formally define baseline risk to be the *risk of the outcome event for a patient under the control condition*, since this indicates the average risk of patient in that trial if they were not treated, then the covariate information would be derived from the outcome data from the control group in each trial. Hence, the same data are used to inform both outcome and covariate values (i.e. both y and x in a regression). This leads to structural dependence within the regression equation. Additionally, both the covariate and outcome are estimated from the trials with finite sample sizes and therefore are estimates rather than true values (i.e. they are measured with error). The issues of structural dependency and measurement error (when combined) present problems associated with regression to the mean, also known as regression dilution bias. If a standard meta-regression model of the form described above is fitted for baseline risk, which ignores regression dilution bias, then the association between covariate and outcome can be overestimated.

The mechanism by which regression dilution bias acts is a little difficult to explain. It is perhaps simplest to imagine a situation where baseline risk does not affect outcome at all, and thus a regression should estimate a slope with a close to zero gradient. Now imagine two particular trials, whose location on an x–y scatter plot (of the form presented in Figure 5.4) should be exactly the same (i.e. the underlying effect sizes and covariate values are identical for both trials). Now imagine in one trial, by chance, the observed event rate in the control group was higher than the true underlying rate. Assuming the event of interest is undesirable, other things being equal this will mean the treatment is estimated to be more effective than it truly is (i.e. if more people on control have the undesirable event, then this should make the treatment look 'better'), which will mean the trial outcome – e.g. OR – is estimated to be lower than it actually is. Thus the play of chance in this example will mean the observed point on the x–y scatter plot will be shifted to the right (due to higher baseline risk) and down (due to smaller OR). Now imagine, by chance, the opposite happens for the second trial, i.e. the observed control group event rate is lower than the true underlying rate. If you think this through, it implies that the OR will be higher due to the treatment being estimated to be less effective than it actually is. This in turn means the observed point on the x–y scatter will be shifted to the left (due to lower baseline risk) and up (due to larger OR). Hence if you connect these two observed points you now have a line with a nonzero gradient, implying a relationship with baseline risk (even though this is observed in a situation where no relationship is assumed).

In the next section we introduce an example and then describe a modified meta-regression model to address these shortcomings.

Example 5.2   BCG TB endoscopic sclerotherapy in the prevention of bleeding for patients with cirrhosis and oesagogastric varices.

Thompson *et al*. [10] have previously considered a meta-analysis of 19 randomised controlled trials assessing the effectiveness of endoscopic sclerotherapy in the prevention of bleeding for patients with cirrhosis and oesagogastric varices. The outcome of interest is the number of patients who go on to develop a bleed. The data for these trials is presented in Table 5.2 and a forest plot of these data with the result of the random effects meta-analysis is presented in Figure 5.9.

Table 5.2   Outcome data from 19 randomised controlled trials of the effectiveness of endoscopic sclerotherapy in the prevention of bleeding for patients with cirrhosis and oesagogastric varices.

	Subjects		Bleeds			Odds of event on
Trials	Control	Treatment	Control	Treatment	OR	control
1	36	35	22	3	0.06	1.57
2	53	56	30	5	0.08	1.30
3	18	16	6	5	0.91	0.50
4	22	23	9	3	0.22	0.69
5	46	49	31	11	0.14	2.07
6	60	53	9	19	3.17	0.18
7	60	53	26	17	0.62	0.76
8	69	71	29	10	0.23	0.73
9	41	41	14	12	0.80	0.52
10	20	21	3	0	0.12	0.20
11	41	42	13	9	0.59	0.46
12	35	33	14	13	0.98	0.67
13	138	143	23	31	1.38	0.20
14	51	55	19	20	0.96	0.59
15	72	73	13	13	0.98	0.22
16	16	13	12	3	0.10	3.00
17	28	21	5	3	0.77	0.22
18	19	18	0	4	12.10	0.03
19	24	22	2	6	4.13	0.09

Of course, this could be achieved by calculating the log odds of an event in the control group and using Equation (5.2) to fit this as a covariate, but this is potentially biased as outlined above, hence the need for the approach described in the next section. From Figure 5.9 it can be seen that, overall, there is a considerable benefit of the treatment with an OR of 0.59. It can also be seen that there is considerable heterogeneity between the different study results. In Table 5.2 OR and odds of an event in the control group are presented. It can be seen that there is some suggestion that the most effective trials are those with the highest probability of events in the control group. Thus, it would seem appropriate to explore the effect of including baseline risk via the fitting of the odds of an event in the control group as a covariate.

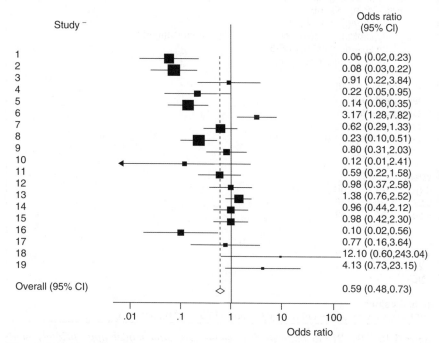

Figure 5.9   Random effects meta-analysis of 19 sclerotherapy trials for the prevention of bleeding for patients with cirrhosis and oesagogastric varices.

5.4.1   Model for including baseline risk in a meta-regression on the (log) OR scale

The model proposed by Thompson *et al.* [10] is used to include baseline risk on a (log) OR scale using a Binomial likelihood, given in Equation (5.3).

$$r_{Ai} \sim \text{Binomial} \ (p_{Ai}, n_{Ai}) \qquad r_{Bi} \sim \text{Binomial} \ (p_{Bi}, n_{Bi})$$
$$\text{logit}(p_{Ai}) = \mu_i \qquad \text{logit}(p_{Bi}) = \mu_i + \delta_i + \beta(\mu_i - \bar{\mu}) \qquad (5.3)$$
$$\delta_i \sim \text{Normal}(d, \tau^2) \qquad i = 1, \dots, k$$

where $\bar{\mu}$ is the mean baseline risk across all studies and is used to centre the covariate (to reduce autocorrelation as described above), and all other quantities have been defined previously. The WinBUGS code which fits this model to the sclerotherapy example is provided in Figure 5.10. The clever/unique aspect of this model is easy to miss, which relates to including μ_i as the covariate. Note

```
Model
{
  for( i in 1 : 19)
    {
          rA[i] ~ dbin(pA[i], nA[i])
        rB[i] ~ dbin(pB[i], nB[i])
          logit(pA[i]) <- mu[i]
          logit(pB[i]) <- mu[i] + delta[i] + beta*(mu[i]-mean(mu[]))
          mu[i] ~ dnorm(0.0,1.0E-5)
          delta[i] ~ dnorm(d, prec)
    }
  d ~ dnorm(0.0,1.0E-6)
  tau~dunif(0,10)
  tau.sq<-tau*tau
  prec<-1 /(tau.sq)
  beta ~ dnorm(0.0,1.0E-6)
}


#Data
rB[]     rA[]     nB[]     nA[]
3 22     35       36
5 30     56       53
. .              .        .

. .              .        .
4 0      18       19
6 2      22       24
END


#Initial Values
list(d = 0, tau = 1, delta = c(0,0,. . .,0,0), mu = c(0,0,. . .,0,0), beta = 0)
```

Figure 5.10   WinBUGS code to fit a meta-regression model appropriately modelling baseline risk for the sclerotherapy trials.

that no separate column of data is specified for this covariate, i.e. it is the same μ_i that has always been included in the modelling and is treated as a random variable (since it is defined as the log odds of p_{Ai}) - thus its value will vary at each iteration of the MCMC simulation. By doing so, the structural dependence between the intercept and slope of this model are correctly accounted for (Note, in other contexts, such a model, which allows for uncertainty in covariate values, is referred to as a measurement error model.)

Example 5.2 (revisited)   BCG TB endoscopic sclerotherapy in the prevention of bleeding for patients with cirrhosis and oesagogastric varices.

The WinBUGS code to adjust for baseline risk (Equation (5.3)) is shown in Figure 5.10. The estimate of the regression slope, β, is -1.01 (95% CrI -1.21 to -0.85), hence there is considerable evidence that the effectiveness of sclerotherapy is associated with the underlying risk of the event in the population. The fitted regression line, together with the study specific estimates, is presented in Figure 5.11.

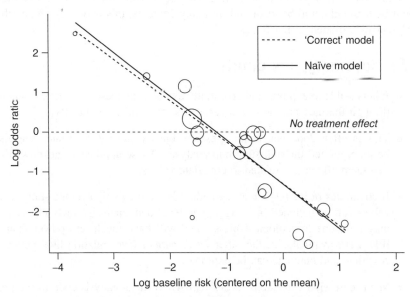

Figure 5.11   Plot of outcome versus baseline risk (log odds of event in the control group) together with fitted regression lines for the sclerotherapy trials.

Also included on this plot are the results that are obtained when fitting a standard regression model to the data [such as Equation (5.2)], ignoring the structural dependence between outcome and covariate. For the standard regression model, the estimate for β is -1.12 (95% CrI -1.45 to -0.79), which is slightly larger than that obtained when the structural dependence between outcome and covariate are taken into account. Hence, as predicted the 'naïve' analysis overestimates the association, although the bias is modest in this example. In instances where there are small numbers of small trials, the bias is potentially much greater [11].

5.4.2   Final comments on including baseline risk as a covariate

This section has illustrated how exploring the relationship between baseline risk and treatment effect can help to explain between study heterogeneity. The ultimate aim of such an analysis would be to identify which patients will benefit (most) from an intervention. However, while knowing treatment effect varies with baseline risk is valuable knowledge to have, it does not directly identify *which* patients would receive most benefit, i.e. you cannot measure an individual's baseline risk. Hence, it would be more valuable still if specific patient characteristics which contribute to an individual's baseline risk could be identified, and these could be included in the analysis. In this way definable subgroups of patients for which the treatment could be targeted could be identified. In many contexts, this may only be possible (or greatly facilitated) using IPD.

5.5 Summary key points

- It is possible to explore, and potentially explain, the reasons for heterogeneity through the incorporation of covariates in meta-analysis models.

- This is often done via meta-regression, but categorical covariates can also be incorporated through subgroup analyses. These approaches acknowledge treatment effects are related to covariate values.

- If covariates of interest are at the patient level, then only average study level values can be included in an aggregate level data analysis. Such an analysis may be prone to ecological biases, and will have much less power than if IPD were available. In the latter case, patient level relationships between covariate and outcome can be explored.

- Meta-regression extensions to the WinBUGS meta-analysis code in the previous chapter are relatively straightforward, however centring of covariates (deleting the mean from all values prior to analysis) is recommended to improve the mixing of the chains.

- Although explaining heterogeneity through meta-regression is potentially a powerful method, its power is often limited due to the number of studies available and other factors.

- It is often of interest to explore how treatment effects vary with the probability of an event in the control group. Such analyses are possible, but the structural dependence between outcome and covariate need accounting for and specific code is provided.

5.6 Further reading

Alternative meta-regression models have been considered elsewhere [1]. Additionally, further baseline risk meta-regression models, making alternative assumptions about the baseline effects across studies, have also been considered elsewhere [11].

5.7 Exercises

We return to the topic of cholesterol lowering, but using a different data set. This data set includes trials of a class of drugs called statins. The data set (shown on next page) is available in an Excel file called *statins.xls*.

The variable names are explained below.

id	ID
name	trial name
nt	total number of patients in treatment arm
nc	total number of patients in control arm
rt	number of deaths (all causes) in the treatment arm
rc	number of deaths (all causes) in the control arm
pubdate	year trial was published
pt_type	patient type – primary (no previous coronary disease)/secondary (previous coronary disease)
fup	duration of study follow-up (in years)
pct_fem	percentage of patients who are female
col_dif	difference in cholesterol level between the two groups at the end of the trial (percentage)
treatment	type of statin given to the treatment group

The statin cholesterol lowering trials data set:

id	name	nt	nc	rt	rc	pubdate	pt_type	fup	pct_fem	col_dif	treatment
1	4S	2221	2223	182	256	1993	Secondary	5.4	19	23.4	Simvastatin
2	Beste-horn	129	125	1	4	1997	Secondary	2.3	0	28.5	Pravastatin
3	Brown	94	52	1	0	1990	Secondary	2.5	0	23.4	Lovastatin
4	CCAIT	165	166	2	2	1994	Secondary	2	18	18.7	Lovastatin
5	Downs	3304	3301	80	77	1998	Primary	5.2	15	16.8	Simvastatin
6	EXCEL	6582	1663	33	3	1991	Primary	.9	41	22.9	Lovastatin
7	Furberg	460	459	1	8	1994	Secondary	3	48	25.5	Lovastatin
8	Haskell	145	155	3	3	1994	Secondary	4	14	15.5	.
9	Jones	83	42	1	0	1991	Secondary	.2	50	16.2	Pravastatin
10	KAPS	224	223	3	4	1995	Primary	3	0	19.5	Pravastatin
11	Kane	48	49	0	1	1990	Diabetic	2	57	22.3	.
12	LIPID	4512	4520	498	633	1998	Secondary	6.1	17	19.9	.
13	MARS	123	124	2	1	1993	Secondary	2	9	30.4	Lovastatin
14	MAAS	193	188	4	11	1994	Secondary	4	12	21.3	Simvastatin
15	PLAC 1	79	78	4	5	1991	Secondary	2	15	12.1	Lovastatin
16	PLAC 2	206	202	4	6	1995	Secondary	3	22.5	20.3	Pravastatin
17	PMSGCRP	530	532	0	3	1993	Primary	.5	24	17.2	Pravastatin
18	Riegger	187	178	2	4	1999	Secondary	1	38.4	12.5	Lovastatin
19	Wein-traub	203	201	3	1	1994	Secondary	.5	28	.	Lovastatin
20	Wscot-land	3305	3293	106	135	1995	Primary	4.9	0	18.6	Pravastatin

A '.' indicates information that was not available from published sources (i.e. it is missing).

Model 5.1: Meta-analysis of statin trials

No files are available for this practical - you have to make your own!

Create a data set in one of the two WinBUGS formats which includes event data necessary for a meta-analysis and in addition the covariate col_diff. Carry out a meta-analysis of the statin drugs in WinBUGS using the direct OR model used in Model 4.3 (Chapter 4 Exercises).

Hint:

(i) You may wish to modify an existing file from a previous practical to speed the process up.

(ii) Delete studies which have missing col_diff data for the purposes of this practical.

(iii) Note also that WinBUGS is very particular on data specified – it complains if data are loaded that is not used. So since we are not using col_diff in this model include the line.temp[i] <-col_diff[i] within the part of the program which loops over studies – this does not interfere with the model and keeps WinBUGS 'happy'.)

• What d o you conclude about the effectiveness of statins?

• Is there evidence of between study heterogeneity?

Model 5.2: Meta-regression on percentage cholesterol reduced

Modify the file you have created in the previous task to include the study level covariate col_diff in a meta-regression.

• Do this initially without centring the covariate. Confirm that this results in high autocorrelation and poor mixing of the chains.

• Then centre the covariate and confirm that autocorrelation has been reduced. Interpret the results of the regression. Does the degree of cholesterol reduced influence the reduction in mortality?

• Calculate the intercept of an uncentred model from the centred one by hand.

• You could create a node in WinBUGS to carry out the uncentring for you.

d.uncent <- d - beta*(mean(col_dif[ ]))

Try this and confirm you get the same results.

• Estimate the predictive interval for the underlying effect in a new study in which the difference in cholesterol reduced between groups is 20%.

Model 5.3: Meta-regression using the discrete covariate patient type

Replace the covariate col_diff with the discrete covariate pt_type coded as 0 for primary and 1 for secondary or diabetic.

- Estimate the pooled mean effect for both groups separately.

- Is there much support for a difference in effect between subgroups of trials?

- An alternative way of calculating the effect in the two subgroups would be to fit two separate (random effect) meta-analysis models to the data. In terms of model specification, how does this approach differ when compared with the regression approach used above?

- Compare the Deviance Information Criterion (DIC) (see Chapter 6) for a (Random Effects) model with and without the covariate pt_type.

Model 5.4: Meta-regression examining the effect of baseline risk on the treatment effect

Modify you existing code to examine the influence of baseline risk using Section 5.4 as guidance. As mentioned in Section 5.2.3 you will need to centre using a constant worked out outside WinBUGS – log((probability of an event given control)/(1-probability of an event given control)).

- Does the treatment effect appear to be influenced by baseline risk?

- Uncentre the regression coefficients as before. It is possible to find the baseline risk value for which the treatment effect goes from beneficial to harmful (with associated uncertainty). This is achieved by adding and monitoring the following node:

eqpoint <-d.uncent/(-beta).

- Can the results of this model be directly used to inform individual patient decisions?

- Fit the standard meta-regression model with baseline risk as a covariate. Do the parameter estimates change?

References

1. Thompson S.G., Sharp S.J. Explaining heterogeneity in meta-analysis: a comparison of methods. *Statistics in Medicine* 1999;**18**:2693–2708.
2. Berkey C.S., Hoaglin D.C., Mosteller F., Colditz G.A. A random-effects regression model for meta-analysis. *Statistics in Medicine* 1995;**14**:395–411.

3. Higgins J.P.T., Thompson S.G. Controlling the risk of spurious findings from meta-regression. *Statistics in Medicine* 2004;**23**:1663–1682.

4. Lambert P., Sutton A.J., Abrams K.R., Jones D.R. A comparison of summary patient level covariates in meta-regression with individual patient data meta-analyses. *Journal of Clinical Epidemiology* 2002;**55**:86–94.

5. Riley R.D., Lambert P.C., Abo-Zaid G. Meta-analysis of individual participant data: rationale, conduct, and reporting. *British Medical Journal* 2010;**340**:c221.

6. Higgins J.P.T., Whitehead A., Turner R.M., *et al*. Meta-analysis of continuous outcome data from individual patients. *Statistics in Medicine* 2001;**20**:2219–2241.

7. Whitehead A., Omar R.Z., Higgins J.P.T., *et al*. Meta-analysis of ordinal outcomes using individual patient data. *Statistics in Medicine* 2001;**20**:2243–2260.

8. Turner R.M., Omar R.Z., Yang M., *et al*. A multilevel model framework for meta-analysis of clinical trials with binary outcomes. *Statistics in Medicine* 2000;**19**:3417–3432.

9. Sutton A.J., Kendrick D., Coupland C.A.C. Meta-analysis of individual- and aggregate-level data. *Statistics in Medicine* 2008;**27**:651–669.

10. Thompson S.G., Smith T.C., Sharp S.J. Investigating underlying risk as a source of heterogeneity in meta-analysis. *Statistics in Medicine* 1997;**16**:2741–2758.

11. Arends L.R., Hoes A.W., Lubsen J., *et al*. Baseline risk as predictor of treatment benefit; three clinical meta-re-analyses. *Statistics in Medicine* 2000;**19**:3497–3518.

6

Model critique and evidence consistency in random effects meta-analysis

6.1 Introduction

An important part of any statistical analysis is an assessment of how well the predictions from a particular model fit with the observed data. Measures of goodness-of-fit can help choose between competing plausible models in a process of model selection. Model critique is not just important for statisticians – it is also important for decision modellers. If the selected model makes predictions that fit poorly with the data, then any outputs from that model, such as parameter estimates, uncertainty in parameters estimates, expected net benefit, resulting optimal treatment strategies and the uncertainty in the optimal strategy, would be a poor reflection of the evidence base. Methods for assessing how well the predictions from a particular model fit the observed data are well established in the field of Frequentist statistics [1], and many of these ideas translate naturally into the Bayesian paradigm.

Typically, decision analysts are concerned with synthesising evidence from different sources to inform parameters in a decision model – for example treatment efficacy informed by a pairwise meta-analysis. This opens up the potential for inconsistencies between the different data sources, where for example one study may find a strong treatment effect whereas the majority of studies find no effect. If the evidence sources are consistent, then this strengthens confidence

Evidence Synthesis for Decision Making in Healthcare, First Edition. Nicky J. Welton,
Alexander J. Sutton, Nicola J. Cooper, Keith R. Abrams and A.E. Ades.
© 2012 John Wiley & Sons, Ltd. Published 2012 by John Wiley & Sons, Ltd.

in any conclusions based on the consistent evidence sources. However, ignoring inconsistency will have implications for model outputs, including the resulting decision analysis. Methods are therefore required to assess, in relation to a particular model, the degree to which the data from different evidence sources are consistent.

We begin with a motivating example of a pairwise meta-analysis of intravenous magnesium vs placebo for patients with myocardial infarction (MI). We then introduce an alternative way to enter data and code in WinBUGS that allows more flexibility and more concise programming, and show the results of the magnesium example meta-analysis. We next introduce the posterior mean residual deviance as a measure of model fit, and the Deviance Information Criteria (DIC) as a basis for model comparison which is particularly useful when dealing with hierarchical (Random Effects) models that are not necessarily nested. We then present exact and approximate methods to explore inconsistency between individual data sources in relation to a given hierarchical (Random Effects) model. The outcome measure in the illustrative example is binary, however all methods can be extended to other types of outcome measures. The only change required in the WinBUGS code is for the likelihood and any measures of fit that rely on the likelihood. An example with continuous data with assumed Normal likelihood is given in Section 9.8.

Example 6.1   Magnesium vs placebo for MI.

We illustrate all of the methods in this chapter in the context of a pairwise meta-analysis of 16 trials of intravenous magnesium vs placebo for patients with acute

Table 6.1   Number of deaths (rt and rc) out of total at risk (nt and nc) from 16 trials of intravenous magnesium vs placebo for treatment of patients with acute MI ordered according to publication date (data from [4]).

| Trial | Trial name | Year | Magnesium | | Placebo | |
			Deaths, rt	Total, nt	Deaths, rc	Total, nc
1	Morton	1984	1	40	2	36
2	Rasmussen	1986	9	135	23	135
3	Smith	1986	2	200	7	200
4	Abraham	1987	1	48	1	46
5	Feldstedt	1988	10	150	8	148
6	Shechter	1989	1	59	9	56
7	Ceremuzynski	1989	1	25	3	23
8	Bertschat	1989	0	22	1	21
9	Singh	1990	6	76	11	75
10	Pereira	1990	1	27	7	27
11	Shechter 1	1991	2	89	12	80
12	Golf	1991	5	23	13	33
13	Thorgersen	1991	4	130	8	122
14	LIMIT-2	1992	90	1159	118	1157
15	Shechter 2	1995	4	107	17	108
16	ISIS-4	1995	2216	29 011	2103	29 039

MI (Table 6.1). The key feature of this meta-analysis is that prior to 1995 there were a lot of small trials that showed magnesium to be effective in preventing mortality in patients with acute MI. In fact, a meta-analysis of intravenous magnesium *vs* placebo was published entitled 'An effective, safe, simple, and inexpensive intervention' [2]. However, in 1995 results from the ISIS-4 (the 4th international study of infarct survival) mega-trial were published which, based on very large numbers, showed no effect of magnesium [3]. The evidence from the ISIS-4 trial appears to be at odds with the earlier evidence. It is therefore of interest to investigate consistency of results from ISIS-4 with results from the earlier trials.

6.2   The Random Effects model revisited

Higgins and Spiegelhalter [5] used the Bayesian random effects meta-analysis model as described in Chapter 4 to analyse and discuss the results from the magnesium example meta-analysis. In this chapter we introduce a different, but equivalent, way to enter the data, write and code the model. This will be useful in later chapters, allows more concise code, and demonstrates the use of nested indexing in the BUGS language. Figure 6.1(a) shows how the magnesium example data were entered into WinBUGS using the method presented in Chapter 3 with each row representing a study. Figure 6.2(b) shows an alternative format where each row, i, represents a single arm of a study, so for each two-arm study there will be two separate rows. We denote the number of deaths in row i by r_i out of a total n_i at risk, however we also need to know which study and which treatment

One row = one study (both arms) 16 rows of data				One row = one arm of a study 32 rows of data			
rt[]	nt[]	rc[]	nc[]	s[]	t[]	r[]	n[]
1	40	2	36	1	2	1	40
9	135	23	135	1	1	2	36
2	200	7	200	2	2	9	135
.	.	.	.	2	1	23	135
.	.	.	.	3	2	2	200
2216	29011	2103	29039	3	1	7	200
END				.	.	.	.
				.	.	.	.
				16	2	2216	29011
				16	1	2103	29039
				END			
(a)				(b)			

Figure 6.1   Two ways to input data in WinBUGS, where each row represents: (a) the data summaries from both active treatment (rt and nt) and placebo (rc and nc) arms of a single study; and (b) the data summaries from a single arm (r and n), with additional indicators (s, study number; t, treatment (2, active treatment; 1, placebo)).

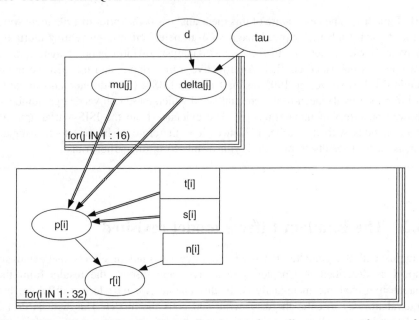

Figure 6.2   Directed Acyclic Graph for the random effects meta-analysis model (Equations (6.1) and (6.2)), where the data are formatted as displayed in Figure 6.1(b).

arm row i represents. We therefore require two new variables, s_i and t_i, which indicate which study number and which treatment arm is represented by row i. So in Figure 6.1(b) row 1 is treatment arm 2 (magnesium) of study 1, row 2 is treatment arm 2 (placebo) of study 1, row 3 is treatment 2 (magnesium) of study 2, and so on. This format allows for easy extension to trials with three or more arms and analysis of more than two treatment options (see Chapter 9).

We can write the Random Effects model (Equation (4.7)) using our new data format:

$$r_i \sim \text{Binomial}(p_i, n_i) \qquad i = 1, \ldots, 32$$

$$\text{logit}(p_i) = \mu_{s_i} + \delta_{s_i} I_{t_i=2} \qquad \text{where } I_{t_i=2} = \begin{cases} 1 & t_i = 2 \\ 0 & t_i = 1 \end{cases} \qquad (6.1)$$

Because we have a generic likelihood statement for each arm, the logistic regression equation needs to pick out the right baseline and treatment parameters. This is done using nested indexing. μ_{s_i} picks out μ_1 when $s_i = 1$ (i.e. rows $i = 1$ and 2), μ_2 when $s_i = 2$ (i.e. rows $i = 3$ and 4) and so on. Similarly for δ_{s_i}, however we only add on a treatment effect for the magnesium arm ($t_i = 2$), which is achieved by multiplying δ_{s_i} by zero when row i represents the placebo arm ($t_i = 1$). The indicator function $I_{t_i=2}$ returns a 1 when the data represent the active arm ($t_i = 2$), and a 0 otherwise.

Suggested exercise *Write out the model for* $i = 1, 2, 3$ *and 4 in the magnesium example and verify that this is identical to that obtained using Equation (4.7).*

The model for study level random effects δ_j is exactly the same as before:

$$\delta_j \sim \text{Normal}(d, \tau^2) \qquad j = 1, \ldots, 16 \qquad (6.2)$$

and we give Normal priors to baseline and mean treatment effect parameters, and a Half-Normal prior to between study standard deviation:

$$\mu_j \sim \text{Normal}(0, 1000^2); \quad d \sim \text{Normal}(0, 1000^2); \quad \tau \sim \text{Half - Normal}(0, 1000^2)$$

The Directed Acyclic Graph (DAG) for the magnesium example is displayed in Figure 6.2. Note the study level parameters μ_j and δ_j lie in a plate (i.e. loop) over study $j = 1, \ldots, 16$, whilst the arm level parameters p_i lie in a plate (i.e. loop) over row $i = 1, \ldots, 32$. The WinBUGS code makes use of the equals(t[i],2) function that returns a 1 if t[i]=2 and a 0 otherwise (in place of the indicator function $I_{t_{i=2}}$):

```
model{
  for (i in 1:32){                              #Loop over data
    r[i] ~ dbin(p[i], n[i])                     #Likelihood
    logit(p[i]) <- mu[s[i]] + delta[s[i]]*equals(t[i],2)   #Logistic regression
  }

  for (j in 1:16){                              #Loop over study
    mu[j] ~ dnorm(0,1.0E-6)                     #Priors for baselines
  }                                             #Random Effects model

  d ~ dnorm(0,1.0E-6)                           #Prior for mean log OR
  tau ~ dnorm(0,1.0E-6)I(0,)                    #Prior for tau
  prec<- 1/(tau*tau)                            #Define precision

  delta.new~dnorm(d,prec)                       #Replicate log OR for
                                                #prediction
  delta[19]<-d                                  #RE mean for plotting
  delta[20] <-delta.new                         #Predictive dist for plotting
}
```

Example 6.1 revisited   Magnesium vs placebo for MI.

The posterior mean for the pooled LogOdds Ratio (LOR) is -0.90 with 95% credible interval $(-1.48, -0.42)$. On the odds-ratio scale the posterior mean is 0.42 with 95% credible interval (0.23, 0.66). These results show a clear treatment effect, with on average the odds of mortality on intravenous magnesium roughly 0.4 times that on placebo. Figure 6.3 shows a caterpillar plot of the shrunken estimates

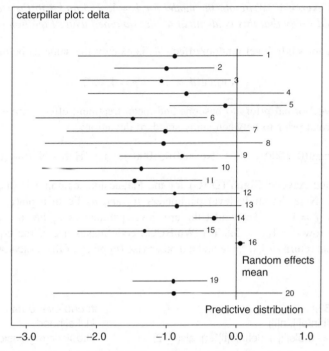

Figure 6.3   Posterior mean and 95% credible intervals for the shrunken LORs for each study in the magnesium example (1–16). The mean LOR (19) and the predictive distribution (20) of a new study from the random effects distribution are also shown. The vertical line indicates 'no effect', i.e. a LOR of 0.

for each study on the log-odds scale, displaying a high degree of heterogeneity between the studies [posterior mean between studies standard deviation 0.72 with 95% credible interval (0.35, 1.3)].

Suggested exercise   *Compare the results from fitting Fixed and Random Effects models to the magnesium example with and without including ISIS-4 (trial number 16). Look at posterior summaries for the mean log-odds ratio and between studies standard deviation.*

Table 6.2 shows that when the ISIS-4 trial is included the Fixed Effect model indicates that there is no effect of magnesium at all (95% credible interval is centred on 0), in contrast with the strong treatment effect seen from the Random Effects model (95% credible range is all negative). However when ISIS-4 is omitted, both models show evidence of a treatment effect of magnesium. The impact of the ISIS-4 mega-trial highlights the key difference between fixed and random effects meta-analyses. The evidence prior to the ISIS-4 trial all supports a protective effect of magnesium on mortality, as shown by both models when ISIS-4 is omitted. However, the ISIS-4 trial provides very strong evidence (based on very

Table 6.2   Posterior mean and 95% credible intervals for the mean LOR, d, and the between studies standard deviation, τ. Results shown for Fixed and Random Effects models including or omitting the results from ISIS-4.

Model	Mean LOR, d	Between studies standard deviation, τ
Fixed Effect (including ISIS-4)	0.01(−0.05, 0.07)	–
Fixed Effect (omitting ISIS-4)	−0.62 (−0.84, −0.40)	
Random Effects (including ISIS-4)	−0.90 (−1.48, −0.42)	0.72 (0.35, 1.29)
Random Effects (omitting ISIS-4)	−1.00 (−1.58, −0.53)	0.61 (0.20, 1.24)

large numbers of patients) that there is no effect of magnesium. The fixed effect analysis is dominated by the very high precision of ISIS-4, giving an estimated mean log-odds ratio close to zero when ISIS-4 is included. The random effects analysis on the other hand assumes that the treatment effects seen in the different studies are drawn from a common distribution effects. The ISIS-4 trial lies in the upper tail of this random effects distribution, and so exerts less influence on the overall estimated mean LOR ratio than for the fixed effect analysis, even though it is a very large study. Instead the inclusion of ISIS-4 leads to greater estimated between study heterogeneity (Table 6.2).

6.3   Assessing model fit

Standard statistical measures of goodness-of-fit such as, residuals, Residual Sum of Squares (RSS) and residual deviance (often called the Likelihood Ratio statistic) can all be calculated within a Bayesian framework to assess the fit of a model. However, instead of point estimates of these statistics, we will obtain posterior distributions for them. These can be summarised in various ways, but typically the posterior mean of these distributions is reported. We will focus on the residual deviance, but other measures of fit can be calculated similarly.

6.3.1   Deviance

The deviance statistic measures the fit of the predictions made by a particular model to the observed data using the likelihood function. The likelihood function measures how 'likely' observed data are given a particular model and so is a natural measure to focus on to assess model fit – in fact Frequentist statistics revolves around maximising the likelihood function. Deviance, D_{model}, is defined as −2 times the log-likelihood, $Loglik_{model}$, for a given model:

$$D_{model} = -2Loglik_{model} \tag{6.3}$$

For a given model and observed data, the larger the likelihood then the closer the model fit. Similarly, the larger the log of the likelihood, $Loglik_{model}$, then the closer the model fit. Multiplying by -2 reverses this, so the smaller the deviance, D_{model}, then the closer the model fit. D_{model} measures how far the model predictions deviate from the observed data. The deviance is simply a function of model parameters that can be written down and calculated for each iteration of a Markov Chain Monte Carlo (MCMC) simulation. Posterior summaries for D_{model} can then be obtained as for other parameters.

The deviance, D_{model}, can be monitored in several ways in WinBUGS. There is always a system node called **deviance** that can be set in **Inference_Samples** that will monitor the relevant deviance formula for a given likelihood. After setting the node and updating, click on the **stats** button to obtain posterior summaries for D_{model}. Alternatively, the posterior mean of the deviance, $\overline{D}_{model}$ can be obtained from the DIC tool. After convergence, set the tool **Inference_DIC_set**. Then, after updating further, click on **DIC**. The posterior mean of the deviance, $\overline{D}_{model}$, is given under the heading **Dbar**. Finally, we could write out the relevant formula as a new node in the WinBUGS code, and then monitor and obtain posterior summaries for this new node.

6.3.2   Residual deviance

The smaller the deviance statistic, D_{model}, then the better the model fit. But how small is small? The disadvantage of using the raw deviance statistic, D_{model}, is that there is no clear answer to this question. Instead we define the residual deviance, D_{res}, which helps us gauge how good the model fit is, by providing a reference point. The residual deviance is equal to the deviance for a given model, D_{model}, minus the deviance for a saturated model, D_{sat}:

$$D_{res} = D_{model} - D_{sat} \qquad (6.4)$$

A saturated model is one where all of the predictions from the model are equal to the observed data values. Formulae for D_{res} based on N data points, for some commonly used likelihood functions, are shown in Table 6.3.

There is no pre-set node for the residual deviance, and it is not included on the DIC tool. Instead we need to write out the relevant formula for a given likelihood, D_{res}, as new nodes in the WinBUGS code. For example, for a Binomial likelihood the formula is:

$$D_{res} = \sum_i 2 \left(r_i \log \left(\frac{r_i}{\hat{r}_i} \right) + (n_i - r_i) \log \left(\frac{n_i - r_i}{n_i - \hat{r}_i} \right) \right) \qquad (6.5)$$

where the model predictions are given by $\hat{r}_i = p_i n_i$, which can be calculated for each iteration of the MCMC simulation. There is a contribution to the residual deviance for each unconstrained data point, i, and the residual deviance is the sum

Table 6.3   Formulae for the residual deviance, D_{res} (Equation (6.4)), for some commonly used likelihood functions.

Likelihood	Model prediction	Residual deviance, D_{res}
$r_i \sim \text{Binomial}(p_i, n_i)$	$\hat{r}_i = n_i p_i$	$\sum_{i=1}^{N} 2 \left(r_i \log \left(\dfrac{r_i}{\hat{r}_i} \right) \right.$ $\left. + (n_i - r_i) \log \left(\dfrac{n_i - r_i}{n_i - \hat{r}_i} \right) \right)$
$r_i \sim \text{Poisson}(\lambda_i E_i)$	$\hat{r}_i = \lambda_i E_i$	$\sum_{i=1}^{N} 2 \left((\hat{r}_i - r_i) + r_i \log \left(\dfrac{r_i}{\hat{r}_i} \right) \right)$
$y_i \sim \text{Normal}(\mu_i, \sigma_i^2) \ \sigma_i^2$ assumed known	$\hat{y}_i = \mu_i$	$\sum_{i=1}^{N} \left(\dfrac{(y_i - \mu_i)^2}{\sigma_i^2} \right)$
$(r_{i,1}, r_{i,2}, \ldots, r_{i,J})$ $\sim \text{Multinomial}$ $(p_{i,1}, p_{i,2}, \ldots, p_{i,J}; n_i)$	$\hat{r}_{i,j} = n_i p_{i,j}$	$\sum_{i=1}^{N} 2 \left(\sum_{j=1}^{J} r_{i,j} \log \left(\dfrac{r_{i,j}}{\hat{r}_{i,j}} \right) \right)$

over these contributions. The WinBUGS code to calculate this consists of two lines of code, the first to calculate the individual contributions to the residual deviance (within a loop over i), and the second to sum over these:

```
for (i in 1:N){                                    #Within loop over data
  rhat[i] <- p[i] * n[i]                           #Model prediction
  dev[i] <- 2 * (r[i] * (log(r[i])-log(rhat[i]))   #Deviance contribution
       + (n[i]-r[i]) * (log(n[i]-r[i]) - log(n[i]-rhat[i])))
}
resdev <- sum(dev[])                               #Outside loop over data
                                                   #Residual deviance
```

For a model that fits the data well, we would expect the individual contributions to the residual deviance to have a roughly chi-squared distribution with degrees of freedom equal to 1. This is exact if the observed data have a Normal likelihood [6]. It follows that if we sum over N unconstrained data points, then we would expect the residual deviance to have a roughly chi-squared distribution with degrees of freedom equal to N. On this basis, we would expect the posterior mean of the residual deviance, $\overline{D}_{res}$, to be close to the number of unconstrained data points, N, if the model predictions are a good fit to the data. If $\overline{D}_{res}$ is much greater than N, then we can examine the contributions to the residual deviance to identify individual data points that are contributing heavily to D_{res}.

Example 6.1 revisited   Magnesium vs placebo for MI.

Figure 6.4 shows the output from the WinBUGS DIC tool for the Random Effects model. The relevant line of Figure 6.4 is that labelled r (our data). If there is more than one variable name for the likelihood statements, then the DIC tool breaks down the results accordingly. For example, if we had written the code as two likelihoods for rc and rt as in Equation (4.7), then there would be a row for rc and another row for rt, and we would want the sum of these (given by total). In this case there is an extra row for tau, because we used the I(0,) notation to obtain a half-normal prior. The I(,) notation is interpreted as censoring by WinBUGS, and so considered to be data. We ignore the line for tau, and just report results from the line for r. The posterior mean deviance is corresponding to our Binomial likelihood for data r is $\overline{D}_{model} = 147.5$. Figure 6.5 shows the posterior density for the residual deviance, D_{res}, which has posterior mean $\overline{D}_{res} = 29.7$ with 95% credible interval (17.1, 46.0). There are 32 unconstrained data points in this example (16 studies × 2 arms), so we would expect the posterior mean of the residual deviance to be close to 32 if the model predictions fit the data well. There is no evidence of lack of fit for the Random Effects model.

Dbar = post.mean of –2logL; Dhat = –2LogL at post.mean of stochastic nodes			
	Dbar	**Dhat**	**pD**	**DIC**
r	147.458	122.905	24.552	172.010
tau	1.386	1.386	–0.000	1.386
total	148.844	124.292	24.552	173.396

Figure 6.4   Output from the DIC tool for the Random Effects model for the magnesium example.

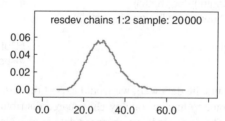

Figure 6.5   Posterior kernel density of the residual deviance for the Random Effects model for the magnesium example.

6.4   Model comparison

A model selection process systematically compares the fit of a set of models. For example, we can simplify our Random Effects model by reducing it to a Fixed

Effect model (model contraction), or we could complicate it further by adding in covariates in a meta-regression (model expansion). Both the deviance and residual deviance statistics can be used to compare the fit of different models. In fact, because the two measures differ only by a constant term, D_{sat}, which does not depend on the model fitted, then when we look at the difference in either measure between two models, we get exactly the same result, i.e.:

$$D_{res1} - D_{res2} = (D_{model1} - D_{sat}) - (D_{model2} - D_{sat}) = D_{model1} - D_{model2}$$

Model fit is not the only consideration to make when selecting a model. The more parameters we include (i.e. the more complicated the model gets), obviously the better the model fit will be. The model that gives the smallest deviance will be one with the same number of parameters as there are unconstrained data points (i.e. a saturated model). But, such a model is of no use for prediction purposes, and cannot be used in a decision analysis (unless making a decision for each study population separately). Instead, we would like to select a model that remains as simple as possible for good predictive power, whilst still fitting well to the observed data – the parsimony principle. Essentially, we wish to make a trade-off between model fit and model complexity. The most commonly used measure to resolve this trade-off in the Frequentist literature is the Akaike Information Criterion (AIC) [7], which simply adds the deviance at the maximum likelihood estimate of parameters, θ, to twice the total number of parameters, k, in a given model:

$$AIC = D(\hat{\theta}) + 2k$$

The AIC can be calculated for non-nested models where it is clear how many parameters there are. However, when there is a hierarchical (random effects) structure, then it is not clear how many parameters there are exactly – it will depend on the degree of between study heterogeneity. The DIC [8] extends the AIC to handle non-nested hierarchical models by defining the effective number of parameters, p_D.

6.4.1 Effective number of parameters, p_D

For a Fixed Effect model it is clear that the number of parameters is equal to the number of study baselines (the μ_j) plus 1 for the single fixed effect, d. So in the magnesium example there are 16 studies, giving 17 parameters in total. At the other extreme, we can fit an independent effects model where each study estimates a treatment effect parameter completely independently of the other studies. In this case the number of parameters is equal to the number of study baselines (the μ_j) plus the number of study treatment effects (the δ_j). So in the magnesium example there are 16 study baselines and 16 study treatment effects, giving 32 parameters in total. The Fixed Effect model is a special case of a Random Effects model when $\tau = 0$, whereas the independent effects model is equivalent to a Random Effects model as $\tau \to \infty$. A Random Effects model with a value of τ between 0 and ∞ lies somewhere between these two extremes and the number of parameters will lie somewhere between these two limits. In the magnesium example the number of parameters will be somewhere between 17 ($\tau = 0$) and 32 ($\tau \to \infty$). If there is very little heterogeneity (i.e. τ close to 0) the number of parameters will be close to 17, and as the heterogeneity, τ, increases, the number of parameters increases towards an upper limit of 32. This is quantified by the effective number of parameters, p_D, which is defined as:

$$p_D = \overline{D}_{model} - D(\hat{\theta}) \qquad (6.6)$$

The effective number of parameters is the posterior mean deviance for a given model, $\overline{D}_{model}$, minus the deviance calculated at some plug-in value for the parameters, $\hat{\theta}$. The DIC tool in WinBUGS uses the posterior mean of the parameters as the plug-in, i.e. $\hat{\theta} = \overline{\theta}$. In the DIC tool output (Fig 6.4) $\overline{D}_{model}$ and $D(\hat{\theta})$ are labelled Dbar and Dhat, respectively.

However, when the relationship between the model predictions and the basic model parameters is highly nonlinear (as is often the case in the multi-parameter evidence syntheses presented later in this book (Chapters 8–11)), then it is more appropriate to use the posterior mean of the model predictions as the plug-in, and calculate p_D externally to WinBUGS (for example in R or Excel).

6.4.2 Deviance Information Criteria

The DIC [8, 9] is equal to the posterior mean deviance, $\overline{D}_{model}$, plus the effective number of parameters, p_D:

$$DIC = D(\hat{\theta}) + 2p_D = \overline{D}_{model} + p_D \qquad (6.7)$$

Either the deviance or the residual deviance can be used in Equations (6.6) and (6.7). Although they lead to different numerical values for the DIC, they only differ by a constant, so that when comparing two different models, the difference in DIC will be the same whether the deviance or residual deviance is used. It has been suggested that differences in DIC over 5 are important (http://www.mrc-bsu.cam.ac.uk/bugs/winbugs/dicpage.shtml), whereas if there are only small differences (less than 3) in DIC there is probably little to choose between two models – although one should check robustness of conclusions to choice of model.

Example 6.1 revisited   Magnesium vs placebo for MI.

Suggested exercise   *Compare the Fixed and Random Effects models for the magnesium example using deviance, residual deviance, effective number of parameters and DIC. Which model would you choose?*

From Table 6.4 the posterior mean deviance for the Random Effects model is 47.8 lower than that for the Fixed Effect model (note that this difference is identical using the residual deviance instead), showing a much greater fit from

Table 6.4   Various model fit summaries for Random Effects and Fixed Effect models for the magnesium example.

Model	$\overline{D}_{res}$	$\overline{D}_{model}$ (Dbar)	$D(\hat{\theta})$ (Dhat)	p_D	DIC
Random Effects	29.7	147.5	122.9	24.6	172.0
Fixed Effect	77.5	195.3	178.5	16.8	212.0

$\overline{D}_{res}$, posterior mean residual deviance; $\overline{D}_{model}$, posterior mean deviance; $D(\hat{\theta})$, deviance at the posterior mean of the parameters; p_D, effective number of parameters; and Deviance Information Criterion, DIC, Deviance Information Criterion.

the Random Effects model. This is not very surprising given the high degree of heterogeneity between studies in this example (Figure 6.3 and Table 6.2). The effective number of parameters p_D is equal to 16.8 for the Fixed Effect model (i.e. 16 baseline parameters and 1 treatment effect parameter), and 24.6 for the Random Effects model - which lies midway between 17 (Fixed Effect model) and 32 (Independent Effects model). The Random Effects model fits better, but is more complex. The DIC provides a trade-off between fit and complexity and is lowest for the Random Effects model, which has a DIC that is 40 lower than that for the Fixed Effect model.

On the basis of the DIC, the model selection process suggests that the Random Effects model is the most parsimonious for the magnesium example. Should we accept this result and proceed with a decision analysis based on the results from the Random Effects model? Recall that the two models give very different results (Table 6.2). The Fixed Effect model fits very well to the ISIS-4 mega-trial (study 16), which dominates the estimated treatment effect for this model. However the Fixed Effect model fits poorly to the other 15 studies, which in turn leads to the high deviance statistic. On the other hand, the Random Effects model fits well to all studies by estimating a large degree of heterogeneity that allows the ISIS-4 trial to be incorporated in the upper tail of the random effects distribution. The fit is good for all studies, but the model predictions are centred on the mean of this random effects distribution, far away from the treatment effect obtained from the ISIS-4 mega-trial. If, for example, we believe the ISIS-4 mega-trial to be providing the most reliable treatment effect estimates, whilst the earlier, smaller studies are more likely to be prone to publishing and other forms of bias, then the Fixed Effect model is the more acceptable – even though it gives a much higher DIC.

6.5   Exploring inconsistency

If the rationale for evidence synthesis is to provide an estimated treatment effect, supported by the evidence, which can be used for inference or decision modelling, then it is crucial that consideration is given to whether the evidence 'fits together' in a coherent picture. In the first instance this means that the process of systematic review that identifies relevant evidence needs to allow for important covariates, patient subgroups, formats of treatment and potential mechanisms for bias. Once the evidence has been assimilated we can statistically assess whether the findings from individual or collections of studies are consistent with the findings from the remaining studies. If we find that the evidence sources provide results that are consistent with each other, then this strengthens conclusions drawn from any pooled summary from the evidence base. If we find that the evidence sources are inconsistent, then we need to go back to the original data sources to explore possible reasons why the evidence sources are giving different results. Note that the statistical methods presented below may be able to identify sets of evidence that give results that are at odds with the remaining evidence, but this does not automatically tell us which piece of evidence is 'wrong'. Typically, smaller studies will be picked out as statistically inconsistent, as these exert less influence on the fitted model. Identifying the causes for inconsistency is however not a statistical issue, and should always be addressed by going back to the original studies.

In this section we describe cross-validation which can be viewed as a gold-standard approach to assessing consistency, then go on to look at mixed predictive *p*-values as an alternative method that approximates cross-validation.

6.5.1   Cross-validation

Cross-validation, commonly used in the Frequentist literature, is a technique whereby an individual data point or subset of data points is omitted from the analysis. The model is then fitted based on the remaining data points, and the results used to predict what we would expect to observe for the omitted data. These predictions are then compared with the actual observed values to assess whether the observations are consistent with the model predictions made based on the remaining evidence. Cross-validation extends naturally to the Bayesian context where the predictions for the omitted data are based on the posterior predictive distributions [10–12].

The key step is how to make predictions for the omitted data. We shall restrict attention to the situation where a single data point is omitted. For a Fixed Effect model we would expect the true treatment effect in an omitted study to be the fixed effect $\delta_{new} = d$, whereas in a Random Effects model we would expect the true treatment effect to be drawn from the random effects distribution of effects, i.e. the predictive distribution:

$$\delta_{new} \sim \text{Normal}(d, \tau^2) \qquad (6.8)$$

The predictive distribution represents two different sources of uncertainty: uncertainty in the mean value, d, and uncertainty as to where in the random effects distribution the new study will lie. This predicts the treatment effect we would expect to see in an infinitely sized new study. However, the omitted study has a (known) finite sample size on each arm, and so there will be an additional element of uncertainty in the observed treatment effect that is due to sampling error. Let the observed data for the omitted study be r_C out of n_C on the control arm and r_T out of n_T on the treatment arm. The predicted number of responders, r_T^{new}, is drawn from a Binomial distribution with the predicted probability of response on the treatment arm, p_T^{new}, and known denominator, n_T:

$$r_T^{new} \sim \text{Binomial}(p_T^{new}, n_T) \tag{6.9}$$

This describes the sampling error that we would expect in a study with n_T on the treatment arm. The predicted probability of response, p_T^{new}, follows the logistic regression relationship (6.1):

$$\text{logit}(p_T^{new}) = \text{logit}(p_C^{new}) + \delta_{new} \tag{6.10}$$

The predicted log-odds on the treatment arm is equal to the predicted log-odds on the control arm plus the predicted treatment effect. The baseline probability of response on the control arm, p_C^{new}, is a nuisance parameter that we need in order to predict the relative treatment effect. We can use the observed data to characterise the baseline probability of response and its uncertainty. We draw the baseline probability of response on the control arm, p_C^{new}, from a Beta distribution:

$$p_C^{new} \sim \text{Beta}(r_C, n_C - r_C) \tag{6.11}$$

The Beta distribution describes the uncertainty in the estimate of a proportion for a given number of responders, r_C, and nonresponders, $(n_C - r_C)$.

Equations (6.8–6.11) provide a method to predict the number of responders on the treatment arm of the omitted study, that allows for the sample size on each arm, the study specific baseline probability of response on the control arm, uncertainty in the mean treatment effect, and the between studies heterogeneity. The predicted number of responders, r_T^{new}, can then be compared with the observed number, r_T. If the observed data, r_T, is supported by the posterior distribution for r_T^{new}, then that data point is consistent with the model predictions based on the remaining data alone. We can compare r_T with r_T^{new} by forming a Bayesian p-value, which measures the probability that r_T^{new} exceeds the observed value r_T, $\text{Pr}(r_T^{new} > r_T)$. This can be achieved using the step(e) function, which records a 1 if its argument $e \geq 0$ and a zero otherwise. So the WinBUGS code

```
p.crossval<- step(r.new-r)
```

creates a node which is a string of 0's (on iterations where $r_T^{new} < r_T$) and 1's (on iterations where $r_T^{new} \geq r_T$). The posterior mean of the node p.crossval gives the posterior probability that the model predictions exceed the observed value. Because the number of responders is discrete (i.e. can only take whole number values), we could get the situation where the model predictions and observed data are equal ($r_T^{new} = r_T$). We can make a continuity correction, where we only record 0.5 rather than 0 or 1 on iterations where $r_T^{new} = r_T$. The WinBUGS code is:

p.crossval<- step(r.new-r) - 0.5*equals(r.new,r)   (6.12)

which uses another WinBUGS function equals(a,b), which records a 1 if its arguments are equal ($a = b$) and a zero otherwise.

Example 6.1 revisited   Magnesium vs placebo for MI.

We are interested in whether the ISIS-4 trial results are consistent with the results from the other 15 trials, so we perform cross-validation on ISIS-4 (conveniently numbered trial 16). ISIS-4 can be omitted from the random effects meta-analysis model in WinBUGS by simply changing the loop over data from 1:32 to 1:30 and the loop over study from 1:16 to 1:15. We do not need to delete the data from the data array. We will also need to adjust the initial values, as we only need 15 deltas and mus rather than 16. The following code is used to form the cross-validation p-value. Note that the observed data from the omitted trial ISIS-4 is r[31] and n[31] from the control arm and r[32] and n[32] from the magnesium arm.

```
delta.new~dnorm(d,prec)                    #Draw new treatment effect
a<- r[31]                                  #No. deaths on control
b<- n[31]-r[31]                            #No. survivors on control
p[31]~dbeta(a,b)                           #Draw new control probability
logit(p[32])<-logit(p[31])+delta.new       #Form new treatment probability
r.new~dbin(p[32],n[32])                    #Draw new no. deaths on treatment
p.isis<- step(r.new-r[32])                 #Record whether predicted no.
      - 0.5*equals(r.new,r[32])            #deaths exceeds observed
```

Figure 6.6 shows that the observed number of deaths on the treatment arm of ISIS-4 is greater than the predicted number of deaths for most iterations of the MCMC simulation, based on a random effects meta-analysis of the remaining 15 studies. This is because the observed treatment effect was much lower on ISIS-4 than for the earlier, smaller trials. The cross-validation p-value is p.isis=0.05042

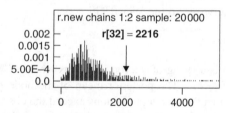

Figure 6.6   Posterior density for the predicted number of deaths on the treatment arm in ISIS-4, r.new, compared with the observed number of deaths r[32]=2216.

which shows that r.new only exceeds r[32] about 5% of the time. There is therefore only weak evidence that the results of ISIS-4 are inconsistent with results from the other 15 studies for a Random Effects model. This result is due to the wide credible interval for the predictive distribution (as a result of the high level of heterogeneity), which still just includes the ISIS-4 result even when based on only the remaining 15 studies. Note that finding evidence of inconsistency does not identify which data point is 'wrong'. For example here, it is perfectly feasible that the ISIS-4 result is showing the real treatment effect, whereas the other 15 studies are in some way biased.

6.5.2 Mixed predictive checks

Cross-validation quickly becomes computationally expensive if we want to find cross-validation p-values for each data point in our meta-analysis. For instance in the magnesium example we would have to run 16 separate models for each of the 16 trials. It is possible to automate the process – for example using the WinBUGS scripting facility or calling WinBUGS from external software such as R. However, we would have to set the number of iterations to be sufficiently high that we are happy that convergence has occurred without manually checking it for each run of the model. An alternative is to find a way to calculate approximate cross-validation p-values in a single run of the MCMC simulation, so that we only need to run the model once. Marshall and Spiegelhalter [13] proposed mixed predictive p-values when working with hierarchical models as approximations to the cross-validation p-values.

The idea is to fit a random effects meta-analysis model to all of the data points. The resulting model is used to make predictions for each of the individual observed data points, which are then compared with the observed data value to form a p-value. Again, the key step is in forming the model predictions. A naïve approach would be to use the study specific treatment and baseline parameters estimated from the model to predict the observed data:

$$r_i^{post} \sim \text{Binomial}(p_i, n_i) \tag{6.13}$$

where the probability of response for data point i is given by the logistic regression (6.1). The posterior probability that r_i^{post} exceeds r_i, $\Pr(r_i^{post} > r_i)$, is known as the posterior predictive p-value [10], however it gives a very conservative estimate of the inconsistency between data point i and the remaining evidence. This is because data point i has been used to inform the model estimate for probability of response p_i. In fact, data point i will have had a particularly strong influence over its own predicted probability of response. If any one study appears to be an outlier, the Random Effects model will typically still give fitted values close to the observations, by providing a higher estimate of between study heterogeneity, τ (as we observed in the magnesium example, Table 6.2).

A less conservative approach is to predict the true treatment effect in each study using the predictive distribution for a 'new' study (Equation (6.8)), as we used in cross-validation. This removes some of the influence of the individual data point on its predicted value – although the observed data will still have some influence on the mean and variance of the random effects distribution. We use the estimated baseline for each study from the model, so that the predicted probability of response is:

$$\text{logit}(p_i^{new}) = \mu_{s_i} + \delta_{new} I_{t_i=2} \quad \text{where } I_{t_i=2} = \begin{cases} 1 & t_i = 2 \\ 0 & t_i = 1 \end{cases} \quad (6.14)$$

Equation (6.14) is identical to the logistic regression (6.1) except that the study specific treatment effect is replaced by the treatment effect predicted in a new distribution from the same random effects population.

The predicted number of responders, r_i^{mxd}, is drawn from a Binomial distribution with the predicted probability of response, p_i^{new}, and known denominator, n_i:

$$r_i^{mxd} \sim \text{Binomial}(p_i^{new}, n_i) \quad (6.15)$$

The posterior probability that r_i^{mxd} exceeds r_i, $\Pr(r_i^{mxd} > r_i)$, is known as the mixed predictive p-value [13]. Mixed predictive p-values can be calculated for each study from a single analysis of the full data set. These will still be conservative compared with the 'gold-standard' method of cross-validation, however can be used as a first step to get an indication of the consistency of the evidence, and guide individual data points on which to run cross-validation. Because we obtain p-values for each study, we are in danger of incorrectly interpreting the significance of these multiple hypothesis tests. If we calculate several p-values on the same data, we would expect these to follow a Uniform distribution on the interval $(0,1)$. Plotting the ordered p-values for each study against the relevant Uniform order statistics provides a tool to gauge whether any of the p-values are unusually small or large.

Example 6.1 revisited   Magnesium vs placebo for MI.

Figure 6.7 shows the DAG for the Random Effects model with mixed prediction for the magnesium example. The WinBUGS code to calculate the mixed predictive p-values is:

```
logit(p.new)<- mu[s[i]]+delta.new*equals(t[i],2)    #Predicted probability of death
r.mxd[i]~dbin(p.new[i],n[i])                         #Predicted no. deaths
p.mxd[i]<- step(r.mxd[i]-r[i])                        #Mixed predictive p-value
          - 0.5*equals(r.mxd[i],r[i])
```

ISIS-4 has a mixed predictive p-value of 0.09, which as we expect is bigger (i.e. more conservative) than the cross-validation p-value of 0.05. Figure 6.8 shows the mixed predictive p-values (for the treatment arms) plotted against Uniform order statistics. The mixed predictive p-values fall close to the line of equality,

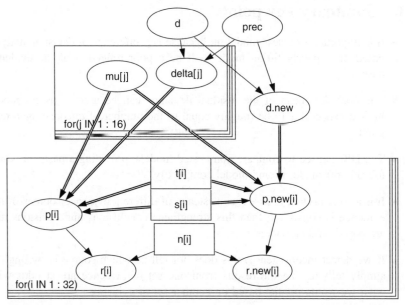

Figure 6.7   Directed Acyclic Graph for the Random Effects model for the magnesium example with mixed prediction.

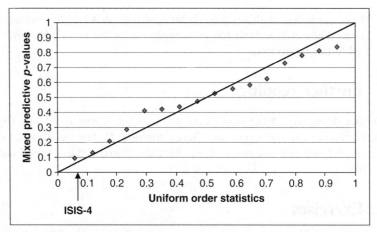

Figure 6.8   Ordered mixed predictive p-values plotted against Uniform order statistics for the magnesium example.

suggesting no evidence of inconsistency. The use of mixed predictive *p*-values leads to lower power to detect inconsistency than cross-validation, and in this example the conclusions using the two different methods (just) lead to different conclusions.

6.6   Summary key points

- It is important to assess model fit, because any inference or decision analysis based on a poorly fitting model will be a poor reflection of the evidence base.

- The posterior mean of the residual deviance can be used to assess model fit. We expect this to be roughly equal to the number of unconstrained data points.

- The DIC is used to compare non-nested models, providing a basis on which to trade-off model fit and model complexity.

- It is also important to assess consistency of different evidence sources. If the evidence is consistent, then this strengthens conclusions and decisions that are based on this evidence.

- If we detect inconsistency, this does not tell us which source is 'wrong'. It simply tells us that the results from one set of evidence are at odds with what we would predict based on another set of evidence.

- Cross-validation is the gold-standard method to assess consistency of evidence sources. However it can be computationally expensive if there are many data points that we want to investigate.

- Mixed predictive p-values provide an approximation to cross-validation p-values that can be calculation in a single run of the model. However they tend to be conservative.

6.7   Further reading

For further discussion of the magnesium example see Sterne *et al*. [4], Higgins and Spiegelhalter [5] and Egger and Davey Smith [14]. For excellent introductions to model selection and model fit see McCullagh and Nelder [1] and Gelman *et al*. [10].

6.8   Exercises

Early Onset Group B Streptococcus (EOGBS) is an infection in newborn babies, which can have serious sequelae including mental retardation and mortality. The infection is passed vertically from mother to child, and so an important part of the disease pathway is to understand the proportion of pregnant women colonised with Group B Streptococcus (GBS) when admitted for labour. Table 6.5 shows the results from 11 different studies that recorded this.

Table 6.5 Number of pregnant women colonised with GBS when admitted for labour out of a total sample (data taken from Colbourn *et al.* [15]).

Study	Year	GBS colonised	Total
Baker	1973	52	205
Dawodu	1983	9	190
Persson	1986	183	366
Joshi	1987	71	3078
Martius	1988	46	212
McDonald	1991	86	994
Citernesi	1996	206	4672
Kubota	1998	85	615
Feikin	2001	34	384
Hammoud	2002	195	1120
Wilk	2003	23	656

6.1 In this example note that the studies have only a single 'arm'. We can think of this as there being only a baseline for each study and no treatment effects, δ. We either put a single fixed effect, $\mu_j = m$, or a random effects distribution on the baselines, $\mu_j \sim N(m, \tau^2)$. The code to do this is for the Random Effects model is:

```
model{
for (i in 1:11) { r[i] ~ dbin(p[i],n[i])
          logit(p[i]) <- mu[s[i]] }
for (j in 1:11) {mu[j] ~dnorm(m,prec) }
m ~ dnorm(0,.001)
tau ~ dunif(0,10)
prec <- 1/(tau*tau)
odds <- exp(m)
logit(prob.GBS) <- m
   }
```

and for a Fixed Effect model:

```
model{
for (i in 1:11) { r[i] ~ dbin(p[i],n[i])
          logit(p[i]) <- mu[s[i]]}
for (j in 1:11) {mu[j] <- m }
m ~ dnorm(0,.001)
odds <- exp(m)
logit(prob.GBS) <- m
   }
```

(a) Fit the Fixed Effect and Random Effects models to estimate the proportion of women colonised with GBS when admitted for labour. Explore the fit of Fixed Effect and Random Effects models using residual deviance, effective number of parameters and the DIC.

(b) Compare the estimated probability of colonisation for both these models.

(c) Assess whether there is any evidence of inconsistency between the studies. Initially use mixed predictive p-values, and then find cross-validation p-value for the most 'extreme' study identified by the mixed predictive p-values.

6.2 The studies in Table 6.5 were actually broken down by whether the woman was at term or pre-term when admitted for labour (Table 6.6).

(a) Re-fit Fixed and Random Effects models on the effect of this covariate on the log-odds of colonisation with GBS (assume the pre-term women are the 'baseline' and the women at term are the 'intervention/ treatment' arm).

(b) Compare the model fit using residual deviance, effective number of parameters and the DIC. Also compare the estimated odds of colonisation for these models.

(c) For the Random Effects model, calculate mixed predictive p-values to assess consistency of individual trials.

Table 6.6 Number of pregnant women colonised with GBS when admitted for labour out of a total sample, broken down by whether the woman was pre-term or at term (data taken from Colbourn *et al.* [15]).

| Study | Year | Pre-term | | Term | |
		GBS colonised	Total	GBS colonised	Total
Baker	1973	2	7	50	198
Dawodu	1983	6	28	3	162
Persson	1986	11	20	172	346
Joshi	1987	17	306	54	2772
Martius	1988	21	61	25	151
McDonald	1991	34	428	52	566
Citernesi	1996	18	311	188	4361
Kubota	1998	7	37	78	578
Feikin	2001	12	84	22	300
Hammoud	2002	28	160	167	960
Wilk	2003	9	143	14	513

References

1. McCullagh P., Nelder J.A. *Generalised Linear Models*. London: Chapman and Hall, 1989.

2. Yusuf S., Koon T., Woods K. An effective, safe, simple, and inexpensive intervention. *Circulation* 1993;**87**:2043–2046.

3. ISIS 4 Collaborative Group. ISIS-4: a randomised factorial trial assessing early oral captopril, oral mononitrate, and intravenous magnesium sulphate in 58 050 patients with suspected acute myocardial infarction. *Lancet* 1995;**345**:669–685.

4. Sterne J.A.C., Bradburn M.J., Egger M. Meta-analysis in Stata. In: Egger M., Davey Smith G., Altman D.G., eds. *Systematic Reviews in Health Care: Meta-Analysis in Context*. London: BMJ Books, 2001;347–369.

5. Higgins J.P.T., Spiegelhalter D.J. Being sceptical about meta-analyses: a Bayesian perspective on magnesium trials in myocardial infarction. *International Journal of Epidemiology* 2002;**31**:96–104.

6. Dempster A.P. The direct use of likelihood for significance testing. *Statistics and Computing* 1997;**7**:247–252.

7. Akaike H. A new look at the statistical model identification. *IEEE Transations on Automatic Control* 1974;**19**:716–723.

8. Spiegelhalter D.J., Best N.G., Carlin B.P., van der Linde A. Bayesian measures of model complexity and fit. *Journal of the Royal Statistical Society, Series B* 2002;**64**:583–616.

9. Spiegelhalter D.J., Thomas A., Best N., Lunn D. *WinBUGS User Manual: Version 1.4*. Cambridge: MRC Biostatistics Unit, 2001.

10. Gelman A., Carlin J.G., Stern H.S., Rubin D.B. *Bayesian Data Analysis*. London: Chapman and Hall, 1995.

11. Stern H.S., Cressie N. Posterior predictive model checks for disease mapping models. *Statistics in Medicine* 2000;**19**:2377–2397.

12. Du Mouchel W. Predictive cross-validation of Bayesian meta-analyses. In: Bernardo J.M., Berger J.O., Dawid A.P., Smith A.F.M., eds. *Bayesian Statistics 5*. Oxford: Oxford University Press, 1996;107–127.

13. Marshall E.C., Spiegelhalter D.J. Approximate cross-validatory predictive checks in disease mapping models. *Statistics in Medicine* 2003;**22**:1649–1660.

14. Egger M., Davey Smith G. Misleading meta-analysis. *British Medical Journal* 1995;**310**:752–754.

15. Colbourn T., Asseburg C., Bojke L., et al. Prenatal screening and treatment strategies to prevent Group B Streptococcal and other bacterial infections in early infancy: coste ffectiveness and expected value of information analysis. *Health Technology Assessment* 2007;**11**(29).

7

Evidence synthesis in a decision modelling framework

7.1 Introduction

Decision models used to evaluate healthcare interventions were introduced in Chapter 3. Data to parameterise such models are sometimes based on primary data collection, but more often rely on published or other secondary sources for cost and effectiveness information [1]. Combining evidence from diverse sources is an essential part of decision modelling – particularly economic evaluations. For example, as defined in Chapter 3, parameters required for such economic models include clinical effectiveness (e.g. from Randomised Controlled Trials, RCTs), resource utilisation with externally derived costs (e.g. from prospective data collection or administrative database), patient outcomes with utility scales (e.g. from prospective data collection), and disease progression rates (e.g. from administrative database).

For the evaluation of healthcare to be truly evidence-based the use of rigorous, transparent and reproducible systematic methods for evidence identification and synthesis are desirable. However, to date very little has been written on the methods of systematic reviews (including meta-analysis) to be used for the synthesis of evidence for an economic decision [1–3]. For example, it is currently unclear what sources of evidence should be included in systematic reviews informing decision model parameters. The potential hierarchy of data sources for economic decision model parameters introduced in Section 3.6, identified meta-analysis of RCTs as the highest ranked evidence for effectiveness parameters but why limit the

Evidence Synthesis for Decision Making in Healthcare, First Edition. Nicky J. Welton, Alexander J. Sutton, Nicola J. Cooper, Keith R. Abrams and A.E. Ades.

data to RCTs. Should *all available evidence* be considered and where appropriate combined? This is also pertinent to other model parameters including probabilities, resource use and utilities where selecting only the best, most relevant, information source for a parameter ignores potentially valuable information from other sources. Methods for combining evidence from different data sources will be addressed in Chapter 11.

In this chapter we extend the decision modelling framework introduced in Chapter 3 to incorporate multiple data for each model parameter. A comprehensive approach to decision modelling is introduced that combines the whole process into a single coherent framework; that is, combines the meta-analyses, estimation of the model parameters, evaluation of the model and sensitivity analysis. The method is demonstrated through the use of a worked example, which evaluates the cost effectiveness of using prophylactic antibiotics in Caesarean section to reduce the incidence of wound infections. This example utilises meta-analysis and model fit methods described in previous chapters. More complex examples, where this method is applied to Markov models, are presented in Chapter 10.

7.2 Evaluation of decision models: One-stage vs two-stage approach

There are two approaches to analysing a decision model with uncertainty – the *two-stage* approach and the *integrated* approach. The two-stage approach first performs the data analysis (e.g. meta-analysis) using the identified evidence on each of the model parameters to obtain distributions. The different model inputs are usually assumed independent and parametric distributions are adopted. For example, probabilities are usually expressed as beta distributions to constrain values between 0 and 1 whilst for costs lognormal or gamma distributions are used to constrain values to be positive. The second stage is to use Monte Carlo simulation [4] to propagate uncertainty through the decision model by drawing values from each of the input parameter distributions thousands of times to obtain the relevant outcomes with uncertainty (e.g. expected Incremental Net Benefit, INB). This two-stage approach is usually implemented using a combination of standard statistical software and spreadsheet programs such as Microsoft Excel® including add-ins Crystal Ball (Oracle, http://www.oracle.com/us/products/applications/crystalball/) or @Risk (Palisade Europe, http://www.palisade.com/risk/).

The integrated approach unifies the two stages described above; that is, the distribution(s) obtained from the data analysis (analyses) is (are) fed directly into the decision model without the need for an intermediate summary stage. This approach adopts a fully Bayesian analysis by updating initial prior opinions on parameters in light of the available evidence using Bayes' theorem to produce posterior distributions. This unified approach ensures that the full joint uncertainty concerning the model parameters is taken into account. Monte Carlo Markov Chain (MCMC) simulation is required to propagate evidence uncertainty 'back' from the data, onto parameters, then 'forward' through the decision model. This modelling

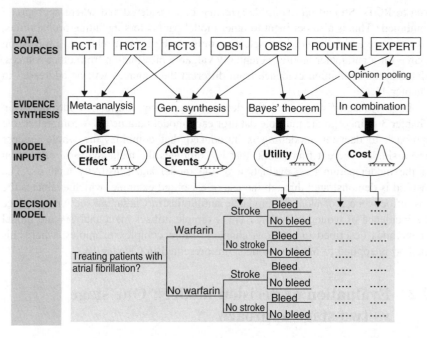

Figure 7.1   Schematic diagram of comprehensive decision modelling.

framework has been termed 'comprehensive decision modelling' [5–10] and a schematic representation is shown in Figure 7.1.

First the structural form of the decision model is established and required model inputs identified. Information about the model inputs is obtained (e.g. from a systematic review of all the available evidence including RCTs, observational studies, routine data sources, and/or expert opinion) and synthesised using the most appropriate methods (e.g. meta-analysis, generalised evidence synthesis, Bayes' theorem, opinion pooling, etc.). Once data analysis is complete the pooled estimates for each of the model parameters, expressed with uncertainty, are either input into the decision analytical model directly, or transformed into the necessary format and then input into the model. Model inputs are derived through transformations of other parameters, themselves estimated with uncertainty and the resulting uncertainty is automatically incorporated into the model. MCMC simulation is used to evaluate the decision model and all preliminary analyses informing the model parameters.

The advantages of this approach compared with a two-stage approach to decision modelling include:

(i) the actual posterior distributions estimated from the meta-analyses, transformed into appropriate format, are input into the model directly thus avoiding the need to make distributional assumptions;

(ii) the incorporation of greater parameter uncertainty (i.e. by allowing for the fact that both the overall population effect and between-study precision in the meta-analyses have both been estimated by the data);

(iii) making full allowance for any potential inter-relationships between model input parameters (e.g. estimates of multiple treatment effects as considered in Chapter 8);

(iv) a more transparent framework, as all analysis is contained within one computer program, thus facilitating sensitivity analysis and updating (i.e. changes in intermediate analyses (e.g. meta-analyses) automatically propagate throughout the model making assessment of the impact on the overall results immediate and transparent);

(v) the ability to make direct probability statements and thus obtain direct answers to the question of interest, e.g. a Bayesian meta-analysis can provide a posterior probability that the effect is above (or below) a particular value, or that one treatment is more cost-effective than another.

This framework also permits greater flexibility in model specification (as will be demonstrated in subsequent chapters).

Example 7.1   Prophylactic antibiotics (cephalosporins) to prevent wound infection following Caesarean section: Stochastic economic evaluation revisited.

Here we extend the analysis presented in Example 3.3 to incorporate all the available evidence on effectiveness of the prophylactic antibiotic cephalosporin (compared with no prophylactic antibiotic treatment) on wound infections in women undergoing Caesarean delivery rather than limiting the analysis to data from one RCT.

Effectiveness data

The effectiveness data for this analysis was extracted from a Cochrane systematic review [11] (Table 7.1) and synthesised using the Bayesian meta-analysis model defined in Equation (4.7). The outcome of interest is the pooled Odds Ratio (OR). Note that meta-analysis of binary outcomes such as the occurrence of wound infections can be analysed on other scales, such as the relative risk or risk difference [12], but thought needs to be given to how the outcome will be used as an input in the decision model.

As can be observed from the data in Table 7.1, the occurrence of wound infection is relatively rare and there are numerous trials in which zero infections were observed in one or both arms of the trials. Such sparse data poses a problem since the OR for these trials is undefined. As discussed in Section 4.3.3, using the Bayesian meta-analysis model specified in Equation (4.7) forgoes the need for continuity corrections by modelling directly the event rates in each arm using

Table 7.1 Prophylactic antibiotics (cephalosporins) in Caesarean section [11].

Study	Events/Total		Study	Events/Total	
	Treatment	Placebo		Treatment	Placebo
Bibi et al. 1994	4/133	28/136	Levin et al. 1983	0/85	3/43
Conover et al. 1984	2/68	1/56	Mallaret et al. 1990	6/136	16/130
Cormier et al. 1989	5/55	8/55	Moro et al. 1974	0/74	2/74
Dashow et al. 1986	3/100	0/33	Phelan et al. 1979	2/61	2/61
Dashow et al. 1986	4/183	3/44	Polk et al. 1982	3/146	9/132
Dillon et al. 1981	0/46	4/55	Roex et al. 1986	1/64	7/65
Elliot et al. 1986	0/119	1/39	Rothbard et al. 1975	0/16	1/16
Fugere et al. 1983	2/60	6/30	Rothbard et al. 1975	2/31	6/37
Gall 1979	1/46	1/49	Saltzman et al. 1985	1/50	2/49
Gibbs et al. 1981	0/50	2/50	Schedvins et al. 1986	2/26	0/27
Hager et al. 1983	1/43	1/47	Stage et al. 1983	3/133	12/66
Hagglund et al. 1989	0/80	3/80	Stiver et al. 1983	6/244	17/117
Harger et al. 1981	2/196	14/190	Tully et al. 1983	1/52	2/61
Hawrylyshyn et al. 1983	2/124	2/58	Tzingounis et al. 1982	2/46	4/50
Ismail et al. 1990	2/74	8/78	Wong et al. 1978	2/48	3/45
Jakobi et al. 1994	4/167	5/140	Work et al. 1977	3/40	1/40
Kreutner et al. 1978	0/48	2/49	Young et al. 1983	1/50	4/50
Kristensen et al. 1990	0/102	1/99			

binomial distributions [13]. It also avoids the assumption of normality of the effect measure in each trial (necessary in the classical analysis), which may be inappropriate when some of the trials included in the meta-analysis are small, or observed risks are close to 0 or 1.

Model parameters

The model parameter estimates used in the evaluation are the same as for Example 3.3 (see Table 3.4).

The probability of a wound infection without prophylactic antibiotics, $p1$, is input into the model with uncertainty by expressing as a beta distribution as described in Example 3.2 (i.e. Beta(41,445)).

The expected probability of contracting influenza if prophylactic antibiotics are introduced ($p2$) can be obtained as follows:

$$\text{logit}(p2) = \text{logit}(p1) + d \tag{7.1}$$

where d is the underlying treatment effect obtained from the meta-analysis. This is particularly appealing since the uncertainty in $p2$ is automatically incorporated into the model and does not have to be calculated.

The costs and Quality Adjusted Life Years (QALYs) in the two groups (i.e. with and without prophylactic antibiotics) are calculated by 'rolling back' the tree as described in Example 3.1. From these quantities the INB can be calculated and cost-effectiveness acceptability curves (CEACs) plotted.

Model evaluation

To evaluate the decision model this comprehensive framework uses Gibbs sampling MCMC simulation methods. All the required WinBUGS code for the whole model is given in the Appendix/web site. Following preliminary test runs, it was decided to use an initial run of 10 000 iterations as a 'burn in' [14], in order to achieve convergence (these values were discarded) with inferences based on a further 20 000 sample iterations. As a further step to ensure model convergence has been achieved, two WinBUGS runs with dispersed starting values (i.e. defining two sets of very different initial values and running two chains simultaneously) are carried out (see Chapter 2).

Meta-analysis results

Thirty-five trials of cephalosporin compared with standard care were identified [11]. Using a random effects meta-analysis model, the pooled OR was estimated to be 0.28 (95% credible interval (CrI) 0.19 to 0.41); that is, the odds of a wound infection in the prophylactic antibiotic treatment group is 28% of that in the standard care group (Figure 7.2).

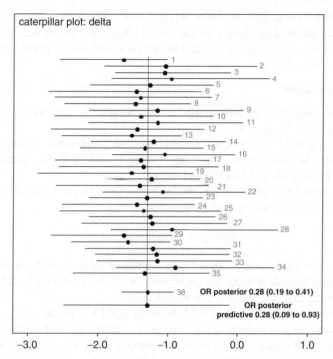

Figure 7.2   Caterpillar plot of the shrunken estimates obtained from the meta-analysis.

The posterior mean of the residual deviance, $\overline{D}_{res} = 78.4$ with 95% CrI (57.8 to 100.6). There are 70 unconstrained data points in this example (35 studies × 2 arms), so we would expect the posterior mean of the residual deviance to be close to 70 if the model predictions fit the data well.

Decision model results

The parameter values, together with their 95% CrI, estimated from the model described above are presented in Table 7.2 together with the results from deterministic (i.e. based on the mean values of the input parameters) and two-stage models. As noted in Section 1.2.2, besides providing us with an analysis of *uncertainty*, probabilistic analysis has the further advantage that it gives a correct computation of expected INB under uncertainty.

The results from the cost-effectiveness analysis are presented graphically in Figure 7.3 based on 20 000 iterations.

Extensions

In the analysis presented above, the posterior distribution for the OR obtained from the meta-analysis has been used to evaluate the decision model. However, the

Table 7.2 Probabilistic decision analysis, based on 20 000 Monte Carlo simulations. We distinguish between the true mean of the input distribution and the estimate based on the simulation.

Parameter	Symbol	Deterministic	Two-stage probabilistic analysis (meta-analysis in Stata, decision model in WinBUGS)[a]	One-stage probabilistic analysis: Estimated mean (95% CrI) from simulation – posterior
Pr(wound infection) standard care	$p1$	0.086	0.084 (0.061 to 0.110)	0.033 (0.061 to 0.110)
ln(Odds Ratio)	d	−1.279	−1.209 (−1.507 to −0.909)	−1.279 (−1.653 to −0.885)
Pr(wound infection) on antibiotics	$p2 = \dfrac{\exp(\text{logit}(p1)+d)}{1+\exp(\text{logit}(p1)+d)}$	0.026	0.027 (0.0172 to 0.040)	0.025 (0.015 to 0.040)
Tau-sq	τ^2	—	—	0.189 (0.000 to 1.086)
Incremental QALYs	Δ_U	3.9102×10^{-4}	3.128×10^{-4} (2.127×10^{-4} to 4.374×10^{-4})	3.198×10^{-4} (2.142×10^{-4} to 4.539×10^{-4})
Incremental cost	Δ_C	−£5.192	−£2.542 (−£23.61 to £15.250)	−£3.566 (−£25.440 to £15.210)
INB (λ = £20 000)	$INB = \lambda\Delta_U - \Delta_C$	13.012	8.773 (−10.690 to 32.000)	9.956 (−10.600 to 34.180)
INB (λ = £30 000)	$INB = \lambda\Delta_U - \Delta_C$	16.922	11.880 (−8.401 to 36.260)	13.160 (−8.304 to 38.570)

[a]Where zero events recorded in a trial for the two-stage analysis need to add a continuity correction.

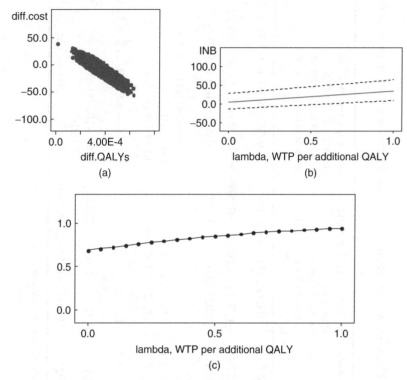

Figure 7.3 WinBUGS graphical output: (a) joint distribution of incremental QALYs, Δ_E and incremental costs, Δ_C; (b) expected incremental net benefit and 95% CrI for a range of λ; (c) cost-effectiveness acceptability curve for a range of λ. WTP, Willing To Pay.

posterior predictive distribution (Section 4.3.1) may be more appropriate given that the main objective is to evaluate the cost-effectiveness of introducing prophylactic antibiotics for Caesarean section patients at a local maternity hospital. The posterior predictive distribution for the OR of having a wound infection has been plotted in Figure 7.2 where it can be observed that although the pooled estimate is the same there is a considerable increase in the level of uncertainty which feeds through to the cost-effectiveness results (i.e. INB ($\lambda = \pounds 20\,000$) = 8.717 ($-34.650$ to 38.970) compared with 9.956 (-10.600 to 34.180) obtained from the original analysis using the posterior mean distribution).

If treatment effect varies with individuals' underlying risk of wound infection then this can also be incorporated into the meta-analysis part of the analysis as described in Chapter 5.

7.3   Sensitivity analyses (of model inputs and model specifications)

An essential tool for studying and validating the behaviour of any model is a sensitivity analysis [15, 16]. Such an analysis assesses the robustness of the results to specific methods used and assumptions made. The more the result obtained is materially unchanged by sensible sensitivity analyses, the more confident we can be in the final results of the model. In addition, assessment of the meta-analysis components of the decision model should also be addressed; for example, the impact of variability in the study populations, interventions administered, outcome measure definitions, and study quality could all have an influence on the model parameter estimates [17]. The comprehensive decision modelling approach facilitates such sensitivity analyses, as changes in intermediate analyses (e.g. meta-analyses) automatically propagate throughout the model making assessment of the impact on the overall results immediate and transparent.

When using Bayesian methods [9] there are additional issues which require exploration; for example, assessment of prior distributions placed on variance components and starting values for the simulation parameters to check convergence of the MCMC sampler (as discussed in Chapter 2).

7.4   Summary key points

The creation of structures in the UK (i.e. National Institute of Health and Clinical Excellence, NICE) and elsewhere to facilitate evidence-based health policy decision making has highlighted the role that systematic reviews and decision models have to play. However, in highlighting their role, numerous methodological challenges have been identified, not least of which is their integration. Whilst we feel the adoption of a comprehensive approach provides a flexible and coherent framework within which to explore and address many of these challenges, it is by no means a panacea and requires careful and critical application, whilst development of these methods will be facilitated by multidisciplinary collaboration between economists, operational researchers and statisticians.

7.5   Further reading

In the literature articles can be found that have applied the comprehensive decision modelling approach [8, 10, 18–24].

7.6   Exercises

These Exercises concern the following decision model (see also Section 3.10) to compare the prophylactic use of neuraminidase inhibitors (NIs) with standard care for influenza:

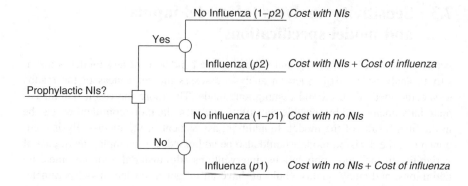

7.1 In the example presented in the Exercises at the end of Chapter 3, it was assumed that all parameters in the decision model were known. This is an unrealistic assumption. An evidence-based approach would be to use the trial evidence to inform the parameters in the model, expressing the parameters with uncertainty in the form of a distribution.

   (a) Combine files *Model 1 decision model.odc* and *meta-analysis.odc* together to obtain Model 2. The treatment effect is calculated from the meta-analysis in terms of the posterior mean distribution, which can then be used to obtain $p2$ (Hint: use Equation (6.1)) and then fed directly into the decision model. Obtain estimates of the mean and associated uncertainty for p2, or and diff.cost.

   (b) Note that in the above models it is assumed that $p1$ is fixed. However, if the data were available (i.e. expressed as 1 out of 20 rather than 0.05) then this parameter could be entered as stochastic – that is, r1~dbin(p1,n1). A vague prior distribution for p1 needs to be specified, i.e. p1~dbeta(1,1).

7.2 Assume the utility for an individual with influenza is 0.5 and without influenza 0.98.

   (a) Extend Model 2 to include equations for calculating the expected utilities for the prophylactic NIs group (utiltrt) and no prophylaxis group (utilctl), and the difference in utilities between the two groups (diff.util).

   (b) Calculate the probability that prophylactic NIs are cost-effective compared with no prophylaxis.

   (c) Paste the values for ProbCE into the yellow shaded cells in the file *Model 3 – CEAC.xls*. Notice the cost-effectiveness acceptability curve appears on the graph.

7.3 Repeat the above analyses using the posterior predictive distribution obtained from the meta-analysis. Compare the results from the two different analyses. In which situations may it be appropriate to use the different estimates of effectiveness to evaluate the decision model?

References

1. Mugford M. Using systematic reviews for economic evaluation. In: Egger M., Davey Smith G., Altman D., eds. *Systematic Reviews in Health Care: Meta-Analysis in Context.* London: BMJ Publishing, 2001;419–428.

2. Hunink M.G.M., Glasziou P., Siegel J., *et al.* Finding and summarizing the evidence. In: *Decision Making in Health and Medicine: Integrating Evidence and Values.* Cambridge: Cambridge University Press, 2001;214–244.

3. Cooper N.J., Sutton A.J., Ades A., Paisley S., Jones D.R., on behalf of the working group on the 'Use of evidence in economic decision models'. Use of evidence in economic decision models: Practical issues and methodological challenges. *Health Economics* 2007;**16**:1277–1286..

4. Sonnenberg F.A., Beck J.R. *Markov* models in medical decision making: a practical guide. *Medical Decision Making* 1993;**13**:322–338.

5. Cooper N.J., Abrams K.R., Sutton A.J., *et al.* Use of Bayesian methods for Markov modelling in cost-effectiveness analysis: an application to taxane use in advanced breast cancer. *Journal of Royal Statistical Society, Series A* 2003;**166**:389–405.

6. Cooper N.J., Sutton A.J., Abrams K.R. Decision analytical economic modelling within a Bayesian framework: Application to prophylactic antibiotics use for caesarean section. *Statistical Methods in Medical Research* 2002;**11**:491–512.

7. Cooper N.J., Sutton A.J., Abrams K.R., *et al.* Comprehensive decision analytical modelling in economic evaluation: a Bayesian approach. *Health Economics* 2004;**13**:203–226.

8. Spiegelhalter D.J., Best N.G. Bayesian approaches to multiple sources of evidence and uncertainty in complex cost-effectiveness modelling. *Statistics in Medicine* 2003;**22**: 3687–3709.

9. Spiegelhalter D.J., Abrams K.R., Myles J.P. *Bayesian Approaches to Clinical Trials and Health-Care Evaluation (Statistics in Practice).* Chichester: John Wiley & Sons, Ltd, 2004.

10. Parmigiani G. Modeling in medical decision making: a Bayesian approach. In: Barnett V., ed. *Statistics in Practice*, Ist edn. Chichester: John Wiley & Sons, Ltd, 2002.

11. Smaill F., Hofmeyr G. Antibiotic prophylaxis for cesarean section. *Cochrane Review* 2001;(3).

12. Deeks J.J., Altman D.G. Effect measures for meta-analysis of trials with binary outcomes. In: Egger M., Davey Smith G., Altman D., eds. *Systematic Reviews in Health Care: Meta-Analysis in Context.* London: BMJ Publishing Group, 2001;313–335.

13. Prevost T.C., Abrams K.R., Jones D.R. Hierarchical models in generalised synthesis of evidence: an example based on studies of breast cancer. *Statistics in Medicine* 2000; **19**:3359–3376.

14. Gilks W.R., Richardson S., Spiegelhalter D.J. *Markov Chain Monte Carlo in Practice: Interdisciplinary Statistics*. London: Chapman and Hall, 1996.

15. Briggs A.H. Handling uncertainty in cost-effectiveness models. *Pharmacoeconomics* 2000;**17**(5):479–500.

16. Brennan A., Akehurst R., Modelling in health economic evaluation: What is its place? What is its value? *Pharmacoeconomics* 2000;**17**:445–459.

17. Sutton A.J., Abrams K.R., Jones D.R., *et al.*, *Methods for Meta-Analysis in Medical Research*. Chichester: John Wiley & Sons, Ltd, 2000.

18. Brown J., Welton N.J., Bankhead C., *et al.* A Bayesian approach to analysing the cost-effectiveness of two primary care interventions aimed at improving attendance for breast screening. *Health Economics* 2006;**15**:435–445.

19. Cooper N.J., Sutton A.J., Abrams K.R., Turner D., Wailoo A. Comprehensive decision analytical modelling in economic evaluation: a Bayesian approach. *Health Economics* 2004; **13**:203–226.

20. Gillies C L, Lambert P.C., Abrams K.R., *et al.* A cost-effectiveness analysis for different strategies for the screening and prevention of type 2 diabetes mellitus. *British Medical Journal* 2008;**336**:1180–1185.

21. Minelli C., Abrams K.R., Sutton A.J., Cooper N.J. Appropriate use of hormone replacement therapy (HRT): A clinical decision analysis. *British Medical Journal* 2004; **328**:371–375.

22. Parmigiani G., Samsa G., Ancukiewicz M., *et al.* Assessing uncertainty in cost-effectiveness analyses. *Medical Decision Making* 1997;**17**:390–401.

23. Sutton A.J., Cooper N., Abrams K.R., Lambert P.C., Jones D.R. Synthesising both benefit and harm: A Bayesian approach to evaluating clinical net benefit. *Journal of Clinical Epidemiology* 2005;**58**:26–40.

24. Vergel Y.B., Palmer S., Asseburg C., *et al.* Is primary angioplasty cost effective in the UK? Results of a comprehensive decision analysis *Heart* 2007;**93**:1238–1243.

8

Multi-parameter
evidence synthesis

8.1 Introduction

So far we have focused on meta-analysis in a relatively simple form, which aims
to combine information from several randomised comparisons of the same two
treatments. We now explore more general approaches to evidence synthesis, suitable
for combining information not only from many studies, but also from different kinds
of studies, and even from studies measuring quite different parameters. What all
the studies have in common is that they must all provide information on one or
more parameters of a common underlying model. To give a simple example, we
might suppose that there is information on the incidence, a, of a certain disease,
and also information about the proportion, b, of incident cases who develop certain
complications. But suppose there was also a study that provided data on the number,
c, of incident patients with these complications that were observed over a period,
T. Based on the information from the first two studies we would expect $c = abT$.
In other words, assuming that T is known, we have three items of data informing
two underlying parameters, a and b. What is needed is a method to combine all
these data, and assess whether they are consistent.

   We have called this more general kind of synthesis Multi-Parameter Evidence
Synthesis (MPES), but the key ideas go back to the Confidence Profile Method
(CPM) of Eddy et al. [1]. The term 'Multi-Parameter Synthesis' was first used
by Hasselblad and McCrory [2]. This kind of synthesis has particular significance for decision modelling. The way decision models are usually 'populated'

Evidence Synthesis for Decision Making in Healthcare, First Edition. Nicky J. Welton,
Alexander J. Sutton, Nicola J. Cooper, Keith R. Abrams and A.E. Ades.
© 2012 John Wiley & Sons, Ltd. Published 2012 by John Wiley & Sons, Ltd.

with parameter values is that each parameter is *separately* given a value, or a distribution, based on the literature. Some parameters may be informed by a meta-analysis, but the parameters are independent, and considered one at a time. This is, however, a highly restrictive approach. In the above example it does not allow us to use the information on *abT* alongside the information on *a* and the information on *b*.

We start the chapter with an example from the CPM literature. As we shall see, this is not a particularly good example of MPES, because it can be computed using forward Monte Carlo (MC) simulation. However, it allows us to clearly contrast Bayesian prior and Bayesian posterior simulation, and to locate standard probabilistic decision modelling within that framework. Later we will move onto examples that better exemplify the main features of MPES, and which require a more powerful engine for Bayesian computation such as Markov Chain Monte Carlo (MCMC).

8.2 Prior and posterior simulation in a probabilistic model: Maple Syrup Urine Disease (MSUD)

MSUD is a very rare inborn error of metabolism that can be detected on new-born 'heel prick' screening. If untreated it carries a high risk of mental retardation (MR). It is *so* rare that trial evidence is never likely to be forthcoming, and evidence on the efficacy of treatment has to be based on historical controls. The analysis below was proposed by Eddy and colleagues [1] as an example of the CPM. From a computational point of view, CPM used different methods, some of which were approximate, others were Bayesian but relying on non-MCMC simulation. This particular problem however can readily be computed with a standard spreadsheet package.

There are five sources of data (Table 8.1), informing, respectively: the birth rate of MSUD (r), the probability of early detection with (ϕ_s) and without (ϕ_n) screening, and the probabilities of MR with (θ_{em}) and without (θ_{lm}) early detection. (We have adopted the notation used in the CPM literature.) The data are all in the form of Binomial likelihoods.

The problem can be set out as a decision tree (Figure 8.1). If screening is implemented, early detection is highly likely, and early intervention can prevent

Table 8.1 Data for the MSUD analysis.

Data	Notation	Outcomes	Obs.
Prob. MSUD	r	7	724 262
Prob. early detection with screening	ϕ_s	253	276
Prob. early detection without screening	ϕ_n	8	18
Prob. retardation with early detection	θ_{em}	2	10
Prob. retardation without early detection	θ_{lm}	10	10

the majority of MR cases. In the absence of screening, early detection is much less likely, but many affected infants can be diagnosed early if MSUD has occurred in other family members. For this reason about 40% of MR cases can be prevented even in the absence of a screening programme, but failure to detect and intervene early has disastrous consequences.

Each of these *basic* parameters requires prior distributions, and as they are probabilities, Beta distributions are a natural choice. We choose minimally informative (uniform) distributions, Beta(1,1). Next we form expressions for the *functional* parameters that can be used to assess the impact of screening on the numbers of MSUD-associated cases of MR. Functional parameters can, by definition, be written as functions of basic parameters.

$\theta_{sm} = \phi_s\theta_{em} + (1 - \phi_s)\theta_{lm}$ Pr (mental retardation in MSUD with screening)

$\theta_{nm} = \phi_n\theta_{em} + (1 - \phi_n)\theta_{lm}$ Pr (mental retardation in MSUD without screening)

$\theta_s = 100,000r\theta_{sm}$ Birth rate of MSUD-associated retardation

with screening

$\theta_n = 100,000r\theta_{nm}$ Birth rate of MSUD-associated retardation

without screening

$e_d = \theta_s - \theta_n$ Reduction in MSUD-associated retardation

due to screening

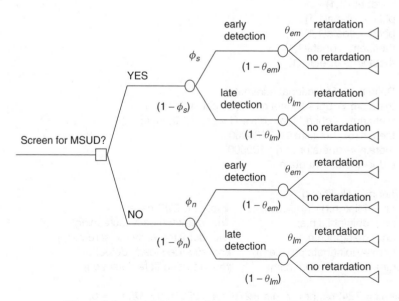

Figure 8.1   Decision tree for screening for MSUD.

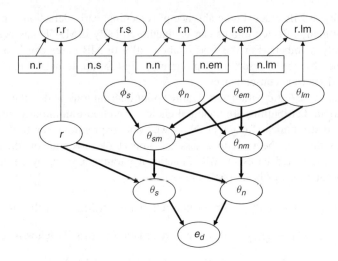

Figure 8.2   Directed Acycylic Graph of the MSUD model.

Figure 8.2 represents the model as a Directed Acycylic Graph. The five basic parameters are those with no parents. The remaining (functional parameters) can be expressed as functions of the basic parameters: these have basic parameters as their parents.

We can set out WinBUGS code and data for this model as follows:

```
model {
# Priors for basic parameters
    r ~ dbeta(1,1)
    phi.s ~ dbeta(1,1)
    phi.n ~ dbeta(1,1)
    theta.em ~ dbeta(1,1)
    theta.lm ~ dbeta(1,1)


# Definition of functional parameters
    theta.sm <- phi.s * theta.em + (1 - phi.s)*theta.lm
    theta.nm <- phi.n * theta.em + (1 - phi.n) * theta.lm
    theta.s <- (theta.sm * r) * 100000
    theta.n <- (theta.nm * r) * 100000
    e.d <- theta.s - theta.n


# Binomial likelihood
    r.r ~ dbin(r,n.r)               #no. of MSUD cases
    r.s ~ dbin(phi.s,n.s)           #no. detected early (screening)
    r.n ~ dbin(phi.n,n.n)           #no. detected early (no screening)
    r.em ~ dbin(theta.em,n.em)      #no. retarded (early detection)
    r.lm ~ dbin(theta.lm,n.lm)      #no. retarded (late detection)
}
list( n.r = 724262, r.r = 7, n.s = 276, r.s = 253, n.n = 18, r.n = 8,
    n.em=10, r.em = 2, n.lm = 10, r.lm = 10)
```

The posterior summary, based on 20 000 samples from each of two chains, after a burn-in of 30 000 samples, gave a mean e.d of −0.34 cases (i.e. a reduction) per 100 000 live births, with a 95% credible interval −0.74 to −0.099.

Note that in this particular case all the data directly informs five basic parameters, and these parameters are sufficient to define the target quantity e.d, the reduction in retardation that would follow screening for MSUD. The simplicity of the problem lies in the fact that there are no data directly informing the functional parameters. Further, because the Beta priors are conjugate with the Binomial likelihood, we can obtain the posterior distributions for the basic parameters in closed form. A Beta(a, b) prior together with binomial data with numerator y and denominator n gives us a Beta($a + y, b + n - y$) posterior. It is this that makes it possible to sample from the Bayesian posterior distributions using standard forward MC simulation. For example, the posterior probability of early detection without screening, given a uniform Beta(1,1) prior, and binomial data 8/18, has a Beta(9,11) distribution. We could therefore use any computer software capable of running simulation, such as Excel, to solve this particular problem.

In practice, the standard method of running a probabilistic decision model for this problem would be to ignore the uniform priors, and simply form Beta distributions from the data provided. For example, the probability of early detection in the absence of screening would be cast as a Beta(8,10) distribution, and forward MC would be used. Technically, one could argue that this is not a Bayesian solution at all as there is no likelihood and no posterior. However, this is a little pedantic and it may be more productive to regard this as forward simulation from an informative Bayesian prior, which has been based on the available data. Further data could be incorporated in principle, but in this case possibly no further data exist.

The MSUD example, therefore, illustrates the relationship between Bayesian posterior simulation and the kind of MC simulation that has dominated probabilistic modelling in the physical, social, and biological sciences for several decades. In this example, simulation from either prior or posterior distributions can be carried out by forward MC, because the posterior can be found in closed form. WinBUGs may be used for this purpose, but so may any spreadsheet or statistical package with random sampling from standard distributions. The same would be true of any model in which all the data points informed basic parameters, and all the likelihoods were conjugate with the priors for those parameters. The MCMC facility of WinBUGS is not, therefore, required. (Exercise 8.1 suggests another approach to the MSUD example, which does require MCMC as the priors are no longer conjugate with the likelihood.) In the next example, however, forward MC simulation would not be sufficient and we must appeal to more powerful methods for Bayesian updating, such as MCMC, which do not rely on conjugacy.

8.3   A model for prenatal HIV testing

This example is based on work originally carried out by Ades and Cliffe [3], and has already been cited extensively in reviews [4], and textbooks [5]. It grew out of a project funded by the UK's Department of Health which was aimed at determining whether prenatal testing for HIV should be offered to all pregnant women (universal testing), or offered only to women in groups at higher risk (targeted testing). The immediate stimulus for this work was the American National Institute of Allergy and Infectious Diseases AIDS Clinical Trials Group 076 trial in 1996 showing that a brief course of zidovudine in pregnancy could lower the risk of transmission of HIV from mother to baby before or during delivery. Drug treatment could therefore be added to other interventions aimed at preventing HIV infection in the newborn, Caesarean section and counselling against breast feeding.

The Bayesian approach presented here post-dated by several years the Department of Health's eventual recommendation that prenatal HIV testing should be offered to all pregnant women, even in areas of lowest prevalence. The analysis is simplified and somewhat stylised, but it illustrates an important characteristic of the data sources that must often be used in studies of screening, namely that data may not be available on the key parameters, but may instead be available on functions of the parameters. Also, and in contrast to the MSUD example, there may be data on more functions of parameters than there are basic parameters, which raises the possibility of conflict between sources of evidence, or – to put it another way – a chance to validate parameter estimates against independent evidence.

The population of pregnant women is split into three mutually exclusive groups: a proportion a consists of women born in Sub-Saharan Africa (SSA), a proportion b are injecting drug users (IDUs), and the rest, who are considered to be Low Risk. Each group can then be HIV infected with probabilities c, d and e, respectively. Infected individuals in each group may then either be already diagnosed prior to their attendance at prenatal clinics, with probabilities f, g and h, respectively, or not. These parameters are significant because women whose infection status has already been established lie outside the target population for screening: higher rates of prior diagnosis will therefore reduce the yield of screening. Figure 8.3 sets out the epidemiological model.

The epidemiological model can be embedded within a decision model (Figure 8.4) which makes explicit the costs and benefits on each outcome. In this simplified analysis we will consider only the costs of a screening test, T, and the Net Benefit of an early maternal diagnosis, M. An economic analysis of this data is presented in Chapter 12.

The critical parameters in an economic analysis of screening are those that relate to the prevalence of the undetected condition. Similarly, in a comparison of universal and targeted testing, the key parameters are those relating to the prevalence of undiagnosed infection in the Low Risk group, as the higher risk groups will be covered by both screening strategies. The crucial parameters are, therefore, e the prevalence of HIV in the Low Risk, and h the proportion of Low Risk HIV infected who are already diagnosed. This intuition is confirmed by the Net Benefit equation. If M is the net monetary benefit of an early diagnosis, T is the cost of an HIV test, then the Incremental Net Benefit (INB) of universal relative to targeted

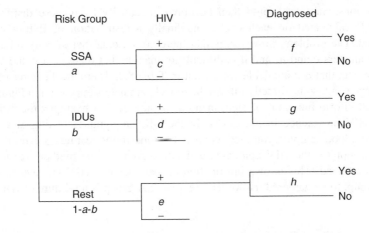

Figure 8.3   Epidemiological model for prenatal HIV screening.

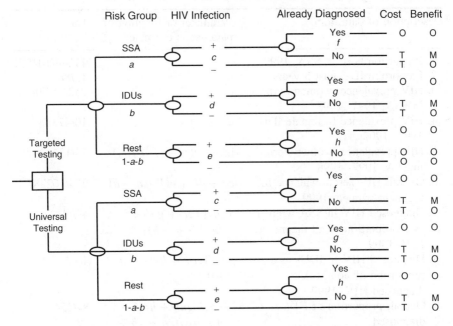

Figure 8.4   Embedding the epidemiology model in a decision tree.

screening for the woman is:

$$\text{INB} = (1\text{-}a\text{-}b)(Me(1\text{-}h) - T(1\text{-}eh))$$

If this example was like MSUD, an investigator would be able to look through the literature and find data sources that informed each of the four parameters in the Net Benefit function. These could then be represented by suitable Beta distributions. Samples would then be drawn repeatedly from these distributions and INB calculated on each cycle, and finally a distribution of INB would be obtained. The problem, however, is that there are no data that directly inform the key parameters e and h, and it is difficult to imagine that there ever could be.

The data that *are* available are set out in Table 8.2. There are 12 items of data, all independent, some directly inform the model parameters appearing in Figure 8.3, but most inform functions of more than one parameter. For example, the fifth item is the HIV prevalence in non-SSAs. In the UK, anonymised testing of residual newborn blood samples, routinely collected for metabolic testing, is carried out in order to monitor the HIV epidemic, and information on the mother's country of birth is retained. This allows information on parameter c, HIV prevalence in the SSA group, to be gathered. However, the *non*-SSA group is a mixture of IDUs and

Table 8.2 Binomial data (numerators and denominators) for the prenatal HIV screening analysis, and the functions of parameters they inform.

Description of data item	Parameter or function of parameters estimated	Data
1. Proportion born in SSA, 1999	a	11044/104577
2. Proportion IDU past 5 years	b	12/882
3. HIV prevalence, women born in SSA, 1997–1998	c	252/15428
4. HIV prevalence in female IDU, 1997–1999	d	10/473
5. HIV prevalence, women born in SSA, 1997–1998	$[db + e(1 - a - b)]/(1 - a)$	74/136139
6. Overall HIV seroprevalence in pregnant women, 1999	$ca + db + e(1 - a - b)$	254/102287
7. Diagnosed HIV in SSA women as a proportion of all diagnosed HIV, 1999	$fca/[fca + gdb + he(1 - a - b)]$	43/60
8. Diagnosed HIV in IDUs as a proportion of non-SSA diagnosed HIV, 1999	$gdb/[gdb + he(1 - a - b)]$	4/17
9. Overall proportion of HIV diagnosed	$[fca + gdb + he(1 - a - b)]/[ca + db + e(1 - a - b)]$	87/254
10. Proportion of infected IDUs diagnosed, 1999	g	12/15
11. Proportion of serotype B in infected women from SSA, 1997–1998	w	14/118
12. Proportion of serotype B in infected women not from SSA, 1997–1998	$[db/[db + e(1 - a - b)]] + we(1 - a - b)/[db + e(1 - a - b)]$	5/31

Low Risk women. Under the epidemiological model of Figure 8.1, HIV prevalence among non-SSAs can be expressed as weighted average of the prevalence in the IDU (d) and Low Risk (e) groups, with the proportions of the population in each group (b) and (1-a-b) as the weights. Similarly the sixth item, the overall HIV prevalence, which is independent as it is based on blood samples in which country of birth information was not retained, is a weighted average of the prevalence in all three groups.

It should be evident that the first five items in Table 8.2 provide enough data to identify the five parameters a−e. When we add item 6, then there are *more* than enough data to identify those five parameters, and in fact there is potential for the different data sources to be *inconsistent*. We might also observe that *any* five of the first six items of data are enough to inform the five parameters a−e. Later we consider how to check for inconsistencies between data sources.

Example 8.1   An introductory synthesis exercise.

We set ourselves the task of writing WinBUGS code to estimate the five parameters a, b, c, d and e from the first six items of data. We begin by assigning priors to these five *basic* parameters. For c, d and e we can straightforwardly assign vague uniform priors Beta(1,1). For a and b we have to add a constraint that ($a + b \leq 1$) because the proportions in each risk group must each be greater or equal to zero, but must always sum to 1. This is a Dirichlet distribution. A convenient way to represent a Dirichlet distribution in WinBUGS is to express it as a series of binomial distributions. For example, the code

```
a ~ dbeta(1,2)
z ~ dbeta(1,1)
b <- z*(1-a)
```

sets up three variables: a, $z = 1 - a$, and $b = z(1 - a)$, where a is a probability, and b is a proportion of $1 - a$, so that the required constraint is satisfied whatever values a and b may take. Note also that the priors give a, b and (1-a-b) equal unit weight, which represents a vague uniform Dirichlet(1,1,1). (Note that, technically, z is a basic parameter because it has a prior, and b is a functional parameter, but we will continue to refer to b as basic for ease of exposition.)

The remaining basic parameters can be given uniform distributions:

```
c ~ dbeta(1,1)
d ~ dbeta(1,1)
e ~ dbeta(1,1)
```

The next step is to define the relationships between the basic parameters and the functional parameters that the data estimates directly. Here it is convenient to create a vector p[ ], which in effect monitors the fitted values:

```
p[1] <- a
p[2] <- b
p[3] <- c
```

```
p[4] <- d
p[5] <- (b*d + (1-a-b)*e/1-a
p[6] <- a*c + b*d + (1-a-b)*e
```

There we are simply writing into WinBUGS code the exact same equations that have already been given in Table 8.2. The final step is to specify the Binomial likelihood, looping over the six items, and then to supply the data, in the form of a vector r[ ] for the numerators and a vector n[ ] for the denominators:

```
for (i in 1:6) {  r[i] ~ dbin(p[i],n[i]) }
```

and to supply the data, in the form of a vector r[ ] for the numerators and a vector n[ ] for the denominators:

```
list(
r=c(11044,    12,    252, 10,    74,    254),
n=c(104577,882,15428,473,136139,102287)
```

When the code is run (file *hivepi-6.odc*), with a burn-in of 10 000, the posterior results shown in Figure 8.5 are obtained based on 50 000 samples from each of two chains.

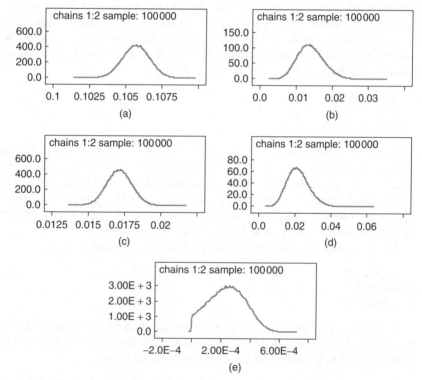

Figure 8.5   Posterior densities for parameters a-e for the introductory synthesis example.

Note that the posterior distribution of e appears to be truncated at zero, indicating that the zero prevalence in the Low Risk group is not entirely ruled out by this subset of the full data set. It is, of course, a major advantage of Bayesian computation that it provides a joint distribution in which all five basic parameters, which are probabilities, must be within the range 0 to 1, whatever the data may be. This follows immediately from specifying them as having Beta priors. But if this was to be programmed for a maximum likelihood solution, range constraints for each parameter would have to be written into the code, and nonstandard constrained optimisation routines would be required.

8.4 Model criticism in multi-parameter models

We now consider how the model criticism tools developed in Chapter 6 can be applied to the more complex kinds of evidence structure found in multi-parameter synthesis applications. We will consider in particular residual deviance, both the deviance attaching to individual data points, which may alert us to which data points are in conflict, and the global deviance as a measure of overall fit. Cross-validation can also be applied, but Mixed Predictive checking is not possible as the HIV data are not in a hierarchical structure.

However, it is worth thinking through at the outset what we mean by 'inconsistency'. Any inconsistency between data sources will manifest itself in the form of discrepancies between data and fitted values under a given model of the data. But does lack of fit always indicate inconsistency? Unlike, for example, a regression model which is regarded as mis-specified if it omits the appropriate covariates, the Figure 8.3 'model' is simply a partition of the population into mutually exclusive and exhaustive groups. Although partitions with other risk groups might be considered preferable or more useful, it is hard to see that the model could be considered to be 'incorrect', or that it could be falsified by any data. If fitted values and data deviate, we would probably therefore conclude that one or more data sources are failing to estimate their target parameters as laid out in Table 8.2. In such cases our interpretation would be that the data sources are *biased*. In other MPES models, however, evidence sources may be inconsistent under one model of how the underlying parameters are related, but not under a different model. As we shall see, statistical investigation can reveal that inconsistency is present, but is unlikely by itself to tell us which data input is the source of that inconsistency.

A further issue to consider in advance of any analysis is the number of potential inconsistencies that there can be. In the MSUD example, there were five basic parameters and five data sources. Inconsistency cannot occur (though see Exercise 8.5). In the full 12-item data set of Table 8.2, there are nine basic parameters, including a parameter w which is not part of the epidemiological model, nor the Net Benefit function: its role, in fact like the roles of c, d, f and g, is simply to make it possible to introduce more data on the key parameters.

In the enlarged data set there is more scope for inconsistency between data sources. A natural approach is to compare the number of parameters (nine) with the number of functions of parameters on which data is available, and regard the difference (three) as a measure of the number of independent inconsistencies there could be in the data set. We might say that there are three degrees of freedom for inconsistency. Applying the same approach to MSUD there are zero inconsistency degrees of freedom, which accords with our intuition. In the six-item HIV data set of Example 8.1, there were five parameters and six data sources, giving one degree of freedom for inconsistency.

Example 8.2   Inconsistency in the HIV data.

The WinBUGS program to synthesise the full 12-item data set (*hivepi-12.odc*) includes code for the Residual Deviance (see Chapter 6). We have run this code with a burn-in of 10 000 and looked at summary statistics of 50 000 samples from each of two chains.

The results (Table 8.3) point to an overall poor fit, with total mean deviance 19.29 compared with an expected 12. Three data points (2, 4, 12) seem to be particularly deviant. These data points provide direct information on b, d, and a function of parameters that carries information on the product bd.

The more formal way to examine this is by cross-validation. Taking as an example, data point 4, we need to form a predictive distribution for the numerator

Table 8.3   Observed data (numerator, denominator and probability), posterior summaries (posterior mean, 2.5% and 97.5% credible limits), and contribution to the posterior mean residual deviance (Dev.) for the HIV example.

Data item	Numerator	Denominator	Prob. data	Post. mean	2.5% credible limit	97.5% credible limit	Dev.
1	11044	104577	0.1056	0.1057	0.1039	0.1076	1.01
2	12	882	0.0136	0.0090	0.00470	0.01503	2.89
3	252	15428	0.0163	0.0172	0.0155	0.0189	1.35
4	10	473	0.0211	0.0124	0.0063	0.0213	3.42
5	74	136139	0.00054	0.00060	0.00048	0.00073	1.50
6	254	102287	0.00248	0.00235	0.00217	0.00255	1.18
7	43	60	0.717	0.688	0.577	0.787	1.02
8	4	17	0.235	0.303	0.165	0.4729	0.84
9	87	254	0.343	0.351	0.295	0.409	1.03
10	12	15	0.8	0.739	0.514	0.915	1.11
11	14	118	0.119	0.113	0.066	0.170	0.94
12	5	31	0.161	0.288	0.200	0.392	2.99
Total mean deviance							19.29

r[4], based only on data points 1–3 and 5–12, that is excluding data point 4, and then compare this predictive distribution with the original data.

To do this the priors and the model sections of the WinBUGS code remain unaltered, but the likelihood is rewritten to exclude r[4]. The data list also remains unaltered. The new likelihood can be coded:

```
for (i in 1:3) { r[i] ~ dbin(p[i],n[i]) }
for (i in 5:12) { r[i] ~ dbin(p[i],n[i]) }
```

The cross-validation method then requires us to create a 'replicate' binomial variable (Figure 8.6), based on the p[4] (*d*), now estimated without the benefit of data point 4, and n[4], and compare this to the original r[4].

```
r.rep ~ dbin(p[4],n[4])
p.xval <- step(r.rep - r[4]) - 0.5 * equals(r.rep,r[4])
```

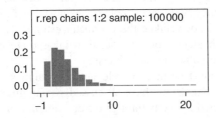

Figure 8.6 Posterior predictive density for the number of events r predicted for data point 4, based on the cross-validation method (i.e. without the benefit of data point 4).

Finally, we must specify dev[4]<-0 in order to sum over the vector dev[ ]. The code for this cross-validation can be found in *hiveip-12-xval4.odc*. The posterior for p.xval and hence the probability of observing a sample r[4] as high as 10 with a sample of n[4], given our model and the remaining data is 0.0048.

Checking on the overall deviance in the absence of data input 4, we find it is 11.5 which is satisfactory for 11 data points. Cross-validation can be carried out for every data point. In some cases the time taken might be prohibitive, but with 12 data points this would still be our recommendation (see Exercise 8.6).

8.5 Evidence-based policy

Politicians increasingly wish to describe their decision making as 'evidence based'. The expression originates, of course, from Evidence-Based Medicine (EBM), a movement which gave rise to the notion that a review of evidence needed to be replicable and based on a protocol. EBM also gave rise to the explosion in meta-analysis as the formal tool for statistically combining the evidence generated by systematic review. But exactly what properties should we, as citizens, expect an evidence-based policy to have? Three desiderata suggest themselves. First, and following EBM, we expect that all the available evidence has been gathered under a replicable protocol, and that it has all been included in the synthesis. Such a rubric ensures both completeness of data and avoids arbitrary selection of evidence, and this would be seen as according exactly with the EBM program. Yet the HIV example shows that the concept 'all available evidence' must be wide enough to include information on functions of parameters. No decision maker, for example, would wish to be accused of basing policy on a subset of the relevant data. To this extent, a synthesis method that is unable to combine *all* the information presented in Table 8.2 cannot be regarded as fit for purpose.

A second principle should be that evidence sources are consistent. This, again, seems hardly controversial. Evidence consistency is an important part of model fit. We would not want policy makers reaching conclusions based on models that did not fit the data, and we would expect models to have been carefully examined and validated for consistency with data. Looking again at the six-item HIV data set, a policy maker who did not validate the parameter estimates against the sixth data item, overall HIV prevalence, or who failed to incorporate it having established consistency, would be vulnerable to criticism.

A final principle must be that the relevant uncertainties are fully represented in the model. The methods we have discussed so far guarantee that sampling uncertainty is propagated correctly through the decision model, and is duly reflected in the posteriors of the parameters, in decision uncertainty, and in key outputs such as the INB. However, this represents sampling variation alone, which is no more than a lower bound on the true uncertainty in parameters. Other sources of uncertainty, such as the bias caused by potential threats to the internal or external validity of the estimates, the impact of heterogeneity due to variation, or structural uncertainty, also need to be considered. Some of these questions are taken up in Section 8.7, and in Chapter 11 we will return to consider bias in the context of treatment effects. Many of these issues are beyond the scope of this book, but some references are given in Section 8.7.

8.6 Summary key points

- We distinguish between forward Monte Carlo simulation from distributions of parameters, and Monte Carlo sampling from the joint posterior distribution of parameters.

- Multi-parameter evidence synthesis combines evidence not just from different sources, but on different parameters, within a coherent overall model. This may often involve more sources of evidence, or more types of sources, than there are parameters, introducing the possibility of inconsistency between different evidence sources.

- But, equally, the possibility of inconsistency is also an opportunity for independent validation of a model.

- We emphasise the advantages of assessing the potential sources of bias in evidence *before* attempting synthesis, due to the dangers of post hoc adjustments.

- Bayesian multi-parameter evidence synthesis meets the requirements we should expect from methods under-pinning 'evidence based' policy: incorporation of all available evidence, assessment of inconsistency, and uncertainty propagation.

8.7 Further reading

The HIV example presented in this chapter was probably the first multi-parameter synthesis to be undertaken using WinBUGs software, though MCMC had already been used in a number of important early papers. Of particular interest are: combining regressions on different subsets of covariates [6]; combination of trial evidence on multiple treatments, reported in an inconsistent way [7]; and synthesis of contingency tables with missing dimensions [8]. Since then a great deal more experience has been gained, not so much with the technique itself, but with how to use it in practice with a wider range of evidence structures, and how to interrogate and understand the results it produces. A greatly expanded version of the HIV analysis, estimating risk group size, HIV prevalence and proportion diagnosed in 13 risk groups [9], now forms the basis for official statistics on HIV prevalence in England and Wales. These models address the fact that, although there is an 'excess' of data in some parts of the network, creating the possibility of inconsistency, in other parts of the network there may be an insufficiency of data to identify all the parameters. The authors introduced hierarchical structures to share the available information more evenly across the parameter space. The extended HIV model had over 100 parameters, and investigators had great difficulty understanding which items of data, or which prior assumptions, were driving the posterior estimates. In such cases it may be necessary to take an empirical approach, varying priors and inputs systematically and observing the effect on posteriors, in order to understand the flow of information through the network.

Deviance and Deviance Information Criterion statistics have been widely used to assess model fit, but a range of other approaches are used. A study of Hepatitis C prevalence in the UK removes each information source in turn and re-examines global and local deviance statistics in each model [10]. Welton and Ades [11] use leverage plots [12] to shed light on what is driving the posterior results in a synthesis of sources of data on toxoplasmosis incidence.

The difficulty in interpreting, or knowing how to respond to, statistical evidence for inconsistency is a theme that runs through much of the research. The data points that 'light up' on statistical probing for inconsistency are simply those where the fitted values are influenced by the other information in the model; they are *not* necessarily the data items that are 'wrong' (see Exercise 8.5). While it may be possible to isolate certain sub-networks as the locus of inconsistency, the identification of which data are 'at fault' is a matter that requires judgement based on epidemiological expertise. A common approach has been to introduce new parameters into the model [9] which can be interpreted as *bias* parameters. If these are given vague priors the effect is to neutralise the inconsistency: the same result would be achieved by removing the data point altogether. In some cases it may be possible to expand the model and at the same time introduce new data to inform the additional parameters while at the same time resolving the inconsistencies [13].

The danger with post hoc adjustments intended to resolve inconsistency is that the same inconsistency can be resolved equally well by removing any one of a number of data points, or adding bias parameters in several different parts of the network. Each different approach constitutes an alternative model with different parameter values, and potentially with fundamentally different public health implications, and yet there is no statistical way of choosing between them. The entire analysis becomes prey to selective interpretation.

It is clearly preferable to identify potential sources of bias attaching to each data point *prior* to putting data together in a synthesis. Turner *et al.* [14] have recently set out a protocol-based approach to eliciting expert opinion on potential biases threatening the internal and external validity of data. While this is oriented to studies of treatment efficacy, similar ideas could perhaps be developed for more general types of synthesis.

For readers interested in what kinds of different evidence structure have been 'synthesised', further references can be found in Ades and Sutton [4], Ades *et al.* [15], and in Eddy *et al.* [1]. An even wider range of synthesis problems, including applications in physics, engineering, education, space and military can be found in a review by Gaver *et al.* [16]. Similar approaches using different forms of Bayesian computation are found in Raftery *et al.* [17] and subsequent papers on Bayesian Synthesis for deterministic population growth models, and the so-called Bayesian Monte Carlo [18], that has been popular in Environmental Health Risk Assessment.

8.8   Exercises

8.1 It is difficult to assign truly vague priors on probabilities using the Beta distribution. Using the MSUD example, compare the account given in this chapter with two alternative approaches: (a) Put vague priors on the logits of the five basic probability parameters; (b) use forward Monte Carlo simulation from Beta priors based on the data. For example, for the probability of early detection without screening, rather than have 8/18 as binomial data, with a Beta(1,1) prior, simulate from a Beta(8,10) distribution. What difficulties have to be faced by the alternative approaches?

8.2 Compare the posterior correlations between the basic parameters in (a) the MSUD problem and (b) the HIV data with six data points. Explain the difference.

8.3 The five-parameter MSUD model gives no scope for examining consistency between the five data sources, as each data source uniquely informs a different parameter. We cannot therefore compare any one data point with predictions based on the remaining data. But, if there was *only* data on the first five data points in Table 8.3, so that we had five parameters informed by five data points, could we ever observe a poor fit between the model and the data?

8.4 Primary toxoplasmosis infection in pregnancy can lead to Congenital Toxoplasmosis (CT) in the infant, and this can result in mental retardation (MR). Some (fictitious) data are available. The model parameters and the data informing them are:

	Parameter	Numerator	Denominator
Proportion of births with CT	p_1	80	200 000
Proportion of CT cases with MR	p_2	10	120
Proportion of birth population	p_3	60	20 000
Proportion of MR population with CT	p_4	2	1200

Use Bayes' rule to verify that $p_4 = p_1.p_2/p_3$. Then write a WinBUGS program that uses all four pieces of information to estimate all the parameters simultaneously, and find the residual deviance at each data point and the overall deviance.

8.5 Carry out cross-validation on data point 4 in Exercise 8.4, and examine the deviance statistics when this data point is removed. Can you determine which data point(s) is, or are, 'wrong'?

*8.6 Write WinBUGS code that carries out cross-validation for each data item in turn, within the same program.

References

1. Eddy D.M., Hasselblad V., Shachter R. *Meta-analysis by the Confidence Profile Method*. London: Academic Press, 1992.

2. Hasselblad V., McCrory D.C. Meta-analytic tools for medical decision making: a practical guide. *Medical Decision Making* 1995;**15**:81–96.

3. Ades A.E., Cliffe S. Markov Chain Monte Carlo estimation of a multi-parameter decision model: consistency of evidence and the accurate assessment of uncertainty. *Medical Decision Making* 2002;**22**:359–371.

4. Ades A.E., Sutton A.J. Multiparameter evidence synthesis in epidemiology and medical decision making: current approaches. *Journal of the Royal Statistical Society, Series A* 2006;**169**:5–35.

5. Spiegelhalter D.J., Abrams K.R., Myles J. *Bayesian Approaches to Clinical Trials and Health-Care Evaluation*. New York: John Wiley & Sons, Ltd, 2004.

6. Dominici F., Parmigiani G., Reckhow K.H., Wolpert R.L. Combining information from related regressions. *Journal of Agricultural, Biological, and Environmental Statistics* 1997;**2**:313–332.

7. Dominici F., Parmigiani G., Wolpert R.L., Hasselblad V. Meta-analysis of migraine headache treatments: combining information from heterogenous designs. *Journal of the American Statistical Association* 1999;**94**:16–28.

8. Dominici F. Combining contingency tables with missing dimensions. *Biometrics* 2000; **56**:546–553.

9. Goubar A., Ades A.E., De Angelis D., *et al.* Bayesian multi-parameter synthesis of HIV surviellance data in England and Wales, 2001. Technical Report. London: Health Protection Agency Centre for Infections, 2006.

10. Sweeting M.J., De Angelis D., Hickman D., Ades A.E. Estimating HCV prevalence in England and Wales by synthesising evidence from multiple data sources: assessing data conflict and model fit. *Biostatistics* 2008;**9**:715–734.

11. Welton N.J., Ades A.E. A model of toxoplasmosis incidence in the UK: evidence synthesis and consistency of evidence. *Applied Statistics* 2005;**54**:385–404.

12. Spiegelhalter D.J., Best N.G., Carlin B.P., van der Linde A. Bayesian measures of model complexity and fit. *Journal of the Royal Statistical Society, Series B* 2002;**64**:583–616.

13. Presanis A., De Angelis D., Spiegelhalter D., *et al.* Conflicting evidence in a Bayesian synthesis of surveillance data to estimate HIV prevalence. *Journal of the Royal Statistical Society, Series A* 2008;**171**:915–937.

14. Turner R.M., Spiegelhalter D.J., Smith G.C.S., Thompson S.G. Bias modelling in evidence synthesis. *Journal of the Royal Statistical Society, Series A* 2009;**172**:21–47.

15. Ades A.E., Welton N., Caldwell D., *et al.* Multiparameter evidence synthesis in epidemiology and medical decision-making. *Journal of Health Services & Research Policy* 2008; **13**(Suppl. 3):12–22.

16. Gaver D., Draper D., Goel P., *et al.* *Combining Information: Statistical Issues and Opportunities for Research*. Washington, DC: National Academy Press, 1992.

17. Raftery A.E., Givens G.H., Zeh J.E. Inference from a deterministic population dynamics model for Bowhead whales (with discussion). *Journal of the American Statistical Association* 1995;**90**:402–430.

18. Brand K.P., Small M.J. Updating uncertainty in an integrated risk assessment: conceptual framework and methods. *Risk Analysis* 1995;**15**:719–731.

9

Mixed and indirect treatment comparisons

We now extend the pairwise meta-analysis methods of Chapter 4 to handle multiple treatment comparisons in a connected network. This will allow us to combine evidence from trials comparing treatments A and B (AB trials), trials comparing A and C (AC trials), and trials of B and C (BC trials), and so on. We will show how to calculate a probability that each treatment is 'best'. If, in addition to the Randomised Control Trial (RCT) data on relative efficacy, we also have information on the costs of each treatment and if the health benefits can be converted into a monetarised form, then the 'Net Benefit' of each treatment can be defined (see Chapter 3). The posterior uncertainty in treatment efficacy can then be propagated through a decision model to generate uncertainty in Net Benefit. This will be portrayed in cost-effectiveness acceptability curves (CEACs) (see Chapters 3 and 7).

Once again, however, the power and convenience of the method must not be allowed to lure the user away from a careful consideration of the assumptions being made, nor from careful attention to convergence.

9.1 Why go beyond 'direct' head-to-head trials?

There is a broad consensus that the 'best' evidence on the effect of treatment B relative to treatment A is provided by head-to-head trials, which provide a 'direct' estimate d_{AB}^{dir}. But, even if this is accepted, several reasons can be advanced for taking a wider view of what the legitimate evidence base should be. First, it may

---

Evidence Synthesis for Decision Making in Healthcare, First Edition. Nicky J. Welton, Alexander J. Sutton, Nicola J. Cooper, Keith R. Abrams and A.E. Ades.
© 2012 John Wiley & Sons, Ltd. Published 2012 by John Wiley & Sons, Ltd.

be that there are no A *vs* B trials, but that instead an 'indirect' estimate can be formed from the results of A *vs* C and B *vs* C trials:

$$\hat{d}_{AB}^{ind} = \hat{d}_{AC}^{dir} - \hat{d}_{BC}^{dir} \tag{9.1}$$

A second reason might be that, even if direct AB evidence exists, it may be sparse; the volume of indirect evidence can be much greater. This is, in fact, a very common situation. Two new active treatments may have been compared with placebo, or to an established standard treatment, but manufacturers have proved reluctant to carry out the head-to-head comparisons that would be of most clinical interest.

This rationale for the indirect estimate is not controversial, but from here forward there is less consensus. The influential Cochrane Collaboration has suggested that direct and indirect estimates should be kept distinct [1]. But once the legitimacy of indirect evidence has been conceded when direct data are lacking or sparse, it is difficult to justify excluding it at all. How sparse must the direct evidence be before we turn to indirect? And if the direct evidence is sparse, why not *pool* the direct and indirect using for example an inverse-variance weighted average? In particular, if indirect evidence is good enough in some cases, why not in every case? After all, the quality of the information in indirect evidence does not change according to the amount of direct evidence that might be available as well!

This pooling of direct and indirect evidence is referred to as a mixed treatment comparison. Using P (precision) to denote the reciprocal of the variance of the estimates [2]:

$$\hat{d}_{AB}^{pooled} = \frac{P_{AB}^{dir} \hat{d}_{AB}^{dir} + P_{AB}^{ind} \hat{d}_{AB}^{dir}}{P_{AB}^{dir} + P_{AB}^{ind}} \tag{9.2}$$

Such pooling can be seen to be no more than an extension of the widely accepted rubric that all the available evidence should be marshalled, to increase precision and to avoid selection biases.

But there is a still more cogent reason for turning to mixed treatment comparison synthesis. Clinicians and national decision-making bodies frequently have to make a choice between several different alternative treatments: in this situation there seems to be no alternative other than to combine the data on all the pairwise comparisons within a single unified analysis, producing an internally consistent set of relative treatment effects. For example, in 2000 a systematic review and economic analysis was published by the National Health Service Health Technology Assessment programme. This compared alternative thrombolytic drugs following heart attacks [3]. The evidence base can be conveniently portrayed in a network diagram (Figure 9.1), in which the nodes are the treatments, and the connecting lines (edges) represent the trial evidence. For example there were eight trials comparing streptokinase (SK) to tissue plasminogen activator (t-PA), two comparing accelerated t-PA (Acc t-PA) to reteplase, and so on.

Clearly, with a network of comparisons to consider it is no longer meaningful to distinguish 'direct' and 'indirect' evidence on each contrast. For any particular

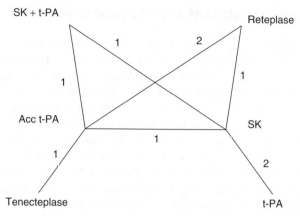

Figure 9.1   Network diagram of the 14 RCTs comparing thrombolytic treatment following myocardial infarction, based on Boland [3].

contrast there may be several different indirect comparisons, and evidence that is direct for one contrast may contribute indirect information for up to 14 others! (If there are K treatments, there are $K(K - 1)/2$ possible pairwise comparisons: so with six treatments there are 15 contrasts of potential interest to a decision maker).

It is possible to restrict all conclusions to the pairwise contrasts on which 'direct' data exist, producing in effect seven separate estimates as if they were not connected in a common network. While it may be possible to piece together a comparative cost-effectiveness analysis of the treatments, based on the pairwise results from the direct evidence, such analyses do not have the properties that decision makers would like them to have. First, this does not lead to an internally consistent rendition of what the evidence base in its entirety is telling us about the relative efficacy of the treatments. Secondly, the uncertainties in the evidence can only be correctly propagated through the model if *all* the data are statistically combined. Nevertheless, *any* use of these data to make a decision about which treatment to use must implicitly make exactly the same assumptions that we will be making in the MTC analyses we will be proposing: namely that the A *vs* B trials estimate the same true effect d_{AB} as would be estimated in the AC, BC, and even CD trials if they had all included treatments A and B.

Eventually, if a comparison must be made between multiple treatments, based on a possibly incomplete set of pairwise comparisons, the data have to be statistically combined in a unified analysis that respects the randomisation. It seems that MTC *in some form* is inevitable. The simple approach suggested by Equation (9.2) is always available, but it cannot be applied in larger networks, and even in three-treatment networks it does not recognise that all three relative treatments effects should pool direct and indirect evidence. Therefore, we now extend the earlier models for pairwise meta-analysis (Chapter 4) so that they can be applied to connected networks of arbitrary size and complexity.

9.2 A fixed treatment effects model for MTC

We will begin with trials generating binomial data. The models are, in fact, recognisable as logistic regression models; however, it is useful to describe the model making use of the terminology of the Confidence Profile Method [4].

Suppose we have four treatments A, B, C and D, where A is the 'reference' or standard treatment. We define three treatment effect parameters representing the Log Odds Ratios (LORs) of B, C and D relative to reference treatment A: d_{AB}, d_{AC}, d_{AD}. These are the *basic* parameters, and they will need to be given priors. There are $4 \times (4 - 1)/2 = 6$ potential contrasts, and in the data set shown in Example 9.1, there is at least one trial directly informing every contrast. The three remaining contrasts, d_{BC}, d_{BD}, d_{CD} are represented by *functional* parameters, and are therefore defined in terms of the basic parameters:

$$d_{BC} = d_{AC} - d_{AB}$$
$$d_{BD} = d_{AD} - d_{AB} \qquad (9.3)$$
$$d_{CD} = d_{AD} - d_{AC}$$

These *consistency equations* [5] capture the idea behind MTC: simply put, if $(b - a) = 2$ and $(c - a) = 3$, then $(c - b)$ must be $= 1$. If we imagine the effects of the four treatments in a single patient population – for example in a 4-arm trial – then it is obvious that the consistency equations must correctly describe the relative efficacies of four treatments in any given target population. If we abandon the consistency relations we would revert to a model in which there were six LORs which are quite unrelated to each other.

First, some notation: we will adopt the convention that d_{XY} is the effect of Y relative to X, and we will always express these relative effects with Y alphabetically following X, because $d_{YX} = -d_{XY}$. The full Fixed Effect model will be as follows. For treatment k in trial j:

$$r_{jk} \sim \text{Binomial}(p_{jk}, n_{jk})$$
$$\text{logit}(p_{jk}) = \mu_j + d_{XY} I(k = Y)$$
$$d_{BC} = d_{AC} - d_{AB}$$
$$d_{BD} = d_{AD} - d_{AB} \qquad (9.4)$$
$$d_{CD} = d_{AD} - d_{AC}$$
$$\mu_j, d_{AB}, d_{AC}, d_{AD} \sim \text{Normal}(0, 100^2)$$

Note that in a trial comparing treatments X and Y, the model statement sets the log-odds of an outcome in trial j on treatment k equal to trial 'baseline' μ_j when $k = X$, and $\mu_j + d_{XY}$ when $k = Y$. The trial baselines are all given unrelated, vague priors. The (basic) parameters for treatment effects relative to the reference treatment A are also given vague priors, while the remaining (functional) parameters are defined in terms of the basic parameters. We now show how this can be coded in WinBUGS.

Example 9.1   Smoking cessation [6]: Mixed treatment comparison.

Our illustrative data set in Table 9.1 is taken from Hasselblad [6]. It is a set of 24 trials comparing four interventions for smoking cessation: no contact (A), self-help (B), individual counselling (C) and group counselling (D).

Table 9.1   Smoking cessation data, from Hasselblad [6]. Number of patients who cease smoking and totals in 24 RCTs.

Comparison	Study number	No contact A	Self-help B	Individual counselling C	Group counselling D
AB (3)	1	79/702	77/694		
	2	18/671	21/535		
	3	8/116	19/146		
AC (15)	4	75/731		363/714	
	5	2/106		9/205	
	6	58/549		237/1561	
	7	0/33		9/48	
	8	3/100		31/98	
	9	1/31		26/95	
	10	6/39		17/77	
	11	64/642		107/761	
	12	5/62		8/90	
	13	20/234		34/237	
	14	95/1107		134/1031	
	15	15/187		35/504	
	16	78/584		73/675	
	17	69/1177		54/888	
ACD (1)	18	9/140		23/140	10/138
AD (1)	19	0/20			9/20
BC (1)	20		20/49	16/43	
BCD (1)	21		11/78	12/85	29/170
BD (1)	22		7/66		32/127
CD (2)	23			12/76	20/74
	24			9/55	3/26

Notice that there is direct evidence on every one of the possible six pairwise contrasts, although the majority of the data compare no contact (A) with individual counselling (C). Figure 9.2 portrays each trial on the log-odds scale. Our objective is to synthesise the data while respecting the randomisation structure in the evidence.

Although we will use the Binomial likelihood attaching to the individual arms, the synthesis itself will only concern the treatment differences, just as was the case for pairwise meta-analysis. In terms of Figure 9.2, this means that each of the lines could be moved up or down by an arbitrary amount without changing the results of the analysis.

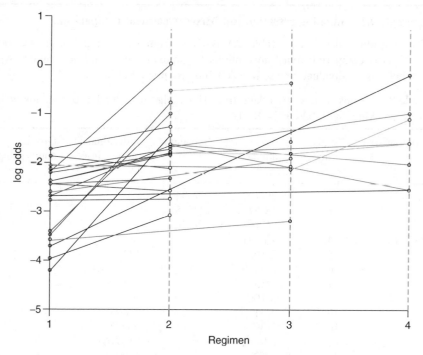

Figure 9.2   Smoking cessation data, based on Hasselblad [6]. Each point repre-sents the log odds of smoking cessation on one arm of a trial. Lines connect arms from the same trial.

Coding for pairwise meta-analysis introduced in Chapter 4 had separate like-lihood statements for treatment and control arms. This would become clumsy with three or more treatments, so we adopt the approach taken in Chapter 6 (Example 6.1), and number the treatments 1, 2, 3,... and so on. d_{AB}, d_{AC}, d_{AD} will now be labelled d[2], d[3], d[4]. d[1] corresponds to d_{AA}, the effect of treatment A relative to itself, and this is set to zero. We also adopt the column format for data entry, as illustrated in Example 6.1, but with an additional variable, b[], which denotes the 'baseline' treatment in each trial, as follows:

s[]	t[]	r[]	n[]	b[]	
1	1	79	702	1	# s[] study number
1	2	77	694	1	# t[] treatment
2	1	18	671	1	# r[] numerator
2	2	21	535	1	# n[] denominator
3	1	8	116	1	# b[] trial 'baseline' treatment
3	2	19	149	1	
...	...	...	...	...	
20	2	20	49	2	
20	3	16	43	2	
...	...	...	...	...	

```
24   4   3   26   3
END
```

Trial 20, for example, compares treatments B and C (treatments 2 and 3), and therefore b[20] is set to 2 for both arms. WinBUGS code for this data set is:

```
for (i in 1:50) { r[i] ~ dbin(p[i],n[i])        #likelihood
logit(p[j,k] <- mu[j] + d[t[i]]-d[b[i]] }       #model
for (j in 1:24) {mu[j] ~ dnorm(0,.0001) }       #priors on baselines
d[1] <- 0
for (k in 2:4) { d[k] ~ dnorm(0,.0001) }        #priors for treatment effects
```

The key to this coding is the d[t[i]] – d[b[i]] in the model statement, which is explained in Table 9.2. This way of writing the code is very compact, and in fact avoids having to specify the functional parameters explicitly at all.

Table 9.2 Coding in the Fixed Effect model, and its relationship to the algebraic representation of the model.

Treatment contrast	t[i]	b[i]		d[t[i]]-d[b[i]]
1,2	2	1	δ_{AB}	d[2]-d[1] = d[2]
1,3	3	1	δ_{AC}	d[3]-d[1] = d[3]
1,4	4	1	δ_{AD}	d[4]-d[1] = d[4]
2,3	3	2	$\delta_{BC} = \delta_{AC} - \delta_{AB}$	d[3]-d[2]
2,4	4	2	$\delta_{BD} = \delta_{AD} - \delta_{AB}$	d[4]-d[2]
3,4	4	3	$\delta_{CD} = \delta_{AD} - \delta_{AC}$	d[4]-d[3]

To run this code, a set of initial values must be provided for the 24 mu[j], and for the three basic treatment effect parameters. d[ ] is a vector length 4, but d[1] is set to a constant (zero) in the code; therefore the first member of the vector is left unspecified in the initial values list, for example (NA,0,0,0). Posterior summaries for the Fixed Effect model are set out in Table 9.3.

Evidently, group counselling is the most effective treatment. To help familiarise yourself with the code and data structure, try Exercise 9.1.

Table 9.3 Posterior summaries of treatment effects in the Fixed Effect model. d[2], d[3], d[4] are the LORs of treatments B (self-help), C (individual counselling) and D (group counselling) relative to treatment A (no treatment), from *mtc-fe.odc*, with a burn-in of 10 000 and 20 000 samples from each of two chains.

Node	Mean	sd	Monte Carlo error	2.50%	Median	97.50%
d[2]	0.2245	0.1253	−0.01986	−0.02111	0.2245	0.4699
d[3]	0.7652	0.05755	0.00685	0.6531	0.7649	0.8796
d[4]	0.8422	0.1753	0.00191	0.4989	84.17%	1.185

9.2.1 Absolute treatment effects

Cost-effectiveness analysis, as explained in the examples presented in Chapters 1, 3 and 7, requires information on the absolute treatment difference on the probability scale. We can generate this from the LORs, but only if we have information on the 'baseline' probability of the outcome. In the context of Example 9.1, the question is: what is the probability of smoking cessation in the 'no treatment' group? This information could be based on one or more cohort studies that are considered to be representative of the target population, or on the more contemporary trials, or a combination of both. The important point is that the issue of a suitable baseline for the treatment A (no contact) strategy should be kept as a separate issue from the calculation of relative treatment effects, which should be based on RCT evidence using methods that respect the randomisation. For the sake of simplicity we assume that a separate analysis has been conducted, which delivers a posterior distribution for the log odds of smoking cessation under treatment A, Normal$(-2.6, 0.38^2)$, which corresponds to a median estimate of 7.5% with a 95% credible interval (3.4 to 14). We can then construct absolute effects for the other treatments as follows, adding the relative treatment effect to this baseline on the log-odds scale, then converting back to the probability scale.

$$A \sim \text{Normal}(-2.6, 0.38^2)$$
$$\text{logit}(T_k) = A + d_k$$

(9.5)

The WinBUGS code that achieves this is:

```
A ~ dnorm(-2.6,precA)              # Generate absolute smoking
precA <- pow(0.38,-2)              # cessation rates
for (k in 1:4) { logit(T[k]) <- A + d[k] }
```

The results are shown in Table 9.4.

9.2.2 Relative treatment efficacy and ranking

The code presented so far delivers posterior LORs for the efficacy of treatments B, C, D relative to A, but it does not address the question of how to make inferences about treatment efficacy. We can clearly generate the LORs for any treatment relative to any other, and also monitor the Odds Ratios:

Table 9.4 Posterior summaries of absolute treatment effects from *mtc-fe.odc*.

Node	Mean	sd	2.50%	Median	97.50%
T[1]	0.07329	0.02625	0.0342	0.06924	0.1357
T[2]	0.09037	0.03324	0.04076	0.08518	0.1687
T[3]	0.1441	0.04745	0.07016	0.138	0.254
T[4]	0.1549	0.05455	0.07091	0.1473	0.2819

Table 9.5 Posterior summaries of Odds Ratios for each pair of treatment comparisons from *mtc-fe.odc*.

Node	Mean	sd	2.50%	Median	97.50%
or[1,2]	1.262	0.1586	0.9791	1.252	1.6
or[1,3]	2.153	0.1241	1.922	2.149	2.41
or[1,4]	2.358	0.4163	1.647	2.32	3.271
or[2,3]	1.732	0.2306	1.326	1.718	2.228
or[2,4]	1.889	0.3651	1.272	1.855	2.698
or[3,4]	1.096	0.1913	0.7711	1.08	1.52

```
for (c in 1:3) { for (k in (c+1):4) {    # All pair-wise log odds ratios
lor[c,k] <- d[k] - d[c] }}               # and odds ratios
```

Posterior results are shown in Table 9.5.

But we are then confronted with a typical multiple comparisons problem. The approach we suggest is to rank the treatments and examine the posterior distributions of the ranks, and also to calculate the probability that each treatment is the best treatment. In the following code the rank(v,s) function returns the number of elements of the vector v whose value is less than or equal to the sth element. Then best[k] takes the value 1 when treatment k has the highest cessation rate and 0 otherwise. We also generate the LORs and Odds Ratios for all six contrasts.

```
for (k in 1:4) {                  # Rank the treatment effects
    rk[k] <- 5 - rank(T[ ],k)     # (with 1=best) & record the
    best[k] <- equals(rk[k],1)}   # best treatment
```

An examination of the posterior densities of the vector rk[ ] (Figure 9.3) shows that treatment 4 (D, group counselling) is ranked best (= 1) most of the time, and treatment 1 (A, no contact) is most often the worst.

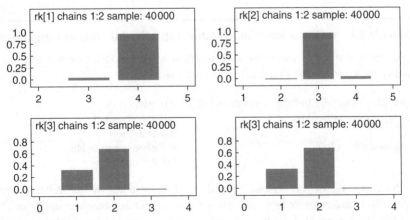

Figure 9.3   Posterior distribution of the ranks of treatment efficacy: Fixed Effect model.

The information in the rankings is neatly summarised in the vector best[k]. The posterior means probabilities are : best[1] = 0, best[2] = 0, best[3] = 0.33, best[4] = 0.67. These results appear to rule out no contact and self-help. Group counselling has the highest probability of being the 'best'.

9.3   Random Effects MTC models

A number of proposals have been made in the literature. Our approach is based on Higgins and Whitehead's work [7] on an AC, AB, ABC network. We have only modified their notation and program code so that it efficiently handles more complex networks with large numbers of treatments. Further, both the model and the code introduced below are the natural extension of the Random Effects model for pairwise comparisons, discussed in Chapter 4, and the Fixed Effect MTC model of the previous section.

In the Random Effects model each trial j on treatment contrast XY estimates a distinct LOR, δ_{jXY}, which is drawn from a common distribution $\delta_{jXY} \sim$ Normal(d_{XY}, σ_{XY}^2). We will make the simplifying assumption that the between-trial variances for all six contrasts are equal, $\sigma_{XY}^2 = \sigma^2$. Adding a vague Uniform prior for σ the full model becomes:

$$r_{jk} \sim \text{Binomial}(p_{jk}, n_{jk})$$
$$\text{logit}(p_{jk}) = \mu_j + \delta_{jXY} I(k = Y)$$
$$\delta_{jXY} \sim N(d_{XY}, \sigma^2)$$
$$d_{BC} = d_{AC} - d_{AB}$$
$$d_{BD} = d_{AD} - d_{AB} \tag{9.6}$$
$$d_{CD} = d_{AD} - d_{AC}$$
$$\mu_j, d_{AB}, d_{AC}, d_{AD} \sim \text{Normal}(0, 100^2)$$
$$\sigma \sim \text{Uniform}(0, 2)$$

Example 9.1   revisited Smoking cessation [6]: Mixed treatment comparison.

There are a number of ways to code a Random Effects model. One approach is to modify the code for the Fixed Effect version, as follows:

```
logit(p[i]) <- mu[s[i]]+ delta[i]*(1-equals(t[i],b[i]))   # model
delta[i] ~ dnorm(md[i],tau)                                # Random effect
                                                           # distribution
md[i] <- d[t[i]] - d[b[i]]                                 #  Define mean of RE
                                                           # distribution
```

Note the use of the equals( ) function. This 'switches in' the relative treatment effect parameter delta[i] only when the treatment and baseline indicators, t[i] and b[i] are not equal. Finally, of course, a prior is needed for the between-trial heterogeneity parameter, for example sd~dunif(0,2).

Results for the Random Effects model are similar to the Fixed Effect model, except as usual the mean treatment effects in the Random Effects model are considerably more uncertain than in a Fixed Effect model (Table 9.6). The probability that each treatment is best is, however, barely changed: best[1] = 0, best[2] = .04, best[3] = 0.19, best[4] = 0.77.

Table 9.6   Posterior summary from Random Effects model of smoking cessation data.

Node	Mean	sd	2.50%	Median	97.50%
D[2]	0.5217	0.3865	−0.2222	0.5148	1.308
D[3]	0.8145	0.2323	0.3718	0.8079	1.293
D[4]	1.176	0.4551	0.3012	1.166	2.106
T[1]	0.07307	2.61×10^{-2}	0.0342	0.06903	0.1345
T[2]	0.1222	5.89×10^{-2}	0.04173	0.1105	0.2694
T[3]	0.1519	5.73×10^{-2}	0.06567	0.1432	0.2874
T[4]	0.2095	9.58×10^{-2}	0.07029	0.1935	0.4384
sd	0.821	0.1845	0.5352	0.796	1.253

9.4   Model choice and consistency of MTC evidence

An important finding from the random effect analysis (Table 9.6) concerns the σ parameter. Not only is its mean value of the same order as the mean treatment effects, but the lower credible limit, 0.54, is so high as to effectively rule out the hypothesis that σ is close to zero. This points us firmly in the direction of the Random Effects model. This can be put on a slightly more formal basis by comparing the Fixed and Random Effects models using some of the model critique methods from Chapter 4. The results (Table 9.7) add very strong support for the choice of a Random Effects model. Even though the number of effective parameters is over 14 points higher in the Random Effects model, this is easily outweighed by the massive improvement in the deviance statistics. Interestingly, the Residual

Table 9.7   Global goodness of fit statistics comparing Fixed Effect and Random Effects models.

	$\bar{D}_{res}$	$\bar{D}$	p_D	DIC
Fixed Effect	267.2	494.8	27.1	521.8
Random Effects	54.2	281.7	44.8	326.6

$\bar{D}_{res}$, posterior mean residual deviance; $\bar{D}$, posterior mean deviance; p_D, effective number of parameters; DIC, Deviance Information Criterion (see Chapter 6 for definitions).

Deviance calculated in WinBUGS, 54.2, is close to the number of observations (50), and we would be justified in concluding that the Random Effects model provides an adequate fit to the data.

Of course, a Random Effects model is extremely tolerant. The variance term will happily stretch to fit trials whose values are far from the mean without producing any sign that the model fit is poor. As we saw with the magnesium meta-analysis (Chapter 6), a globally poor fit can only be obtained if one or two very large trials are distinctly far from the mean of the others. Therefore, the comparison of Fixed and Random Effects models tells us mostly about the level of between-trial heterogeneity *within* the different comparison types. It may not tell us much about whether the key consistency assumptions are being met.

9.4.1 Techniques for presenting and understanding the results of MTC

A healthy sceptic will not, therefore, feel fully comfortable with the results of MTC on the basis of goodness of fit statistics alone. The output from the MTC is, furthermore, rather remote from the original data. Users often report 'not knowing what is going on'. Here we will suggest some additional tabulations and analyses that can be useful.

First, it is useful to examine every pairwise comparison on which there is direct data, and then compare the posterior LOR from the MTC analysis with the estimates produced by a standard pairwise meta-analysis, using Fixed Effect or Random Effects models as appropriate. Careful examination of these results – both central estimates and confidence intervals – can be extremely informative. Carrying out such a comparison also throws light on the main 'drivers' of the posterior results. For example, in the smoking cessation data set, readers will be able to confirm that the MTC analysis contributes relatively very little to the AC comparison. This is simply because of the large amount of direct data on this comparison. By contrast, posteriors for several of the other contrasts supported by only small numbers of trials tend to be 'pushed around' and forced to conform with the AC information. Other useful approaches can be found in some of the recent applied publications. For example, Cipriani *et al.* [8] plot the probabilities of each ranking for every treatment; an effective way of contrasting the alternative treatments on each outcome.

A second procedure is to examine the deviance contributions attaching to each data point. If there are any with high values (say over 2.0), it may be worth checking that they do not all arise from trials within one particular comparison (say AB). If so, it is quite likely that the AB data are inconsistent with the AC and BC. In this particular data set the deviant observations tend to be ones with zero cell counts.

There have been a number of more technical papers on inconsistency in MTC, and this is still an area of active research. Some further pointers to the literature are given in Section 9.10. A further possibility is a direct comparison between a model based on the consistency equations, and one that is not (see Exercise 9.4).

9.5 Multi-arm trials

In a multi-arm trial j comparing, say, treatments A, B and C, the posterior distributions of δ_{jAB} and δ_{jAC} should be correlated because both depend on the same trial baseline μ_j. Given the homogeneous variance model assumed so far, it can be shown that the trial-specific treatment effects are drawn from a Multi-Variate Normal (MVN) distribution [7]:

$$
\begin{pmatrix} \delta_{jAB} \\ \delta_{jAC} \end{pmatrix} \sim MVN \left(\begin{pmatrix} d_{AB} \\ d_{AC} \end{pmatrix}, \begin{pmatrix} \sigma^2 & \sigma^2/2 \\ \sigma^2/2 & \sigma^2 \end{pmatrix} \right)
\tag{9.7}
$$

In order to capture this correctly the code needs to be amended. This can be done in a variety of ways. The first method we suggest is designed for a data set with 2- or at most 3-arm trials, but maintains the arm-based data structure. We parameterise the bivariate normal as a made up of a univariate normal for δ_{jAB}, and a second univariate normal for δ_{jAC}, conditional upon δ_{jAB}:

$$
\delta_{jAB} \sim \text{Normal}(d_{AB}, \sigma^2)
$$

$$
\delta_{jAC}|\delta_{jAB} \sim \text{Normal}\left(d_{AC} + \frac{\delta_{jAB} - d_{AB}}{2}, \frac{3\sigma^2}{4} \right)
\tag{9.8}
$$

Code to carry out this analysis can be found in the file mtc-re-3arm. It relies on an additional vector m[ ] in the data that carries the arm number, 1, 2 or 3. When m[ ] takes the value 3, the mean and precision of the random effect distribution are adjusted:

s[ ]	t[ ]	r[ ]	n[ ]	b[ ]	m[ ]	
1	1	79	702	1	1	# s[ ] study number
1	2	77	694	1	2	# t[ ] treatment
2	1	18	671	1	1	# r[ ] numerator
2	2	21	535	1	2	# n[ ] denominator
...	...	...	...	...	...	# b[ ] trial 'baseline'
21	2	11	78	2	1	# m[ ] arm number
21	3	12	85	2	2	
21	4	29	170	2	3	
...	...	...	...	...	...	
24	4	3	26	3	2	
END						

In fact, the conditional univariate approach suggests a more general coding, which is appropriate for multi-arm trials without limit on the numbers of arms. However, this form of coding (*mtc-re-multiarm.odc*) requires a quite different data structure in which each record refers to a trial, not to an arm.

r[,1]	n[,1]	r[,2]	n[,2]	r[,3]	n[,3]	t[,1]	t[,2]	t[,3]	na[ ]
9	140	23	140	10	138	1	3	4	3
11	78	12	85	29	170	2	3	4	3

| 75 | 731 | 363 | 714 | NA | 1 | 1 | 3 | NA | 2 |
| ... | ... | ... | ... | ... | ... | | | | |

END

These records represent, in order, a 3-arm trial of treatments 1, 2 and 3; a 3-arm trial of treatments 2, 3 and 4; and a 2-arm trial of treatments 1 and 3. The vector na[ ] carries the number of arms, and the matrix t[,] identifies which arm has which treatment. Note that 'empty' positions must be filled out with 'NA'. The number of vectors needed is determined by the maximum number of arms.

This coding is actually both revealing and flexible. First, it makes the point that *every* trial is a sample from a multi-variate normal distribution with the absent arms 'missing at random'. That is, if we are considering an MTC with, say, five treatments, then every trial samples the four relative treatment effects from a 4-way multivariate distribution:

$$
\begin{pmatrix} \delta_{i12} \\ \delta_{i13} \\ \delta_{i14} \\ \delta_{i15} \end{pmatrix} \sim MVN \left(\begin{pmatrix} d_2 \\ d_3 \\ d_4 \\ d_5 \end{pmatrix} \begin{pmatrix} \sigma^2 & 0.5\sigma^2 & 0.5\sigma^2 & 0.5\sigma^2 \\ 0.5\sigma^2 & \sigma^2 & 0.5\sigma^2 & 0.5\sigma^2 \\ 0.5\sigma^2 & 0.5\sigma^2 & \sigma^2 & 0.5\sigma^2 \\ 0.5\sigma^2 & 0.5\sigma^2 & 0.5\sigma^2 & \sigma^2 \end{pmatrix} \right)
$$

With this structure it is possible to 'trick' WinBUGS into generating predictive distributions for every treatment in every trial, regardless of which treatments appeared in which. This is done by simply including that treatment in the data structure, but giving its numerator as 'NA'. The same manoeuvre also allows the user to obtain posterior predictions for the absolute effect of any treatment in any trial. This coding is recommended for applications where a model for the baseline is being considered.

9.6 Assumptions made in mixed treatment comparisons

The assumptions can be stated in a variety of ways. The key assumption is that the treatment effect being estimated in, say, AB trials is the same (Fixed Effect models), or exchangeable with (Random Effects models) with the treatment effects that would be estimated in AC, BC, or even CD trials, if these also included treatments A and B. Another way of putting this is that every trial can be considered as a multi-arm trial including all the treatments, but that not all the treatments are reported. Those that are not reported are *missing at random*. This means that their 'missing-ness' is not related to the results.

There is an empirical literature (see Section 9.10) that generally supports the assumption, though networks with sufficient numbers of trials to test this, particularly within a random effects framework, are relatively unusual. There have been reports where the consistency assumption has been shown to *not* be met [9, 10], but in these cases authors had 'lumped' together treatment regimes with different doses or treatments combined in different combinations. Pooling results from treatments which are *known* or suspected to have different efficacy is risky: in pairwise meta-analysis this leads to heterogeneity and difficulties of interpretation, while in MTC it can cause conflict between direct and indirect evidence. In a decision-making context, where both the target patient group and the treatments tend to be very tightly defined, the introduction of covariates that can modify relative treatment effects is probably much less likely to occur. Factors that interact with the treatment effects are, of course, the origin of heterogeneity in pairwise meta-analysis and inconsistency between direct and indirect evidence.

The use of MTC certainly raises a wide range of questions about trial inclusion criteria, treatment definition, and potential relative effect modifiers that all require very careful thought. What is often overlooked is that these same factors are no less important in pairwise meta-analysis. Unfortunately, a Random Effects model can always be fitted to the data, however extreme the heterogeneity, and the difficulty of interpreting the pooled effect from such models is not always appreciated.

9.7 Embedding an MTC within a cost-effectiveness analysis

In this section we pick up the earlier theme of integrating evidence synthesis with cost-effectiveness analysis (Chapter 7), and extend it a little further to show how WinBUGS can be easily programmed to produce CEACs where there are more than two strategies.

The economic part of the model is kept deliberately simple: Figure 9.4 depicts the decision tree, and shows that benefits in the form of life years gained only accrues with the proportion who quit smoking, while the treatment costs accrue

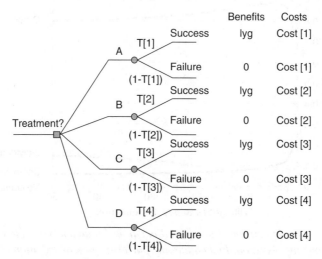

Figure 9.4   Decision tree for a cost-effectiveness analysis of four treatment strategies for smoking cessation. See text and Table 9.8 for details.

Table 9.8 Parameters for a cost-effectiveness analysis on smoking cessation.

Parameter	Code	Value
Prob (smoking cessation)	T[1], T[2], T[3], T[4]	WinBUGS joint posterior
Cost treatment 1	C[1]	0
Cost treatment 2	C[2]	200
Cost treatment 3	C[3]	6000
Cost treatment 4	C[4]	600
Life years gained per cessation	lyg	$\sim$ Normal(15,4^2)

whether or not the treatment is successful. The analysis is therefore based on our Bayesian joint posterior distribution of the relative treatment effects from Win-BUGS, combined with costs for each of the treatments and an estimate of the additional life years gained by an individual who gives up smoking (Table 9.8). The latter is estimated to be 15 years with a standard error of 4 years.

If a decision maker is willing to pay £w to gain an additional life year, the Net Benefit for each strategy k can be coded as follows:

NB{k,w} = w*T[k] * lyg−C[k]

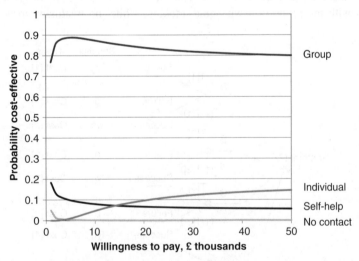

Figure 9.5 Cost-effectiveness acceptability curves for an analysis of four interventions for smoking cessation. Embedding the posterior joint distribution of treatment effects from an MTC analysis of the Hasselblad [6] data within a probabilistic cost-effectiveness analysis.

The additional code required includes a variable p.ce[k,w] the probability that treatment k is cost-effective at willingness to pay w. The following allows us to plot the CEACs for willingness to pay from £1000 to £50 000:

```
for (w in 1:50){                          # Loop over willingness to pay, w
  for (k in 1:4){                         # Loop over intervention, k
    nb[k,w]<- T[k]*lyg*w*1000 - cost[k]   # Net benefit function
    p.ce[k,w]<-equals(rank(nb[,w],k),4)   # Probability most cost-effective
}}
```

Note that in this code the absolute probability of smoking cessation on treatment k, T[k] is formed by adding the *mean* LOR to the log odds of smoking cessation on 'no contact', T[1]. (See Exercise 9.7 for the use of the predictive distribution.) The file *mtc-re-ceac.odc* contains the code for this analysis. To produce the CEACs shown in Figure 9.5, the matrix p.ce must be monitored, and then its posterior mean must be copied and pasted as four columns into Excel. Treatment 4 (group counselling) comes out as cost-effective at almost any willingness to pay. This is expected as it is the most effective treatment while also being less expensive than its main competitor, treatment 3 (individual counselling).

9.8 Extension to continuous, rate and other outcomes

The MTC example data set in this chapter has, like most meta-analyses, been based on trials that report binary outcomes. Here we show that the same MTC structures can be analysed when the trial outcomes are continuous, rate or other outcomes. As we shall see, the underlying models for all these outcomes are identical. The essential differences lie in the likelihood, as set out in Table 6.3, and therefore also in the deviance functions, and in the 'linking' functions, such as log or logit, which specify the relationship between the outcome variable and the scale of what is sometimes called the 'linear predictor'.

The invariance of the MTC model can best be seen by a comparison of the Win-BUGS code required for each outcome. For binomial data we coded the Random Effects model as follows:

```
r[i] ~ dbin(p[i],n[i])                              #binomial likelihood
logit(p[i]) <- mu[s[i]] + delta[i] * (1-equals(t[i],b[i]))   #model
delta[i] ~ dnorm(md[i],prec[i])
md[i] <- d[t[i]]−d[b[i]]
```

For continuous outcome data, for example blood pressure, we would have a mean for each arm, Y[i] and a precision P[i] of that mean. The precision of course is the inverse of the variance, which is the square of the standard error of the mean. Usually the standard error is based on the pooled standard deviation, pooling across treatment arms. The only changes are in the likelihood and in the left-hand side of the model statement: the right-hand side consists of the linear predictor, which remains unchanged:

```
Y[I] ~ dnorm(theta[i],P[i])                              #normal likelihood
theta[i] <- mu[s[i]] + delta[i] * (1-equals(t[i],b[i]))  #model
```

The same approach is used where trial summaries are reported, such as LORs $Y[i]$ for study i, with precision $P[i]$ (see Chapter 4).

Another common reporting format is a number of individuals experiencing an event (death, healing and so on) in each arm $e[i]$, and the number of person years at risk $R[i]$. The number of events can be assumed to be drawn from a Poisson distribution on the expected number of events: this is the hazard multiplied by the time at risk:

```
exp.e(i) <- theta[i] * R[i]        #expected number of events
e[i] ~ dpoiss(exp.e[i])            #poisson likelihood
log(theta[i]) <- mu[s[i]] + delta[i] *   #model
           (1-equals(t[i],b[i]))
```

This model assumes a constant hazard rate during follow-up in each trial arm. Trials quite often report numbers of patients in whom the event has occurred by a specified follow-up time, of say $T[i]$ years, with each trial possibly having a different follow-up time. If the hazard rate is λ, then the probability of the event not occurring is $\exp(-\lambda T)$, and the probability, p, that it does occur is $1- \exp(-\lambda T)$. This leads to models of the form: $1 - p = \exp(-\lambda T)$, or $-\log(1 - p) = \lambda T$, or $\log(-\log(1 - p)) = \log(T) + \log(\lambda)$. This is the so-called complementary log–log transformation. This can be coded directly in WinBUGS, modelling on the log hazard scale, i.e. $\log(\lambda)$, and $\log(T)$ as an 'offset' on the right-hand side:

```
r[i] ~ dbin(p[i],n[i])             # binomial likelihood,
                                   # p[i] prob event
cloglog(p[i]) <- log(T[i]) + mu[s[i]]
          + delta[i] * (1-equals(t[i],b[i]))   #model
```

Finally, we mention analyses which are based on differences between arms, rather than the arm-based analyses. The data then consist of the difference $D[i]$ and its precision $P[i]$:

```
D[i] ~ dnorm(delta[i],P[i])        #normal likelihood
```

There is no need to specify trial baselines mu[j]. Note that this formulation would work for continuous outcomes or in cases where the $D[i]$ is the log of the empirical LOR and $P[i]$ the reciprocal of its variance. The same code can be used for log relative risk or log hazard ratios.

All the above models are intended for a random effect formulation, with a mean specified by md[i]<- d[t[i]] - d[b[i]], and a precision parameter prec. As ever, care must be taken when putting priors on prec. With continuous outcomes, the outcome scale must be taken into account: for logistic analyses, Uniform(0,2) priors on the between-trial standard deviation may be adequate, but Uniform (0,100) may be more suitable with continuous outcomes such as IQ.

9.9 Summary key points

- Models for indirect comparisons and mixed treatment comparisons have been introduced which are extensions of the 'standard' methods for pairwise meta-analysis introduced in Chapter 4.

- Both fixed and random effect versions have been presented, and the latter has been shown to be, in effect, identical to its pairwise equivalent, but with the univariate normal distribution of the trial-specific relative treatment effect δ_j replaced by a multivariate normal of dimension $(K - 1)$, for a K-treatment MTC.

- MTC makes the same exchangeability assumptions as pairwise meta-analysis, but requires them to hold over the entire ensemble of studies, not just within the studies making the same comparison. The consistency assumptions should be checked, while recognising there are seldom enough data to rule out inconsistency. Careful attention to trial inclusion criteria, to the uniform definition of treatments, and to the potential presence of effect-modifying covariates, is strongly recommended, to limit heterogeneity.

- MTC extends naturally to continuous and hazard rate outcomes, and to analyses based on between-treatment differences.

9.10 Further reading

There has been continued debate about the extent to which the assumptions behind MTC models are met, and therefore how suitable they are for routine use. Recent papers can be consulted for slightly different opinions [11–13]. Some of the concern has been expressed through empirical studies of consistency in simple evidence networks [9, 10, 14], but it is important to remember that Equation (9.1) tells us that if indirect evidence is 'biased' in some way, this can only arise if the direct evidence on which it is based is also biased [15, 16].

Although producers of 'official' guidance on synthesis methodology adopt a relatively cautious tone [1, 17] the methods are being used at an increasing rate in practical decision-making applications, such as cost-effectiveness analyses submitted to the National Institute of Health and Clinical Excellence (NICE), and in leading clinical journals. Recently, an ISPOR Task Force (International Society for Pharmacoeconomics and Outcomes Research) on Network Meta-Analysis delivered a strong endorsement [18, 19].

Inconsistency has been a continuing focus. An interesting way of extending these models is to relax the consistency equations by adding additional parameters.

One approach is to add an 'inconsistency factor' to each consistency equation. This was the approach adopted by Lu and Ades [5]. In their formulation the inconsistency factors were drawn from a higher level distribution, the variance of which represented the variation between direct and indirect estimates. Lumley's earlier paper [20], where the expression 'network meta-analysis' was used for the first time, proposed what was effectively the same idea using the term incoherence. Lu and Ades [5] also give an explicit rationale for the number of inconsistency factors in a given network, and relates this to the degrees of freedom for inconsistency. Adding an 'inconsistency factor' to each consistency equation is equivalent to a model in which, for example, the AB, AC and BC effects are entirely unrelated (see Exercise 9.4). Another approach is 'node-splitting' [21]. Applied to MTC networks this method allows the direct evidence on any contrast to be compared with all the other evidence on that contrast [22].

There have also been further developments to the underpinning of MTC. Lu and Ades [23] have extended the homogeneous variance models used in this chapter to consider heterogeneous variance models. The consistency relation forces certain relationships between the between-study variances of the AB, AC and BC effects, which give rise to interesting problems in estimation. Another development has been the demonstration that MTC estimates are, like standard meta-analytic estimates, linear combinations of the original study-specific estimates [24].

For those seeking practical help in applying Bayesian MTC models, a wide range of worked examples, including WinBUGS computer code, can be found on the NICE Decision Support Unit (DSU) web site (http://www.nicedsu.org.uk/). These comprise the basic MTC models, including extensions to rate models, competing risk models, and probit models; inconsistency analysis; and meta-regression and regression on baseline and bias models.

A further source of worked examples on somewhat more advanced applications can be found in methodology journals. Many of these involve multiple outcomes as well as mixed treatment comparisons. Ades [25] explores a 'chain of evidence' structure (see also Eddy et al. [4]), in which evidence is available on (a) treatment effects on an intermediate outcome (coronary patency), (b) the relation between coronary patency and mortality, and (c) treatment effects on mortality. Clearly, given any two of these evidence sources it should be possible to predict the third, creating a possibility of cross-validation, and also a possibility of synthesis within a single coherent model. Another kind of multi-outcome structure is when a binary outcome, such as proportion healed, is reported at multiple follow-up times. Lu et al. [26] develop extensions to the basic MTC code for this situation.

Statistical combination of outcomes reported in different ways represents another challenge for evidence synthesis, but also an opportunity to illustrate the flexibility of Bayesian MCMC with WinBUGS. The NICE DSU web site includes examples of 'shared parameter' models that can synthesis rate parameter whether reported as binomial outcomes in a cloglog analysis, log hazard ratios and their variances, or Poisson outcomes with time at risk. In a more complex example [27], from trials on treatments for influenza, some trials reported time to end influenza while others reported time to end symptoms, and others both. In addition some reported mean time to survival and others median time, and some reported the probability of remaining with influenza up to 28 days. A synthesis was achieved using a Weibull model, with each different outcome informing a different function of the underlying parameters.

A similar situation arises in cancer trials which usually report some combination: per cent 'responders' – i.e. per cent whose tumour progression is delayed, time to tumour, and time to death. Welton *et al.* [28] show how these outcomes, which are clearly correlated as well as structurally related, can be synthesised.

A final example concerns Markov models in the context of clinical trials. According to the approach adopted in Briggs *et al.* [29] (Section 10.4), a separate Markov model is estimated for each treatment. This almost certainly represents a major over-parameterisation of the model. A more interesting alternative is to consider which transition or transitions the treatment acts on. Price *et al.* [30] look at an indirect comparison of several treatments for asthma. The treatment effect is put on the log transition rate, and the transition rates are estimated from the data, taking into account that patients may have moved between several states between the times when observations are made. This effectively embeds a conventional relative treatment effect model within a multi-parameter evidence synthesis problem of the type described in Chapter 8. This approach not only produces parameter estimates and cost-effectiveness analyses with considerably less uncertainty than are obtained by estimating a separate transition matrix for each treatment, but it can also be used to throw light on underlying mechanisms [31]. For example, it was possible to show that treatments in which patients spent more time 'successfully treated' worked by speeding recovery exacerbations, rather than by delaying the onset of an exacerbation.

9.11 Exercises

9.1 A new, 25th trial is added to the smoking cessation data. Eighteen out of 80 stop smoking on treatment 4, 14 out of 96 on new treatment 5. Adjust the *mtc-fe.odc* code to incorporate this trial. Which is the most effective treatment now? Why are the posterior results for d[2],d[3] and d[4] altered when the new evidence is added ?

9.2 Use the Monte Carlo error (MC error) summary to confirm the answer to Exercise 9.1.

9.3 Fit a Random Effects model with $\sigma \sim$ Uniform(0,0.01) and interpret the Residual Deviance and the Deviance Information Criterion (DIC) results.

9.4 Starting from the WinBUGS code mtc-re, code an alternative model in which there are separate parameters for d_{AB}, d_{AC}, d_{AD}, d_{BC}, d_{BD}, d_{CD}. This model abandons the consistency equations, but fits a Random Effects model with a 'shared' variance parameter to what is in effect a 'model' in which there are six otherwise unrelated meta-analyses. Use Residual

Deviance and DIC statistics to comment on the consistency assumptions, and compare the posterior results on the treatment effect parameters.

9.5 What are the posterior correlations between d[2], d[3], and d[4]?

9.6 Suppose we had not integrated the WinBUGS code into the cost-effectiveness analysis, but had instead programmed the cost-effectiveness analysis in a spreadsheet package, and added the posterior mean and standard deviations for the four T[k] based on WinBUGS posterior summaries. Would this give the same CEACs?

9.7 Modify the code in *mtc-re-ceac.odc* so that the economic analysis is based not on the distributions of mean treatment effects, but on the predictive distributions of treatment effects that might be expected in a new trial. Produce CEACs. Bearing in mind that the 24 RCTs in the original analyses were carried out on a range of different patient groups, which of the two alternative analyses do you think most appropriate if you had to recommend that one of the four treatments should be offered routinely by a healthcare provider?

References

1. Higgins J.P.T., Green S. *Cochrane Handbook for Systematic Reviews of Interventions Version 5.0.0 [updated February 2008]*. Chichester: The Cochrane Collaboration, John Wiley & Sons, Ltd, 2008.

2. Bucher H.C., Guyatt G.H., Griffith L.E., Walter S.D. The results of direct and indirect treatment comparisons in meta-analysis of Randomized Controlled Trials. *Journal of Clinical Epidemiology* 1997;**50**:683–691.

3. Boland A., Dundar Y., Bagust A., *et al.* Early thrombolysis for the treatment of acute myocardial infarction: a systematic review and economic evaluation. *Health Technology Assessment* 2003;**7**:1–136.

4. Eddy D.M., Hasselblad V., Shachter R. *Meta-Analysis by the Confidence Profile Method*. London: Academic Press, 1992.

5. Lu G., Ades A. Assessing evidence consistency in mixed treatment comparisons. *Journal of the American Statistical Association* 2006;**101**:447–459.

6. Hasselblad V. Meta-analysis of multi-treatment studies. *Medical Decision Making* 1998;**18**:37–43.

7. Higgins J.P.T., Whitehead A. Borrowing strength from external trials in a meta-analysis. *Statistics in Medicine* 1996;**15**:2733–2749.

8. Cipriani A., Furukawa T.A., Salanti G., *et al.* Comparative efficacy and acceptability of 12 new generation antidepressants: a multiple-treatments meta-analysis. *Lancet* 2009;**373**:746–758.

9. Song F., Altman D., Glenny A-M, Deeks J. Validity of indirect comparison for estimating efficacy of competing interventions: evidence from published meta-analyses. *British Medical Journal* 2003;**326**:472–476.

10. Chou R., Fu R., Hoyt Huffman L., Korthuis P.T. Initial highly-active antiretroviral therapy with a protease inhibitor versus non-nucleoside reverse transcriptase inhibitor: discrepancies between direct and indirect meta-analyses. *Lancet* 2006;**368**: 1503–1515.

11. Caldwell D.M., Ades A.E., Higgins J.P.T. Simultaneous comparison of multiple treatments: combining direct and indirect evidence. *British Medical Journal* 2005;**331**:897–900.

12. Salanti G., Higgins J.P.T., Ades A.E., Ioannidis J P A. Evaluation of networks of randomised trials. *Statistical Methods in Medical Research* 2008;**17**:279–301.

13. Sutton A.J., Ades A.E., Cooper N., Abrams K.R. Use of mixed and indirect comparisons in technology assessment. *Pharmacoeconomics* 2008;**26**:753–767.

14. Song F., Xiong T., Parekh-Bhurke S., *et al*. Inconsistency between direct and indirect comparisons of competing interventions: meta-epidemiological study. *British Medical Journal* 2011;**343**: d4909.

15. Caldwell D.M., Gibb D.M., Ades A.E. Validity of indirect comparisons in meta-analysis.[Letter.] *Lancet* 2007;**369**: 270.

16. Ades A.E., Dias S., Welton N.J. Song *et al* have not demonstrated inconsistency between direct and indirect comparisons (online letter). 2011. *British Medical Journal* 2011.

17. Pharmaceutical Benefits Advisory Committee. *Guidelines for preparing submissions to the Pharmaceutical Benefits Advisory Committee, Version 4.3*. Canberra: Australian Government, Department of Health and Aging, 2008.

18. Jansen J., Fleurence R., Devine B., *et al*. Interpreting indirect treatment comparisons and network meta-analysis for health-care decision making: Report of the ISPOR Task Force on Indirect Treatment Comparisons Good Research Practices: Part 1. *Value in Health* 2011;**14**:417–428.

19. Hoaglin D.C., Hawkins N., Jansen J.P., *et al*. Conducting indirect-treatment-comparison and network-meta-analysis studies: Report of the ISPOR Task Force on Indirect Treatment Comparisons Good Research Practices: Part 2. *Value in Health* 2011;**14**: 429–437.

20. Lumley T. Network meta-analysis for indirect treatment comparisons. *Statistics in Medicine* 2002;**21**:2313–2324.

21. O'Hagan A. HSSS model criticism (with discussion). In: Green P.J., Hjort N.L., Richardson S.T., eds. *Highly Structured Stochastic Systems*. Oxford: Oxford University Press, 2002; 423–453.

22. Dias S., Welton N.J., Caldwell D.M., Ades A.E. Checking consistency in mixed treatment comparison meta-analysis. *Statistics in Medicine* 2010;**29**:932–944.

23. Lu G., Ades A.E. Modelling between-trial variance structure in mixed treatment comparisons. *Biostatistics* 2009;**10**:792–805.

24. Lu G., Welton N.J., Higgins J.P.T., White I.R., Ades A.E. Linear inference for mixed treatment comparison meta-analysis: a two-stage approach. *Research Synthesis Methods* 2011;**2**:43–60.

25. Ades A.E. A chain of evidence with mixed comparisons: models for multi-parameter evidence synthesis and consistency of evidence. *Statistics in Medicine* 2003;**22**:2995–3016.

26. Lu G., Ades A.E., Sutton A.J., *et al.* Meta-analysis of mixed treatment comparisons at multiple follow-up times. *Statistics in Medicine* 2007;**26**:3681–3699.

27. Welton N.J., Cooper N.J., Ades A.E., Lu G., Sutton A.J. Mixed treatment comparison with multiple outcomes reported inconsistently across trials: evaluation of antivirals for treatment of influenza A and B. *Statistics in Medicine* 2008;**27**:5620–5639.

28. Welton N.J., Willis S.R., Ades A.E. Synthesis of survival and disease progression outcomes for health technology assessment of cancer therapies. *Research Synthesis Methods* 2010;**1**:239–257.

29. Briggs A.H., Ades A.E., Price M.J. Probabilistic sensitivity analysis for decision trees with multiple branches: Use of the Dirichlet distribution in a Bayesian framework. *Medical Decision Making* 2003;**23**:341–350.

30. Price M., Welton N., Ades A.E. Parameterisation of treatment effects for meta-analysis in multi-state Markov models. *Statistics in Medicine* 2011;**30**:140–151.

31. Price M.J., Welton N.J., Briggs A.H., Ades A.E. Model averaging in the presence of structural uncertainty about treatment effects: inflence on treatment decision and expected value of information. *Value in Health* 2011;**14**:205–218.

10

Markov models

10.1 Introduction

In Chapters 1–9 we have primarily focused on situations where there is a binary
outcome, for example survival. In pure survival models there are only two possible states that an individual can be in – alive and dead. This is illustrated in
Figure 10.1(a), where individuals in the *Alive* state may make a transition to the
Dead state, and once there they remain dead. Death is an *absorbing* state, because
it is not possible to leave that state. In models of disease progression, it is common
for there to be several possible health states, and for individuals to move between
these states over time. Figure 10.1(b) shows a common such structure where individuals move between remission and relapse states of disease, and can move to the
absorbing Dead state from either one of these health states.

In Chapter 7 an integrated approach to decision modelling was introduced and
the method demonstrated for binary outcomes using a decision tree model. In fact
this approach can readily be extended to models where there are several (multinomial) competing outcomes, as long as events are assumed not to repeat over time.
Figure 10.1(c) shows one such example where newborns that develop meningitis may go on to one of three possible health states: *OK, Disability*, and *Dead*.
However, for events that may occur repeatedly (for example transitions between
manic and depressive episodes for bipolar disorders illustrated in Figure 10.1(d)),
or over a prolonged time period (for example HIV illustrated in Figure 10.1(e),
cancer, or heart disease), the decision tree becomes 'bushy' and the approach cum-
bersome [1]. For this reason, the use of decision trees is most suited to problems
that involve chance events that occur over a relatively short time period, so that
only one possible state transition may occur.

Evidence Synthesis for Decision Making in Healthcare, First Edition. Nicky J. Welton,
Alexander J. Sutton, Nicola J. Cooper, Keith R. Abrams and A.E. Ades.
© 2012 John Wiley & Sons, Ltd. Published 2012 by John Wiley & Sons, Ltd.

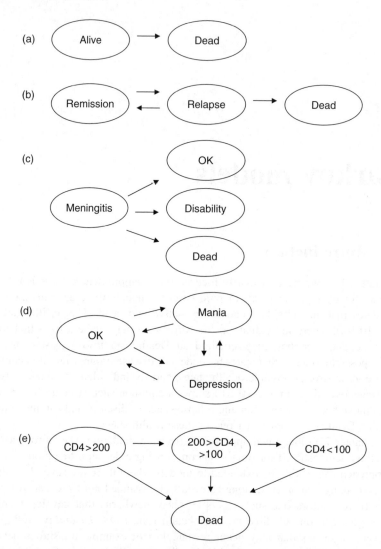

Figure 10.1   Three examples of multi-state models, where the different states are shown in ovals, and the arrows indicate possible transitions between states for: (a) pure survival model; (b) disease remission model where individuals cycle between remission and recurrence states, and can die when in either state; (c) competing risk model where newborns with meningitis, if they survive, are left with either no, mild, moderate, or severe disabilities; (d) repeating events in bipolar disorders; and (e) progression through CD4 states for HIV patients in the absence of treatment.

In this chapter we introduce Markov models, which can be used to describe transitions between states where events can repeat over time. We extend the ideas in Chapter 7 to present an integrated approach for decision analysis for these more complex models that avoids 'bushy' decision trees [2]. We begin by describing Markov models, how they can be viewed in both continuous and discrete time, and how to build a decision analysis around a Markov model. We then illustrate, using an example data set on treatments for asthma in children, how the state transition parameters can be estimated from a single trial and the results integrated in a decision model. Finally we discuss how transition parameters can be estimated from a synthesis of available evidence, in particular focusing on different formats for reporting results that may have been used in different studies.

10.2 Continuous and discrete time Markov models

A multi-state model is one in which at any one point in time individuals are in one of a finite set of health states and progression between the health states over time occurs according to a set of transition parameters. Time is therefore a key aspect of these models. We can view time in two different ways. We can think of time as a continuum, in which case the relevant transition parameters are transition *rates*. For example, in a survival analysis the relevant transition parameter would be the mortality rate for a given degree of exposure to risk, such as annual mortality rate per 100 000 capita. Alternatively, we can think of time chopped up into equal discrete time periods. For example, we may consider transitions from one week to the next, so that each week is a different time period and the cycle length of the process is 1 week. In this case, the relevant transition parameters are transition *probabilities*. For example, in a survival analysis the relevant transition parameter may be the probability of death over a 1-month time period. Clearly, transition rates and transition probabilities are related quantities, and generally one can be derived from the other through a system of differential equations (see Section 10.6.2). Typically, discrete time models are used in decision analysis where, for computational convenience, movement between the states is assumed to occur at fixed increments of time (e.g. daily, weekly, monthly, yearly), usually chosen to represent a clinically meaningful time interval.

In a general multi-state model the transition rates and probabilities for each individual can depend on the complete history of previous transitions between states. For example, the probability of a remission could be different for an individual who has previously had a remission than for an individual who has never had a remission. Markov models make the simplifying assumption that the transition rates and probabilities only depend on the current state that an individual is in. In other words, all previous transitions are 'forgotten'. This special property is called the Markov property or Memoryless property. Markov models provide a powerful modelling tool because they build in time dependence, whilst at the same time remaining simple enough to compute.

10.3 Decision analysis with Markov models

Figure 10.2 illustrates a discrete time decision model for the disease remission example. This simple model consists of three health states – *Well, Recurrence* and *Dead*. The arrows indicate possible pathways through the model and each is assigned a probability, π. These transition probabilities form the matrix presented in Table 10.1. Note that each row of the matrix must sum to one as in each cycle of the model an individual in, say, the Well state must either remain in Well or move to Recurrence or Dead. Also as Dead is obviously an absorbing state (a state from which it is impossible to return), the probability of remaining in Dead is one. Zeros in the transition matrix indicate pathways that are not possible given the model (for example Dead to Well). In a fully probabilistic model, the transition probabilities will be expressed with uncertainty by specifying relevant distributions (see Section 10.4). Each health state is assigned a set of outcomes, costs (C) and utilities (U), which can be summarised as an expected *payoff* associated with a single cycle spent in that health state.

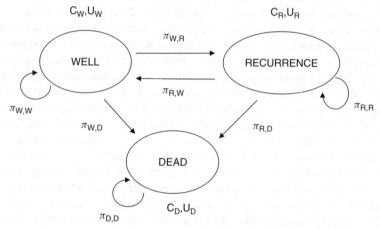

Figure 10.2   A discrete time decision model for the disease remission example, where the πs denote transition probabilities, the costs per cycle are denoted by C and the utilities by U.

Table 10.1   Transition probability matrix for example presented in Figure 10.2.

		Time, $t+1$		
		Well	Recurrence	Dead
Time, t	Well	$0.7\ (\pi_{W,W})$	$0.2\ (\pi_{W,R})$	$0.1\ (\pi_{W,D})$
	Recurrence	$0.2\ (\pi_{R,W})$	$0.6\ (\pi_{R,R})$	$0.2\ (\pi_{R,D})$
	Dead	0	0	$1\ (\pi_{D})$

10.3.1   Evaluating Markov models

Typically, economic Markov models are evaluated using cohort simulation as this focuses on the average individual experience [3]. Micro-simulation methods may be more appropriate where the focus is on characterising variability between individuals, but these methods are not discussed here.

Cohort simulation considers a hypothetical cohort of individuals distributed among the different health states and follows their movement between health states from cycle to cycle based on the specified transition probabilities [4]. Figure 10.3 illustrates the first two time cycles of a cohort simulation for the above example model assuming a cohort size of 1000 all starting in the Well state. At each time cycle, the number of individuals in each state is multiplied by the relevant transition probability (specified in Table 10.1) to calculate individuals' movement between states. The model is usually run until all (or nearly all) individuals reach the absorbing state; in this case Dead.

Expected payoffs are calculated for each cycle of the model by multiplying the number of individuals in each health state by the relevant cost and utility. This process is illustrated in Table 10.2 for expected costs, but is the same for utilities. Summing the cycle costs and dividing by 1000 individuals in the cohort gives the average cost for each individual (£2900). Note that for economic models it is usual practice to discount costs and utilities that occur in the future. This can be achieved by weighting each of the cycle costs by a factor that reflects how far it is into the future. The discount factor for the nth cycle can be calculated as $1/(1+r)^n$ where

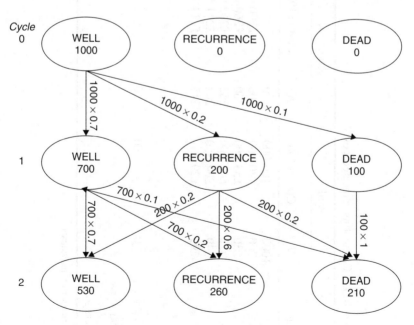

Figure 10.3   Cohort simulation.

Table 10.2 Calculating expected costs.

Cycle	Well		Recurrence		Dead		Cycle cost	Discounted cycle cost
	N	Cost (£100)	N	Cost (£1000)	N	Cost (£0)		
0	1000	£100 000	0	£0	0	£0		
1	700	£70 000	200	£200 000	100	£0	£270 000	£262 135.92
2	530	£53 000	260	£260 000	210	£0	£313 000	£295 032.52
3	423	£42 300	262	£262 000	315	£0	£304 300	£278 477.61
4	349	£34 850	242	£241 800	410	£0	£276 650	£245 799.94
5	292	£29 231	215	£214 780	493	£0	£244 011	£210 486.03
.	.		.		.		.	
.	.		.		.		.	
.	.		.		.		.	
90	0	£0	0	£0	1000	£0	£0	£0.03
Total							£2 899 997	£2 356 231
Average							£2900	£2356

N, number of individuals.

r denotes the discount rate. The discounted cost is presented in the last column of Table 10.2, where the discount rate, r, has been set to 3%.

Note that in this illustrative example the model parameters (i.e. transition probabilities and costs) are assumed fixed. As described in Chapter 7, a probabilistic model can be fitted by expressing the model parameters as distributions and then using Monte Carlo or Monte Carlo Markov Chain (MCMC) simulation to evaluate the model. With Markov models care needs to be taken when defining uncertainty in the transition probability matrix to ensure that the rows sum to one at each iteration of the sampler. This, along with other issues, is addressed in the following sections of this chapter.

10.4 Estimating transition parameters from a single study

The decision analysis presented in Section 10.3 relies on having estimated values for the transition parameters together with the uncertainties in these estimates. Typically, these parameters are estimated independently of each other either using evidence on specific transitions from a single study or meta-analysis of studies, or by using different evidence sources for different transitions. However, for a given current state occupied by an individual, the state transitions by the next time cycle are not independent. This is because transition probabilities must sum to one (or equivalently the rates must sum to zero). In this section we illustrate how the transitions probability parameters may be estimated jointly from a single study, together with uncertainties in the parameter estimates.

Example 10.1   Prophylactic treatments for asthma [5].

We use as an example data from two arms of a 4-arm clinical trial comparing prophylactic treatment for asthma in children. Each week the patients were defined to be one of five health states:

1. STW: successfully treated week

2. UTW: unsuccessfully treated week

3. Hex: hospital treated exacerbation

4. Pex: primary care treated exacerbation

5. TF: treatment failure (absorbing state)

When a patient experienced treatment failure, they were taken off the treatment and remained in treatment failure for the remaining follow-up in the trial, so that treatment failure is an absorbing state. Figure 10.4 shows the Markov transition model for progression between these five health states, where the 1-week transition

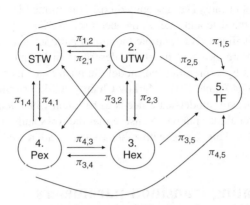

Figure 10.4 Markov model showing possible 1-week transitions between health states STW, UTW, Pex, Hex and TF in the asthma example. The probability of making the transition from state i to state j in a 1-week time period is denoted by $\pi_{i,j}$.

probability that a patient moves from state i to state j in a 1-week time period is denoted by $\pi_{i,j}$.

We shall concentrate on the joint estimation of transition parameters in a single arm, so although the trial compared four treatments, to keep the example simple we restrict attention to just two of the trial arms:

1. Seretide[TM]: salmeterol/fluticasone propionate combination 50/100 mcg bid

2. Fluticasone: fluticasone propionate 100 mcg bid

We model the two arms independently, but in Section 10.5 outline how the arms can be jointly estimated and the methods extended to mixed treatment comparison meta-analysis.

Table 10.3 shows the data reported from the Seretide[TM] and Fluticasone arms over a 12-week follow-up period. The observed transitions are summarised into aggregate form. For example, the first row of the Seretide[TM] arm shows that there were 210 observations where a STW state was followed by another STW state, 60 observations where a STW state was followed by an UTW state and so on. The second row of the Seretide[TM] arm shows that there were 88 observations where an UTW state was followed by a STW state, 641 observations where an UTW state was followed by another UST state, and so on. Note that there are 12 observed transitions for each patient for each of the 12 weeks follow-up, but it is not possible to see the exact sequence of transitions from the reported data. Under the Markov assumption, each transition depends only on the current state and not on the history of transitions prior to the current state. The reported data are therefore sufficient to estimate Markov transition parameters, but there is not enough information reported to investigate more complex models or to assess whether the Markov assumption holds in this example.

Table 10.3   Numbers of observed transitions, $r_{i,j}$, between pairs of states i and j over a 12-week follow-up period for treatment arms Seretide™ and Fluticasone in the asthma example. The row total, n_i, represents the total number of observations where patients had previously spent a week in state i (note that each patient may count more than once to each transition count and row total).

Observed no. of transitions, $r_{i,j}$	STW, $j=1$	UTW, $j=2$	Hex, $j=3$	Pex, $j=4$	TF, $j=5$	Row total, n_i
Seretide^{TM} (12 weeks follow-up)						
STW, $i=1$	210	60	0	1	1	272
UTW, $i=2$	88	641	0	4	13	746
Hex, $i=3$	0	0	0	0	0	0
Pex, $i=4$	1	0	0	0	1	2
TF, $i=5$	0	0	0	0	81	81
Fluticasone (12 weeks follow-up)						
STW, $i=1$	66	32	0	0	2	100
UTW, $i=2$	42	752	0	5	20	819
Hex, $i=3$	0	0	0	0	0	0
Pex, $i=4$	0	4	0	1	0	5
TF, $i=5$	0	0	0	0	156	156

10.4.1 Likelihood

Each row of data, in the format displayed in Table 10.3, has a multinomial likelihood. Given the row total, n_i, starting a week having previously spent a week in state i, there are five possible subsequent states: STW, UTW, Hex, Pex or TF, each with a corresponding transition probability: $\pi_{i,1}, \pi_{i,2}, \pi_{i,3}, \pi_{i,4}, \pi_{i,5}$, where these probabilities are constrained to sum to 1. We write this likelihood as:

$$(r_{i,1}, r_{i,2}, r_{i,3}, r_{i,4}, r_{i,5}) \sim \text{Multinomial}(\pi_{i,1}, \pi_{i,2}, \pi_{i,3}, \pi_{i,4}, \pi_{i,5}; n_i)$$

The multinomial distribution is the extension of the Binomial for when there are more than two possible outcomes – five in the asthma example.

Each row of Table 10.3 is independent, but the counts *within* rows are not independent. This is because each individual starting in state i must make a transition to one of the five states. If there is a high probability that they go to STW, then there will be correspondingly lower probabilities of going to the other states. There is no likelihood for the absorbing state because all transitions from this state are to the absorbing state with certainty (probability $\pi_{5,5} = 1$).

10.4.2 Priors and posteriors for multinomial probabilities

The Dirichlet is the natural prior distribution to use for multinomial probabilities. The Dirichlet is the extension of the Beta distribution for more than two probabilities that are constrained to sum to 1, and is conjugate to the multinomial likelihood. This means that the posterior distribution for the transition probabilities is also Dirichlet. The Dirichlet distribution has the same number of parameters as there are states (five in the asthma example):

$$(\pi_{i,1}, \pi_{i,2}, \pi_{i,3}, \pi_{i,4}, \pi_{i,5}) \sim \text{Dirichlet}(d_{i,1}, d_{i,2}, d_{i,3}, d_{i,4}, d_{i,5})$$

The prior values for the d's represent the prior number expected in each state for a given prior sample size [6]. For example, if we believe a priori that each transition is equally likely, then each of the d's will be equal, and the larger the d's the more certain we are of this assertion. Typically, all the d's are set equal to 1 for a flat prior.

Because the Dirichlet distribution is conjugate to the Multinomial, we can write down the posterior distribution for the transition probabilities in closed form:

$$(\pi_{i,1}, \pi_{i,2}, \pi_{i,3}, \pi_{i,4}, \pi_{i,5}) \sim \text{Dirichlet}(d_{i,1} + r_{i,1}, d_{i,2} + r_{i,2}, d_{i,3} + r_{i,3},$$
$$d_{i,4} + r_{i,4}, d_{i,5} + r_{i,5})$$

We shall, however, illustrate how to find this posterior distribution in WinBUGS, as this provides a useful simulation framework for propagating the joint parameter uncertainties into a decision model (see Section 10.5).

Example 10.2 revisited   Prophylactic treatments for asthma [5].

The WinBUGS code to estimate the transition parameters for the asthma example is:

```
model{                                         # Treatments: tmt=1 (Seretide™),
   for (tmt in 1:2){                           # tmt=2 (Fluticasone)
      for (i in 1:4){                          # There are 4 non-absorbing states
         r[tmt,i,1:5] ~ dmulti(pi[tmt,i,1:5],n[tmt,i])   # Multinomial data
         pi[tmt,i,1:5] ~ ddirch(prior[tmt,i,1:5])        # Dirichlet prior for probabilities
      }
   }
}
```

We use the structure format for inputting data to enter matrices:

```
#Data

list(                                                          # Seretide
     r=structure(.Data=c(210,   60,   0,   1,   1,             # Row 1 (STW)
                          88,  641,   0,   4,  13,             # Row 2 (UTW)
                           0,    0,   0,   0,   0,             # Row 3 (Hex)
                           1,    0,   0,   0,   1,             # Row 4 (Pex)
                                                               # Fluticasone
                          66,   32,   0,   0,   2,             # Row 1 (STW)
                          42,  752,   0,   5,  20,             # Row 2 (UTW)
                           0,    0,   0,   0,   0,             # Row 3 (Hex)
                           0,    4,   0,   1,   0),            # Row 4 (Pex)
                        .Dim=c(2,4,5)),                        # Matrix
                                                               # dimensions
     n=structure(.Data=c(272,746,0,2,  100,819,0,5), .Dim=c(2,4)),   # Row totals

     prior=structure(.Data=c(1,1,1,1,1,   1,1,1,1,1,   1,1,1,1,1,    # Dirichlet priors,
     1,1,1,1,1,   1,1,1,1,1,   1,1,1,1,1,   1,1,1,1,1,   1,1,1,1,1),  # all set = 1
                     .Dim=c(2,4,5))
)
```

Table 10.4 shows the resulting posterior means for the transition probabilities with 95% credible intervals. Note that where there are no data (on transitions from Hex) the posterior distribution is equal to the prior (i.e. each destination state has equal probability = 0.2).

Table 10.4 Posterior means for the transition probabilities with 95% credible intervals for treatment arms Seretide™ and Fluticasone in the asthma example.

Posterior mean for $\pi_{i,j}$ (95% credible interval)	STW, $j = 1$	UTW, $j = 2$	Hex, $j = 3$	Pex, $j = 4$	TF, $j = 5$
Seretide™					
STW, $i = 1$	0.762 (0.71,0.81)	0.220 (0.17,0.27)	0.004 (0.00,0.01)	0.007 (0.00,0.02)	0.007 (0.00,0.02)
UTW, $i = 2$	0.119 (0.10,0.14)	0.855 (0.83,0.88)	0.001 (0.00,0.01)	0.007 (0.00,0.01)	0.019 (0.01,0.03)
Hex, $i = 3$	0.200 (0.01,0.61)	0.200 (0.01,0.61)	0.200 (0.01,0.61)	0.200 (0.01,0.61)	0.200 (0.01,0.61)
Pex, $i = 4$	0.286 (0.04,0.64)	0.144 (0.00,0.47)	0.144 (0.00,0.46)	0.142 (0.00,0.46)	0.284 (0.04,0.64)
TF, $i = 5$	0	0	0	0	1
Fluticasone					
STW, $i = 1$	0.638 (0.54,0.73)	0.314 (0.23,0.41)	0.010 (0.00,0.03)	0.009 (0.00,0.03)	0.029 (0.01,0.07)
UTW, $i = 2$	0.052 (0.04,0.07)	0.914 (0.89,0.93)	0.001 (0.00,0.00)	0.007 (0.00,0.01)	0.026 (0.02,0.04)
Hex, $i = 3$	0.200 (0.01,0.60)	0.200 (0.01,0.60)	0.200 (0.01,0.60)	0.200 (0.01,0.60)	0.200 (0.01,0.60)
Pex, $i = 4$	0.101 (0.00,0.34)	0.500 (0.21,0.79)	0.100 (0.00,0.34)	0.199 (0.03,0.48)	0.100 (0.00,0.33)
TF, $i = 5$	0	0	0	0	1

The following code calculates Residual Deviance for multinomial likelihood (see Table 6.3):

```
for (tmt in 1:2){                           # Loop over treatments
   for (i in 1:4){                          # Loop over starting states
      for (j in 1:5){                       # Loop over destination states
         rhat[tmt,i,j]<- pi[tmt,i,j]*n[tmt,i]    # Predicted no. given model
         dev[tmt,i,j]<-                          # residual deviance for each cell
            2*r[tmt,i,j]*log(r[tmt,i,j]/rhat[tmt,i,j])
      }
      resdev[tmt,i]<- sum(dev[tmt,i,1:5])   # residual deviance for each row
   }
}
resdevtot<- sum(resdev[1:2,1:4])            # total residual deviance
```

The resulting posterior summaries for the residual deviance are shown in Table 10.5.

Table 10.5   Posterior summaries for the residual deviance in the prophylactic treatments for the asthma example.

Node	Mean	sd	MC error	2.5%	Median	97.5%	Start	Sample
resdev[1, 1]	5.238	3.325	0.02319	0.8928	4.548	13.5	10 001	20 000
resdev[1, 2]	5.039	3.165	0.02315	0.8708	4.398	12.93	10 001	20 000
resdev[1, 4]	3.042	1.676	0.01229	0.7141	2.736	7.192	10 001	20 000
resdev[2, 1]	5.893	3.377	0.02482	1.202	5.269	14.04	10 001	20 000
resdev[2, 2]	5.022	3.168	0.02111	0.8541	4.376	13.02	10 001	20 000
resdev[2, 4]	4.614	2.483	0.01644	1.104	4.184	10.57	10 001	20 000
resdevtot	28.85	7.152	0.04939	16.6	28.14	44.52	10 001	20 000

There are four unconstrained data points for each row of data, so we expect the posterior mean for the total residual deviance to be roughly equal to 32. However, there was no evidence at all for the Hex state, so in fact there are also two redundant rows of data. We therefore expect a value closer to 24. In the asthma example the posterior mean for the total residual deviance is 29, showing that the model predictions fit fairly well to the observed data, and there is little evidence of extra-multinomial variation.

The shade of each square on the grid in Figure 10.5 shows the strength of correlation between two transition probabilities, and the direction of the line shows whether it is a positive or negative correlation. We can see that there are only correlations between probabilities in the same row of data. In other words the estimated transition probabilities are independent *between* rows. However, there are negative correlations between transition probabilities for a given treatment and intial state (i.e. *within* rows of data). This is because the probabilities must sum to one. If on a given iteration of the MCMC simulation one particular transition probability is high, then the other transition probabilities from that row must be lower to ensure they still sum to one. This imposes the negative correlations. Any resulting inference or decision analysis made on these estimated transition probabilities should incorporate the correlations resulting from their joint estimation.

10.5 Propagating uncertainty in Markov parameters into a decision model

We can obtain summaries from a Markov model by repeatedly applying the transition parameters over time to find the expected number or proportion of individuals in each state after a certain number of time periods have elapsed. For example, we can find the proportion of individuals in each state in the asthma model over a 12-week period. Various summaries can then be calculated to compare the performance of the two treatments. The key outcome of interest in this analysis was the expected number of successfully treated weeks (i.e. time spent in STW, state 1). If we perform these calculations in WinBUGS then they can be evaluated for each iteration of the MCMC simulation, so that we obtain posterior summaries that incorporate all uncertainties, dependencies and correlations in the transition parameters that feed into the decision model. We can also obtain Bayesian p-values that tell us the proportion of simulations when the expected time in STW was greatest under Seretide^{TM} compared with Fluticasone (i.e. the probability that Seretide^{TM} is 'best' according to this criterion).

Let $s_{i,t}$ be the proportion of individuals in state i at time t. This needs to be initialised at time $t = 1$. For example, we could suppose that all individuals put on treatment are initially in state STW ($i = 1$), in which case $s_{1,1} = 1$ and $s_{2,1} = s_{3,1} = s_{4,1} = s_{5,1} = 0$. The proportion in each state at time t can be found from the proportions in each state at time $(t - 1)$ and the transition probabilities:

$$s_{i,t} = s_{1,(t-1)}\pi_{1,i} + s_{2,(t-1)}\pi_{2,i} + s_{3,(t-1)}\pi_{3,i} + s_{4,(t-1)}\pi_{4,i} \qquad (10.1)$$

Of the proportion of individuals in state $i = 1$ at time $(t - 1)$, a proportion $\pi_{1,i}$ will move from state 1 to state i by time t. Similarly, of the proportion of individuals in state $i = 2$ at time $(t - 1)$, a proportion $\pi_{2,i}$ will move from state 2 to state i by time t, and so on. Equation (10.1) is known mathematically as an *inner product* between $s_{(t-1)}$, the vector of proportions in each state at time $(t - 1)$, and π_i, the vector of transition probabilities to destination state i. WinBUGS has an inner product function that can be used to easily calculate summaries from Markov models.

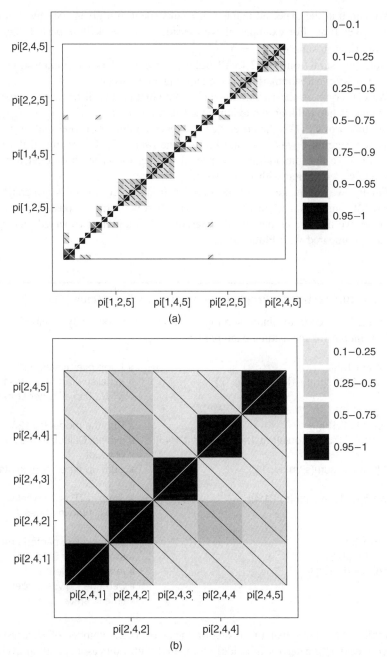

Figure 10.5   Correlation matrix for: (a) all transition probabilities and (b) focusing on transitions from Pex (state 4) for Fluticasone (treatment 2). The line in each square in the grid represents the direction of correlation (all negative given treatment and starting state), and the shading represents the strength of the correlation (see key).

We can find the expected number of weeks spent in a given state by summing the $s_{i,t}$ over time. For example, if we consider a 12-week time period, then the expected time in state i is $E_i = \sum_{t=2}^{13} s_{i,t}$.

Note, we sum from $t = 2$ to 13 because time $t = 1$ is the initialisation time point, and we want summaries for the subsequent 12 weeks.

We can compare the two treatments by calculating the difference in expected time in each state (adding in a treatment subscript, tmt), $D_i = E_{tmt=1,i} - E_{tmt=2,i}$.

In other words, D_i is the difference in expected number of weeks spent in state i between Seretide™ ($tmt = 1$) and Fluticasone ($tmt = 2$). For example, if we set $i = 1$, then we find the additional expected number of successfully treated weeks on Seretide™ compared with Fluticasone.

Finally, we can make use of the step function to record a 1 every iteration of the MCMC simulation when $D_i > 0$, so that when we form the posterior mean of this node, we find the probability that Seretide™ has a greater expected time spent in state i compared with Fluticasone.

Example 10.3 revisited   Prophylactic treatments for asthma [5].

The WinBUGS code to obtain summaries from a decision analysis based on the Markov model for the asthma example is:

```
for (tmt in 1:2){                               # Loop over treatment
  for (i in 1:5){ s[tmt,i,1]<- equals(i,1) }    # Initialise starting state: 1 in
                                                # STW,  0 in all other states
  for (i in 1:4){
    for (t in 2:13){                            # Run the model for 12
      s[tmt,i,t]<- inprod(s[tmt,1:4,t-1], pi[tmt,1:4,i])   # cycles. Calculate the inner-
    }                                           # product
    E[tmt,i]<- sum(s[tmt,i,2:13])               # Sum up time spent in state i
  }
  E[tmt,5]<- 12-sum(E[tmt,1:4])                 # Time in TF is 12 weeks
}                                               # minus time in states 1 to 4

for (i in 1:5){                                 # Additional expected time in
  D[i]<- E[1,i]-E[2,i]                          # state i under Seretide™
  prob[i]<- step(D[i])                          # Indicates whether
}                                               # Seretide™ gives longer
                                                # time in state i
```

Table 10.6 shows that the posterior mean expected number of successfully treated weeks is greater for Seretide™ compared with Fluticasone, and on average less time is spent in the other health states (UTW, Hex, Pex, and TF). There are on average two additional successfully treated weeks on Seretide™, and the probability of the number of successfully treated weeks on Seretide™ compared with Fluticasone is practically 1.

Table 10.6   Posterior summaries for the expected time spent in each health state for the two treatments in the asthma example.

Posterior mean (95% credible interval)	STW, $(i = 1)$	UTW, $(i = 2)$	Hex, $(i = 3)$	Pex, $(i = 4)$	TF, $(i = 5)$
Expected no. of weeks in state i					
Seretide™	5.03	5.75	0.05	0.10	1.06
Fluticasone	2.64	7.17	0.07	0.12	2.00

Additional expected time in state i for Seretide™ compared with Fluticasone

2.39	−1.42	−0.02	−0.02	−0.94
(1.2, 3.5)	(−2.7, −0.0)	(−0.2, 0.1)	(−0.2, 0.1)	(−2.1, 0.1)

Probability that expected time in state i is greater for Seretide™ than Fluticasone

0.999	0.022	0.414	0.411	0.037

10.6   Estimating transition parameters from a synthesis of several studies

10.6.1   Challenges for meta-analysis of evidence on Markov transition parameters

In Section 10.4 we saw how to estimate Markov transition parameters from a single study reporting data in aggregate summary form. The approach allowed the uncertainty and correlations inherent from the joint estimation of related parameters to be characterised. Extending the approach to meta-analysis of evidence from several studies that provide information on Markov transition parameters is challenging for a number of reasons.

Studies may report results in different formats at different observation times and for different outcomes. Some studies may report aggregate summaries in the same format as described in Section 10.4 (Table 10.3), which provide information directly on transition probabilities. We can think of these data as *partially observed* because we only know state occupancy at specific points in time, and do not have information on any intervening transitions between those two time points. Other studies may report detailed event history data giving the number of events and time at risk, which provide information directly on transition rates, rather than probabilities. We can think of these data as *continuously observed* because we have information on all transitions that occur. Studies reporting aggregate data may report transitions for different cycle lengths – for example one study may inform 1-week transition probabilities, whereas another may tell us directly about 1-month transition probabilities. Also, different studies may report results for different states. For example, some studies may only provide information on survival rather than detailed disease progression, whereas other studies may only be concerned with particular disease specific end-points. It may seem impossible to combine information in the face of such heterogeneously reported results. However, the underlying process of disease progression is the same in all of the studies, it is just that they provide information on different functions of the underlying basic model parameters, as was the case in Chapter 8. Therefore the studies can be statistically combined, but this needs to be done with care, exploiting mathematical relationships between the Markov transition parameters (see Sections 10.6.2–10.6.7).

The objective of synthesising evidence from different studies is to obtain combined estimates of Markov transition parameters that reflect the available body of evidence. These estimates may in turn input into downstream analyses, such as a cost-effectiveness analysis. It is of little value to obtain different estimates in each study and in each arm of each study, with no pooled estimates that can be used to summarise the evidence. We therefore cannot consider different studies or arms of studies independently, and must impose structured models on the baseline progression of disease and impact of treatment on disease progression. Because there are multiple states, this process is more complex than for meta-analysis with a single outcome – for example, we need to consider which transitions the treatment effect may be acting on. Modelling the transition parameters also allows the mixed treatment comparison models presented in Chapter 9 to be extended to Markov models.

Unfortunately, when modelling transition parameters, it is rare that we can work directly with transition probabilities. Although logistic regression models that are typically used with binary data can be extended to multinomial outcomes, the necessity for transition probabilities to sum to 1 leads to model parameters that do not have a natural interpretation. Instead, it is much more convenient to model transition rates, which are only constrained to be positive. Log-linear models can then be used to model the rates, and regression parameters can be interpreted as hazard ratios.

Evidence reported in an event history format directly informs rate parameters through Poisson likelihoods. Evidence reported in aggregate format informs transition probabilities for a given observation cycle length, which in turn can be written down as functions of the underlying rate parameters. In the terminology introduced in Chapters 8 and 9, the transition rates are the *basic* parameters, and the transition probabilities are the *functional* parameters. The transition rates and probabilities are functionally related through a system of differential equations – see Section 10.6.2

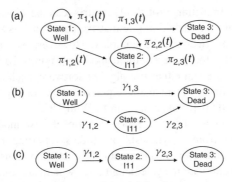

Figure 10.6 Three-state Markov models: (a) in discrete time with transition prob-abilities $\pi_{i,j}(t)$ from state i to state j with observed cycle length t; (b) in continuous time with transition rates $\gamma_{i,j}$; (c) in continuous time where all transitions from state 1 to state 3 occur via tunnel state 2.

for more details. Treating transition rates, rather than transition probabilities, as the basic parameters has the added advantage that we can fit models with fewer parameters. To illustrate suppose we had aggregate data on all three of the transitions displayed in Figure 10.6(a). By modelling transition probabilities we would be obliged to include three transition probability parameters. However, if we model transition rates, then both the models displayed in Figure 10.6(b) and 10.6(c) are possible, with either three or two rate parameters. Figure 10.6(c) is a feasible alternative because all of the observed transitions from state 1 to state 3 may have gone via state 2.

In the remainder of this section we show how studies reporting aggregate data can be combined to indirectly inform transition rates, demonstrate how studies reporting event history data can directly inform transition rates, and finally outline how treatment effects can be incorporated in this framework. The material is based on Welton and Ades [7] and is reasonably technical, and can be omitted without losing continuity for the remainder of the book.

10.6.2* The relationship between probabilities and rates

Transition probabilities and rates are mathematically related through a system of differential equations, known as Kolmorgorov's forward equations [8]:

$$P'(t) = P(t)G \qquad (10.2)$$

where $P(t)$ is the matrix of transition probabilities with cycle length t, and G is the matrix of transition rates. Equation (10.2) can be solved to give

$$P(t) = e^{tG} \qquad (10.3)$$

In other words the transition probability matrix can be obtained by taking the exponential of t times the transition rate matrix. This is not as simple as it sounds, as exponentials of matrices can be complex. However, we can write down the solutions algebraically for some common models (Figures 10.7–10.9). For more complicated models, we can either use algebra software, such as Maple, to obtain solutions in closed form, or solve the equations numerically within an MCMC simulation using WBDiff [9] as an add-on to WinBUGS.

Figure 10.10 gives a schematic representation of how model parameters can be jointly estimated from a synthesis of studies reporting results in different formats. Aggregate data provide information directly on transition probabilities, $P(t_e)$ for a given observation cycle length, t_e, which are functions of the rate parameters, G, via the forward equations. Event history data provide information directly on the rate parameters, G. The forward equations can then be invoked again to obtain estimates for transition probabilities at any cycle time, t, required for a decision analysis. We illustrate how this can be achieved in WinBUGS in Sections 10.6.3–10.6.7.

State 1 $\xrightarrow{\gamma_{1,2}}$ State 2

$$G = \begin{bmatrix} -\gamma_{1,2} & \gamma_{1,2} \\ 0 & 0 \end{bmatrix}$$

$$P(t) = \begin{bmatrix} e^{-(\gamma_{1,2})t} & 1 - e^{-(\gamma_{1,2})t} \\ 0 & 1 \end{bmatrix}$$

Figure 10.7 Two-state forwards model, rate matrix G, and corresponding transition probability matrix, $P(t)$ that solves Kolmorgorov's forward equations.

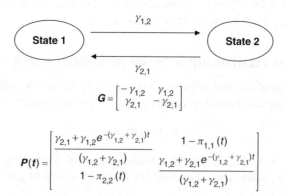

State 1 $\xrightarrow{\gamma_{1,2}}$ State 2
$\xleftarrow{\gamma_{2,1}}$

$$G = \begin{bmatrix} -\gamma_{1,2} & \gamma_{1,2} \\ \gamma_{2,1} & -\gamma_{2,1} \end{bmatrix}$$

$$P(t) = \begin{bmatrix} \dfrac{\gamma_{2,1} + \gamma_{1,2} e^{-(\gamma_{1,2} + \gamma_{2,1})t}}{(\gamma_{1,2} + \gamma_{2,1})} & 1 - \pi_{1,1}(t) \\ 1 - \pi_{2,2}(t) & \dfrac{\gamma_{1,2} + \gamma_{2,1} e^{-(\gamma_{1,2} + \gamma_{2,1})t}}{(\gamma_{1,2} + \gamma_{2,1})} \end{bmatrix}$$

Figure 10.8 Two-state forwards and backwards model, rate matrix G, and corresponding transition probability matrix, $P(t)$ that solves Kolmorgorov's forward equations.

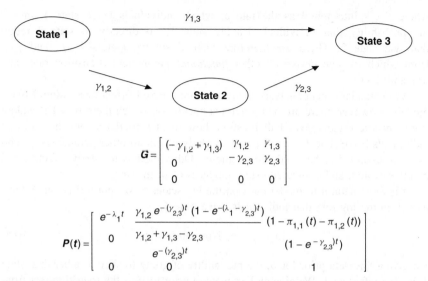

$$G = \begin{bmatrix} (-\gamma_{1,2} + \gamma_{1,3}) & \gamma_{1,2} & \gamma_{1,3} \\ 0 & -\gamma_{2,3} & \gamma_{2,3} \\ 0 & 0 & 0 \end{bmatrix}$$

$$P(t) = \begin{bmatrix} e^{-\lambda_1 t} & \dfrac{\gamma_{1,2}\, e^{-(\gamma_{2,3})t}\, (1 - e^{-(\lambda_1 - \gamma_{2,3})t})}{\gamma_{1,2} + \gamma_{1,3} - \gamma_{2,3}} & (1 - \pi_{1,1}(t) - \pi_{1,2}(t)) \\ 0 & e^{-(\gamma_{2,3})t} & (1 - e^{-\gamma_{2,3})t}) \\ 0 & 0 & 1 \end{bmatrix}$$

*Figure 10.9   Three-state forwards model, rate matrix **G**, and corresponding transition probability matrix, **P(t)** that solves Kolmorgorov's forward equations.*

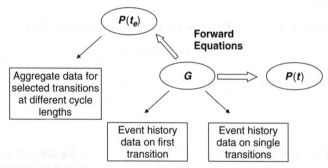

*Figure 10.10   Aggregate data provide information directly on transition probabilities, **P(t_e)** for a given observation cycle length, t_e, which are functions of the rate parameters, **G**, via the forward equations. Event history data provides information directly on the rate parameters, **G**.*

10.6.3* Modelling study effects

We use as an example the three-state forwards model illustrated in Figure 10.9. There are three transition rate parameters, $\gamma_{1,2}$, $\gamma_{1,3}$, and $\gamma_{2,3}$, and the transition probability parameters can be written in terms of these three rates, for given observed cycle length, T, using the solution to the forward equations given in Figure 10.9. It is useful to re-parameterise the rates from state 1 as follows:

$$\gamma_{1,2} = \lambda_1(1 - \rho); \qquad \gamma_{1,3} = \lambda_1 \rho \qquad (10.4)$$

where λ_1 is interpreted as the rate at which individuals leave state 1, and ρ the probability that individuals leaving state 1, go directly to state 3 rather than via state 2. There are therefore three *basic* parameters λ_1, ρ, and $\gamma_{2,3}$, from which we can derive all other *functional* parameters (transition rates and probabilities).

As in standard meta-analysis, we can fit either Fixed Effect or Random Effects models. However, there are now three parameters on which there may be random study-specific effects. We shall illustrate how to fit a model where the rate that individuals leave state 1, $\lambda_{1,s}$, depends on study, s, but all other parameters, ρ, and $\gamma_{2,3}$, are assumed to be fixed across studies. Other models for study effects could be investigated, and compared using goodness of fit measures.

It is most natural to model rates on the log scale, so we put a Random Effects model on the log rate that individuals leave state 1:

$$\log(\lambda_{1,s}) \sim \text{Normal}(L, \tau^2) \qquad (10.5)$$

We give a flat Beta prior for ρ, the probability of going to state 3 rather than state 2, having left state 1. We give an Exponential prior to $\gamma_{2,3}$, the transition rate from state 2 to state 3. Finally, we give a flat Normal prior for the random effects mean, L, and a uniform prior on τ, the between study standard deviation in the log rate of leaving state 1.

$$\rho \sim \text{Beta}(1, 1); \ \gamma_{2,3} \sim \text{Exponential}(.001); \ L \sim \text{Normal}(0, 100^2);$$

$$\tau \sim \text{Uniform}(0, 1)$$

The WinBUGS code for this model is:

```
model{

for (s in 1:5) {
   loglam1[s] ~ dnorm(L,prec)         # Random effects model
                                      # on log(lambda1)
   log(lambda1[s]) <- loglam1[s]      # Derive lambda1 and
   gamma12[i]<-lambda1[i]*(1-rho)     # transition rates 1 to 2
   gamma13[i]<-lambda1[i]*rho         # and 1 to 3
}
                                      # Priors for:
gamma23 ~ dexp(.001)                  # transition rate 2 to 3
L ~ dnorm(0,.00001)                   # Random effects mean
tau ~ dunif(0,1)                      # Between study sd
prec <- 1/(tau*tau)
rho ~ dbeta(1,1)                      # Prob go to 3 rather
}                                     # than 2, having left 1
```

10.6.4*   Synthesis of studies reporting aggregate data

Table 10.7 shows illustrative data from two studies that report aggregated data on all possible transitions for the three-state forwards model illustrated in Figure 10.9. As for the analysis of a single study reporting results in this format, each row of data for study s has a Multinomial likelihood:

$$(r_{s,i,1}, r_{s,i,2}, r_{s,i,3}) \sim \text{Multinomial}(\pi_{s,i,1}(T), \pi_{s,i,2}(T), \pi_{s,i,3}(T); n_{s,i})$$

where the $\pi_{s,i,j}(T)$ are the study specific transition probabilities for observation cycle length, T, and are functions of the basic rate parameters as given in Figure 10.9.

Table 10.8 shows illustrative data from three studies that report aggregated data, but only on transitions to death (state 3). These studies tell us about the transition probability from state 1 to state 3 for observation cycle T.

Table 10.7   Studies 1 and 2 reported the aggregated number of observed transitions, $r_{s,i,j}$, from state i to state j in study s, with observation cycle length $T = 1$.

			Destination state, j	
	Starting state, i	State $j = 1$	State $j = 2$	State $j = 3$
Study $s = 1$	State $i = 1$	87	4	9
	State $i = 2$	0	3	1
Study $s = 2$	State $i = 1$	210	8	15
	State $i = 2$	0	5	3

Table 10.8   Studies 3–5 reported only transitions to death (state 3). Each study reported a different observation cycle length, T, and study 4 followed up some individuals at $T = 1.5$ and others at $T = 2$, giving two independent observations.

Study, s	Number of transitions to state 3, $r_s(T)$	Number starting in state 1, $n_s(T)$	Observation cycle length, T
3	38	181	2
4	15	177	1.5
4	11	103	2
5	13	335	5

The data have a Binomial likelihood, because only two possible outcomes are recorded, transition to state 3 or not:

$$r_s(T) \sim \text{Binomial}(\pi_{s,1,3}(T), n_s(T))$$

Note that study 4 has two observations. The transition probabilities for these two observations will differ only through the different observation cycle length, T. The WinBUGS code to incorporate these data is:

```
for (s in 1:2){
    for (i in 1:2){                                        # Multinomial likelihood for
        r.agg[s,i,1:3]~dmulti(pi.agg[s,i,1:3],n.agg[s,i])  # studies 1 & 2 reporting
    }                                                      # aggregated no. of
                                                           # transitions
}

for (obs in 1:6){
    pi.agg[obs,1,1]<- exp(-(gamma12[study[obs]]+          # Calculate transition
gamma13[study[obs]])*T[obs])                              # probabilities relevant to
    pi.agg[obs,1,2]<- gamma12[study[obs]]*(exp(-          # each observation
gamma23 * T[obs]) - exp(-(gamma12[study[obs]]+            # (study and cycle length
gamma13[study[obs]])*T[obs] ) )                           #  specific). These are
/(gamma12[study[obs]]+ gamma13[study[obs]] -             #  functions of basic
gamma23                                                   # parameters via
    pi.agg[obs,1,3]<- 1 - pi.agg[obs,1,1] - pi.agg[obs,1,2] # equations in Fig. 8.9
                                                           #  and equation (8.4)
    pi.agg[obs,2,1]<- 0
    pi.agg[obs,2,2]<- exp(-gamma23)
    pi.agg[obs,2,3]<- 1 - pi.agg[obs,2,2]
}

for (i in 1 : 4) {                                         # Studies 3-5 (4 data
    r.d[i] ~ dbin(pi.agg[(i+2),1,3],n.d[i])               # points) reported no.
    }                                                      # transitions from
                                                           # state 1 to state 3.
```

where the data is entered in the following way:

```
list(                                    # Studies 1 & 2 report
r.agg=structure(.Data=c(87,   4,    9,   # aggregate data for all
                         0,   3,    1,   # states, for given
                                         # observation cycle
                       210, 8,   15,     # length T
                         0,   5,   3),.Dim=c(2,2,3)),
n.agg=structure(.Data=c(100,  4,
                       233,   8),.Dim=c(2,2)),
```

```
                                        # Studies 3-5 (4 obsns)
r.d=c(38,15,11,60),    n.d=c(181,177,103,335),    # report no. transitions to
                                        # death for given observation
                                        # cycle length, T

                                        #Cycle length, T, & study
T=c(1,1, 2,1.5,2,5), study=c(1,2,3,4,4,5)    # number for 6 aggregate
)                                       # data observations
```

10.6.5* Incorporating studies that provide event history data

Table 10.9 gives data from eight studies that observe transitions and the timing of those transitions, so that transition rates can be estimated directly from the observed number of transitions for given person years at risk. Studies 6 and 7 focused on transitions from state 1 to state 2, studies 8 and 9 focused on transitions from state 1 to state 3, and studies 10–13 focused on transitions from state 2 to state 3. Each of these observations has a Poisson likelihood, with mean equal to the person years at risk multiplied by the relevant transition rate, which becomes additive on the log scale:

- Studies 6 and 7 on transitions from state 1 to state 2:

$$r_{s,1,2} \sim \text{Poisson}(\mu_s)$$

$$\log(\mu_s) = \log(E_s) + \log\left(\underbrace{\lambda_{1,s}(1 - \rho)}_{\gamma_{s,1,2}}\right)$$

- Studies 8 and 9 on transitions from state 1 to state 3:

$$r_{s,1,3} \sim \text{Poisson}(\mu_s)$$

$$\log(\mu_s) = \log(E_s) + \log\left(\underbrace{\lambda_{1,s}\rho}_{\gamma_{s,1,3}}\right)$$

- Studies 10–13 on transitions from state 2 to state 3:

$$r_{s,2,3} \sim \text{Poisson}(\mu_s)$$
$$\log(\mu_s) = \log(E_s) + \log(\gamma_{2,3})$$

Table 10.10 shows two studies that report event history data (i.e. number of transitions and person years at risk), but only recorded the first transition that

Table 10.9 Studies 6–13 reported event history data, giving the number of observed transitions and person years at risk, E. Studies 6 and 7 report results for transitions from state 1 to state 2; studies 8 and 9 for transitions from state 1 to state 3; and studies 10–13 for transitions from state 2 to state 3.

Study, s	Number of observed transitions			Person years at risk, E
	$r_{1,2}$	$r_{1,3}$	$r_{2,3}$	
6	8			120
7	20			620
8		12		140
9		44		677
10			9	34
11			12	35
12			5	15
13			6	25

Table 10.10 Studies 14 and 15 reported event history data, giving the number of observed first transitions from state 1 and person years at risk, E.

Study, s	Number of observed transitions		Person years at risk, E
	$m_{1,2}$	$m_{1,3}$	
14	18	40	380
15	30	75	1169

occurred. Each study therefore reports the total number of transitions that went directly from state 1 to state 2, $m_{s,1,2}$, and the total number of transitions that went directly from state 1 to state 3, $m_{s,1,3}$. The sum of these, $n_s = m_{s,1,2} + m_{s,1,3}$, is the total number of transitions from state 1, and has a Poisson likelihood, providing information on the rate of leaving state 1, $\lambda_{1,s}$:

$$n_s \sim \text{Poisson}(\nu_s)$$

$$\log(\nu_s) = \log(E_s) + \log(\lambda_{1,s})$$

Given individuals have left state 1, the split between those whose destination was state 3 rather than state 2 has a Binomial likelihood with probability, ρ:

$$m_{s,1,3} \sim \text{Binomial}(\rho, n_s)$$

The WinBUGS code to incorporate these data is:

```
for (i in 1:2) {                                    # Studies 6-7 report event
  r12[i] ~dpois(mu[i+5])                            # history data on transition 1->2
  log(mu[i+5]) <- log(E12[i]) + log(gamma12[i+5])   # Poison likelihood


}
for (i in 1:2) {                                    # Studies 8-9 report event
  r13[i] ~dpois(mu[i+7])                            # history data on transition 1->3
  log(mu[i+7]) <- log(E13[i]) + log(gamma13[i+7])   # Poison likelihood
}
for (i in 1:4) {                                    # Studies 10-13 report event
  r23[i] ~dpois(mu[i+9])                            # history data on transition 2->3
  log(mu[i+9]) <- log(E23[i]) + log(gamma23)        # Poison likelihood
}
                                                    # 2 studies reporting event
for (i in 1:2) {                                    # history data on first tranistion
  n[i] <- m12[i] + m13[i]                           # from state 1
  n[i] ~ dpois(nu[i])                               # likelihood for Poisson rate
  log(nu[i]) <- log(E[i]) + loglam1[i+13]

  m13[i] ~ dbin(rho,n[i])                           # likelihood for binomial
}                                                   # proportion going to state 3
```

Note that the indexing is adjusted to obtain the appropriate study number. The data are entered in the following way:

```
r12=c(8,20),        E12=c(120,620),              # STUDIES 6-7
r13=c( 12,44),      E13=c(140,677),              # STUDIES 8-9
r23=c(9,12,5,6),    E23=c(34,35,15,25),          # STUDIES 10-13
m12=c(18,30),   m13=c(40,75),   E=c(380,1169)    #STUDIES 14-15
```

10.6.6*   Reporting results from a Random Effects model

Table 10.11 shows posterior summaries for the model parameters. However, it is not immediately clear how to report results for the random effects parameters, λ_1, $\gamma_{1,2}$, and $\gamma_{1,3}$. Figure 10.11 shows the heterogeneity between studies in the estimated rate of leaving state 1, λ_1. Note that studies 10–13, which provide information on the transition from state 2 to state 3, provides no information on the rate of leaving state 1. The estimate for these studies is simply the predictive distribution of the rate leaving state 1 that we would expect to see in a new study.

There are several possible ways to summarise the Random Effects model for the rate of leaving state 1. We illustrate three of these here:

- The random effects mean (on a log-scale), L, giving rate parameters:

$$\gamma_{1,2} = e^L(1 - \rho); \text{ and } \gamma_{1,3} = e^L \rho$$

- The predictive distribution for the log rate of leaving state 1 in a new study, giving rate parameters:

$$\gamma_{1,2} = \lambda_1^{pred}(1 - \rho); \text{ and } \gamma_{1,3} = \lambda_1^{pred}\rho$$

$$\text{where, } \log(\lambda_1^{pred}) \sim N(L, \tau^2)$$

- Calibrate to a representative study – for example the most recent, or in the relevant country (for illustration we shall calibrate to study 15), giving rate parameters

$$\gamma_{1,2} = \lambda_{1,15}(1 - \rho); \text{ and } \gamma_{1,3} = \lambda_{1,15}\rho$$

The WinBUGS code to calculate these summaries is:

```
g12[1] <- (1-rho) * exp(L)              #1. Random effects mean, L
g13[1] <-  rho * exp(L)


loglam1.pred~dnorm(L,prec)              #2. Predictive distribution
log(lambda1.pred)<-loglam1.pred        # for loglam1
g12[2] <- (1-rho) * lambda1.pred
g13[2] <- rho * lambda1.pred


g12[3] <- (1-rho) * lambda1[15]         #3. Calibrate to study 15
g13[3] <- rho * lambda1[15]
```

Table 10.12 shows posterior summaries for the transition rate parameters for each of these three scenarios. Using the predictive distribution leads to wider credible intervals than using the random effects mean. Calibrating to study 15 leads to lower estimated rate parameters, because the study-specific rate of leaving state 1 was lower than average for this particular study population.

Finally, we can reapply the forward equations to obtain estimates transition probabilities at a given cycle length, T. Table 10.13 shows the results for a cycle length of $T = 1$, obtained from the following WinBUGS code:

```
for (j in 1:3){                        #Transition probabilities over
  P11[j]<-exp(-(g12[j]+g13[j]))         #cycle length T=1, from the
  P12[j]<-g12[j]*(exp(-gamma23)-exp(-   #Forwards equations (Fig.
(g12[j]+g13[j])))/(g12[j]+g13[j]-gamma23)  #10.9). Calculated for the
  P13[j]<- (1-P11[j]-P12[j])            #three methods of
  P22[j]<- exp(-gamma23)                #summarizing the random
  P23[j]<- 1-P22[j]                     #effects distribution for the
}                                       #rate of leaving State 1
```

10.6.7* Incorporating treatment effects

Suppose that studies 1 and 2 also had a treatment arm, producing the aggregate data shown in Table 10.14.

Table 10.11   Posterior summaries for the model parameters from the three-state forwards model shown in Figure 10.9 from a synthesis of the data in Tables 10.7–10.10.

Parameter	L	τ	ρ	$\gamma_{2,3}$
Posterior mean	−2.25	0.41	0.68	0.30
(95% credible interval)	(−2.54, −1.96)	(0.22, 0.73)	(0.62 0.74)	(.21,. 41)

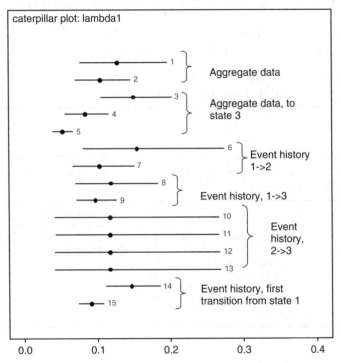

Figure 10.11   Posterior mean rate of leaving state 1, with 95% credible intervals for studies 1–15.

Table 10.12   Posterior summaries for the transition rate parameters from state 1 for three different summaries of the random effects distribution on the rate of leaving state 1.

Posterior mean (95% credible interval)	$\gamma_{1,2}$	$\gamma_{1,3}$
Random effects mean, L	0.034 (0.024, 0.047)	0.072 (0.053, 0.097)
Predictive distribution	0.037 (0.013, 0.086)	0.079 (0.028, 0.183)
Calibrate to study 15	0.029 (0.022, 0.037)	0.062 (0.050, 0.075)

Table 10.13   Posterior summaries for the transition probability parameters for cycle length $T = 1$, and for three different summaries of the random effects distribution on the rate of leaving state 1. Note that transitions from state 2 do not depend on the rate of leaving state 1, and so only one set of results is shown.

Posterior mean (95% credible interval)	$\pi_{1,1}$	$\pi_{1,2}$	$\pi_{1,3}$	$\pi_{2,2}$	$\pi_{2,3}$
Random effects mean, L	0.90 (0.87,0.92)	0.03 (0.02,0.04)	0.07 (0.05,0.10)	0.74 (0.66,0.81)	0.26 (0.19,0.34)
Predictive distribution	0.89 (0.77,0.96)	0.03 (0.01,0.06)	0.08 (0.03,0.17)	-	-
Calibrate to study 15	0.91 (0.90,0.93)	0.02 (0.02,0.03)	0.06 (0.05,0.08)	-	-

Table 10.14   Treatment arms for studies 1 and 2, which reported the aggregated number of observed transitions, $r_{s,i,j}$, from state i to state j in study s, with observation cycle length $T = 1$.

		Destination state, j		
	Starting state, i	State $j = 1$	State $j = 2$	State $j = 3$
Study $s = 1$	State $i = 1$	140	2	14
	State $i = 2$	0	2	0
Study $s = 2$	State $i = 1$	264	5	27
	State $i = 2$	0	3	2

The treatment arm data have the same likelihood format as the control arms, however the transition rates and hence also the transition probabilities are assumed to be effected by treatment. We can model the impact of treatment on the transition rate parameters in a variety of models. For example, Figure 10.12 shows two possible mechanisms through which the treatment may affect the underlying rate parameters. Figure 10.12(a) shows the treatment effect acting on transitions from state 1 to state 2, but not effecting any other transitions, whereas Figure 10.12(b) shows the treatment effect acting equally on all transitions. The parameter h can be interpreted as the hazard ratio of making a particular transition under treatment

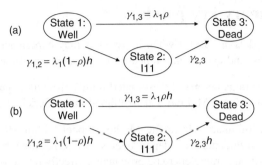

Figure 10.12   Two possible parameterisations of treatment effect for the three-state forwards model: (a) treatment effect, h, acts on transitions from state 1 to state 2 only; (b) treatment effect, h, acts on all transition equally.

relative to control. Of course more complex models could be investigated, such as random treatment effects rather than assuming a single fixed treatment effect, and also different treatment effect parameters on different transitions.

We shall use the model shown in Figure 10.12(a) for illustration, and the WinBUGS code required to fit this model is:

```
for (s in 1:2){                                          # STUDIES 1 & 2
  for (i in 1:2){
    r.agg[s,i,1:3]~dmulti(pi.agg[s,i,1:3],n.agg[s,i])     # Treatment arm
    r.aggt[s,i,1:3]~dmulti(pi.aggt[s,i,1:3],n.aggt[s,i])  # likelihood
  }
  pi.aggt[s,1,1]<- exp(-(gamma12[s]*h+gamma13[s])*T[s])   # Forward
  pi.aggt[s,1,2]<- gamma12[s]*h*(exp(-gamma23 * T[s])     # equations for
- exp(-(gamma12[s]*h+gamma13[s])*T[s] ) )                 # treatment arms
/(gamma12[s]*h+gamma13[s] - gamma23 )                     # −including
  pi.aggt[s,1,3]<- 1 - pi.aggt[s,1,1] - pi.aggt[s,1,2]    # treatment
  pi.aggt[s,2,1]<- 0                                      #effects h
  pi.aggt[s,2,2]<- exp(-gamma23)
  pi.aggt[s,2,3]<- 1 - pi.aggt[s,2,2]
}
                                                          #Normal prior
logh~dnorm(0,.00001)                                      #on log-hazard
log(h)<- logh                                             #ratio
```

The posterior mean hazard ratio is 0.525 with 95% credible interval (0.020, 1.04), suggesting there is some evidence that the treatment reduces the rate at which individuals move from state 1 to state 2.

10.7 Summary key points

- Markov models are useful when individuals may experience one of several health states, and events may repeat or occur over long time periods.

- Transition parameters may be estimated jointly from aggregated data from a single study using a Multinomial likelihood and a Dirichlet prior.

- Calculating summaries from the Markov model within MCMC simulation allows for all uncertainties, dependencies and correlations between the estimated transition parameters to be propagated directly into a decision analysis.

- Modelling transition rates rather than transition probabilities allows us to carry out a synthesis of different studies reporting different summaries of Markov model parameters; model disease progression and treatment effects; and may lead to simpler models with fewer parameters.

- Transition probabilities can be obtained from the basic parameters (transition rates) by solving Kolmorgorov's forward equations.

- Different plausible pathways for the disease progression and treatment effect can be explored using model fit methods.

- Models for treatment effects can readily be incorporated, including mixed treatment comparison evidence structures.

10.8 Further reading

Welton and Ades [7] give more details on the synthesis of studies on Markov parameters, and in particular provide code to find numerical solutions to the forward equations, using WBDiff [9] an add-on to WinBUGS, on their web site (http://www.bris.ac.uk/cobm/research/mpes/mdpm.html).

The methods have since been used to parameterise treatment effects for the asthma example [10], and also for the HIV example shown in Figure10.1(e) where there is individual patient data with left, right and interval censoring [11].

10.9 Exercises

10.1 Run the model for the asthma example (*asthma.odc*), and produce a matrix of correlations between the transition probabilities by choosing *Inference_ Correlations*. Enter pi in both boxes, and *click on matrix*. You can home in on parts of this graph, for example if we want correlations between transitions from state 4, for Fluticasone (treatment 2), type in pi[2,4,] into the two boxes rather than just pi.

10.2 For the three-state model and aggregated 2-monthly transitions data table given below:

(a) Estimate the 2-month Markov transition probabilities.

(b) Find the expected time spent in state 1 over a 1-year period.

$r_{i,j}$	$j = 1$	$j = 2$	$j = 3$	n_i
$i = 1$	20	3	7	30
$i = 2$	0	5	5	10

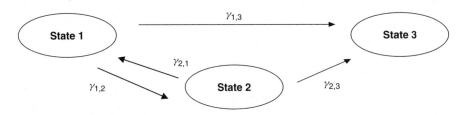

References

1. Keeler E. Decision trees and Markov models in cost-effectiveness research. In: Sloan F., ed. *Valuing Health Care*. Cambridge: Cambridge University Press, 1996; 185–205.

2. Sonnenberg F.A., Beck J.R. Markov models in medical decision making: a practical guide. *Medical Decision Making* 1993;**13**:322–338.

3. Briggs A., Sculpher M., Claxton K. *Decision Modelling for Health Economic Evaluation*. Oxford: Oxford University Press, 2006.

4. Hunink M., Glasziou P., Siegel J., *et al*. *Decision Making in Health and Medicine: Integrating Evidence and Values*. Cambridge: Cambridge University Press, 2001.

5. Briggs A.H., Ades A.E., Price M.J. Probabilistic sensitivity analysis for decision trees with multiple branches: Use of the Dirichlet distribution in a Bayesian framework. *Medical Decision Making* 2003;**23**:341–350.

6. Gelman A., Carlin J.G., Stern H.S., Rubin D.B. *Bayesian Data Analysis*. London: Chapman and Hall, 1995.

7. Welton N.J., Ades A.E. Estimation of Markov chain transition probabilities and rates from fully and partially observed data: Uncertainty propagation, evidence synthesis and model calibration. *Medical Decision Making* 2005;**25**:633–645.

8. Grimmett G.D.R., Stirzaker D.R. *Probability and Random Processes*. Oxford: Oxford University Press, 1992.

9. Lunn D. WinBUGS Differential Interface (WBDiff). http://www.winbugs-development.org.uk/. 2004.

10. Price M., Welton N., Ades A.E. Parameterisation of treatment effects for meta-analysis in multi-state Markov models. *Statistics in Medicine* 2011;**30**:140–151.

11. Price M.J., Welton N.J., Ades A.E. Parameterising the effect of cotrimoxazole prophylaxis in a multi-state Markov model of HIV disease progression in African children. International Society for Clinical Biostatistics, 28th Annual Conference, Alexandroupolis, Greece, 2007; Abstract.

11

Generalised evidence synthesis

11.1 Introduction

There is no doubt that the Randomised Controlled Trial (RCT) produces the most reliable evidence on the comparative effectiveness of interventions; however, good, conclusive randomised evidence may not exist for every treatment decision. Also, it may not exist in the future due to economic, ethical or organisational considerations [1]. Therefore, there are occasions when it will be necessary to consider forms of nonrandomised (observational) data on which to estimate effectiveness. In other contexts, there may be some randomised evidence, but for various reasons including concerns about its quality (internal validity), generalisability (external validity) and size (i.e. estimates are imprecise) or extent (i.e. only available for certain treatments in the decision space), a decision is taken to consider further observational evidence in addition to the randomised evidence.

When observational evidence is considered either instead of, or in combination with, randomised evidence, the question arises as to whether we need to apply new methodology in order to sensibly synthesise it. It is possible to perform a meta-analysis of the observational evidence, and it is also possible to perform a meta-analysis of all of the observational and randomised evidence combined. As before (Chapter 4), each study, irrespective of design, would estimate a treatment effect with a given precision. However, such an approach would ignore the commonly held belief that observational data potentially produce more biased estimates than data from trials (which is the whole premise for doing costly trial based experiments

Evidence Synthesis for Decision Making in Healthcare, First Edition. Nicky J. Welton,
Alexander J. Sutton, Nicola J. Cooper, Keith R. Abrams and A.E. Ades.
© 2012 John Wiley & Sons, Ltd. Published 2012 by John Wiley & Sons, Ltd.

in the first place). For this reason, many analysts are understandably reticent about using observational evidence uncritically in this way. This is further confounded by the fact that even data generated from the same type of study design may not be of equal quality and may also be at risk of biases. There are good RCTs and poorly conducted RCTs and the situation is the same for observational studies of the same design (although further issues of the relative merits of different observational designs compound things even more).

Therefore, a strong case could be made for considering the risk of bias of each study in the synthesis, randomised or observational [2]. If it were possible to identify and quantify all the biases, then methods for adjusting each study for these in the synthesis could be developed [2, 3]. Methods are emerging for doing this, either based on large databases of empirical data [3] or using expert opinion [2]. However, these methods are still very much at the experimental stage, particularly if observational and randomised evidence is being considered, although such methods may become proceduralised and recommended in the future.

In this chapter we do not consider methods to adjust individual studies for biases, but rather consider approaches to combining randomised and observational evidence, acknowledging that the observational data are potentially more biased than the randomised. In this way, issues of differential quality of the evidence type (rather than study level) are considered. Although somewhat more complex than standard meta-analysis, this approach to bias adjustment is less involved than methods for adjusting individual studies for biases.

Example 11.1   Hormone replacement therapy.

Hormone replacement therapy (HRT) is used for the relief of menopausal symptoms. It has also been shown to provide a benefit for the prevention of bone fractures, particularly for women with osteoporosis and low bone mineral density. However, around the year 2000, concerns were raised over possible increased risk of breast cancer with HRT use. Figure 11.1 presents a random effects meta-analysis of the randomised evidence available on the risk of breast cancer with HRT by 2002. The resulting pooled estimate of 0.97 (0.67 to 1.39), while being quite uncertain, provides little concern that HRT increases the risk of breast cancer significantly. However, the individual trials were originally designed to detect differences in either menopausal symptoms or vertebral/nonvertebral fractures [4, 5].

In Figure 11.2 the observational data on the use of HRT and risk of breast cancer adjusted for known confounders, available around the same time, is presented [6]. Here the observational data, stratified by design (case-control study with hospital or population based controls, and cohort studies) suggests an increased risk of breast cancer with HRT use (Odds Ratio (OR) 1.18 (1.10 to 1.26)).

Systematic differences in duration of HRT use and follow-up duration between the observational and randomised evidence were identified, and before considering the evidence further both sources of evidence were adjusted for these using meta-regression. This adjustment resulted in an OR of 0.89 (0.39 to 1.44) and

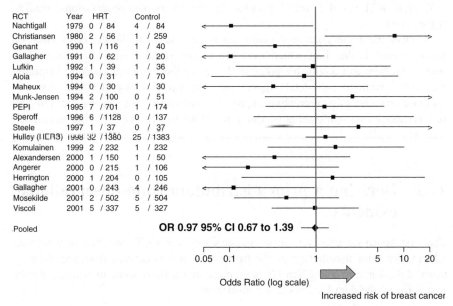

Figure 11.1 Forest plot (Random Effects model) of the randomised evidence of HRT vs *control for breast cancer outcome.*

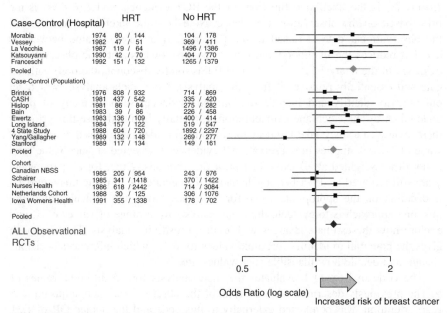

Figure 11.2 Forest plot of the observational evidence, stratified by design, for risk of breast cancer with HRT (evidence adjusted for known confounders).

1.31 (1.16 to 1.47) at 5 years' duration for the RCTs and observational studies, respectively.

Hence, the issue here in deciding on an estimate for the effect of HRT on breast cancer is deciding which evidence to use (randomised, observational or both), and how to account for potential biases in the evidence chosen. Assuming we do not want to completely ignore the observational evidence, the next two sections consider two alternative approaches to using both the randomised and observational data while acknowledging the latter source may be more biased.

11.2   Deriving a prior distribution from observational evidence

The first approach considers a meta-analysis of the RCT evidence in which an informative prior distribution on the treatment effect is derived from the observational data. Ibrahim and Chen [7] have presented a framework in which a power transform of the data likelihood is considered:

$$P(\theta|Data) = L(\theta|RCTs) \times [L(\theta|Obs)]^{\alpha} \times P(\theta) \qquad (11.1)$$

where $P(\theta|Data)$ is the posterior distribution for set of model parameters, $L(\theta|RCTs)$ is the likelihood function for the RCT evidence, and $L(\theta|Obs)$ is the prior based on the observational evidence. Note how the likelihood function for the observational data is raised to the power α. If α takes a value between 0 and 1 it reduces the likelihood and thus discounts/downweights the observational evidence in the analysis. If α is set to be 0 this totally discounts the observational data and essentially removes it from the analysis. Note, meta-analyses which set out only to identify and include randomised evidence, such as many of those undertaken by the Cochrane Collaboration, essentially implicitly use this prior for their reviews, i.e. they take the decision to only consider randomised evidence. A value of 1 for α implies the observational evidence is accepted at 'face value' and is not downweighted at all. Note that prior distributions, $P(\theta)$, for all parameters q are still required as described in Chapter 4. The challenge in using this approach is deciding on the appropriate value for α to use. Given the difficulty of doing this, one approach is to evaluate the meta-analysis for a range of values of α, and explore how the estimate changes with α in a sensitivity analysis. This approach gives the potential to identify threshold values for α for which inferences/decisions change and decide how plausible such values are.

The code in Box 11.1 evaluates the meta-analysis for 12 different values of α. The previously described meta-analysis of the observational data, adjusted to 5 years' duration, was conducted externally to this code and the pooled OR of 1.31 (1.61 to 1.46) was transformed to a ln(OR) of 0.27 with associated standard error of 0.061 which translates to a precision of 271.3. How these data are used in the code is described below.

```
# Prior based on distribution of pooled effect (21)

model {

# (a) Create multiple datasets
for (i in 1:19){
        for(k in 1:12){
                rc[i,k] < rc.dat[i]
                rt[i,k] <- rt.dat[i]
                nc[i,k] <- nc.dat[i]
                nt[i,k] <- nt.dat[i]
                }
        }

# (b) Estimate RCT meta-analysis model for each value of alpha
for (k in 1: 12) {
        for( i in 1 : 19 ) {
        rc[i,k] ~ dbin(pc[i,k], nc[i,k])
                rt[i,k] ~ dbin(pt[i,k], nt[i,k])
                logit(pc[i,k]) <- mu[i,k]
                logit(pt[i,k]) <- mu[i,k] + delta[i,k]+ beta*(duration[i]-5)
                mu[i,k] ~ dnorm(0.0,1.0E-6)
                delta[i,k] ~ dnorm(d[k], prec[k])
                }
        d[k] ~ dnorm(0.270, prec.d[k])  # Use of
                                        # meta-analysis of obs data
        OR.5years[k]<- exp(d[k])
        prec[k] <- 1/tau.sq[k]
        tau.sq[k] <- tau[k]*tau[k]
        tau[k] ~ dunif(0,5)
                }
        beta ~ dnorm(0.0,1.0E-6)

# (c) Calculate precision of prior (from Lancet meta-analysis of
# observational studies) downweighted using alpha

for (k in 1:12) {
        prec.d[k] <- alpha[k]*271.3
        }    }


# Data

list(rt.dat = c(0,2,1,0,1,0,0,2,7,6,1,32,2,1,0,1,0,2,5),
nt.dat = c(84,56,116,62,39,31,30,100,701,1128,37,1380,232,150,215,
        204,243,502,337),
```

```
rc.dat = c(4,1,1,1,1,1,1,0,1,0,0,25,1,1,1,0,4,5,5),
nc.dat = c(84,259,40,20,36,70,30,51,174,137,37,1383,232,50,106,105,
      246,504,327),
duration=c(10,2,1,2,1,2.92,1,2,3,2,2,4.08,5,2,1,3.17,3,4.58,2.83),
alpha=c(0.000001,0.001,0.1,0.2,0.3,0.4,0.5,0.6,0.7,0.8,0.9,1.0)
)


# Starting/Initial Values


list(mu=structure( .Data=c( ** place 19 * 12 = 228 initial values here **),
            .Dim=c(19,12)),
delta=structure( .Data=c(** place 19 * 12 = 228 initial values here **),
            .Dim=c(19,12)),
d = c(0,0,0,0,0,0,0,0,0,0,0,0,0),
beta=0,
tau=c(1,1,1,1,1,1,1,1,1,1,1,1))
```

Box 11.1   Code implementing a range of power priors to discount the observational evidence in the HRT and risk of breast cancer example.

In Box 11.1, the WinBUGS code is broken down into three parts, (a), (b) and (c). Part (a) of the code simply duplicates the data from the 19 RCTs in the meta-analysis 12 times; once for each value of α used to downweight the observational data. Part (b) is the meta-analysis code itself, which is a slight adaption of the meta-regression code described in detail in Section 5.2.3 (the covariate included here is duration of HRT use). In this code, i indexes studies and k indexes each of the (12) meta-analyses. The only difference between each of the 12 meta-analyses is the prior distribution placed on the overall pooled effect, d, which is dictated by the line:

$$d[k] \sim dnorm(0.270, prec.d[k])$$

Here the mean of the prior distribution is the mean Log Odds Ratio (LOR) estimate from the meta-analyses of the observational data as described earlier. The precision of this prior distribution, prec.d[k], is defined in part (c) of the code. Here the estimated precision of the pooled ln(OR) for the observational studies, 271.3, is multiplied sequentially by each of the 12 values for α supplied in the data. Recall, that since we are working on the log scale and assuming Normality, multiplying the precision like this is equivalent to raising the likelihood to the equivalent power. (Note some of the initial values have been omitted for space reasons but the structure required for these is retained.)

Using this code, the value for the pooled OR and its uncertainty can be examined. These values are displayed graphically in Figure 11.3. In this plot, the OR and 95% credible interval (CrI) associated with ignoring the observational data are presented on the left-hand side of the plot. The values, including the observational

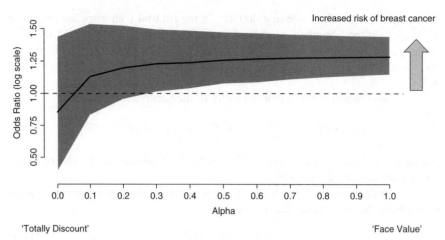

Figure 11.3 Mean OR and 95% CrI for different power transform priors to discount the observational evidence on the risk of breast cancer with HRT.

data at face value and not discounting at all are on the right-hand side. If decisions were being based on uncertainty, i.e. 95% CrIs, then this would change at a value of α of approximately 0.3 where the CrI no longer includes an OR of 1. Hence, you have to discount the observational evidence considerably before you would conclude that HRT did not increase the risk of breast cancer.

11.3 Bias allowance model for the observational data

There have been several empirical investigations reported in which the results of randomised and observational studies on the same question have been systematically compared to establish, on average, how biased the observational studies are assuming that the randomised studies are unbiased. These investigations have reported varying potential extent of bias from $+/- 30\%$ [8], through $+/- 50\%$ [9] to $+/- 100\%$ [10]. Thus these studies suggest observational studies are potentially biased, although the direction of the bias is largely unpredictable. Such data, being external to future research topics, could potentially be utilised in informative priors informing likely bias in future studies.

In the account which follows, the potential bias in the observational studies is modelled using an extra variance component which represents the bias. Values for the variance used are based on those being reported in the empirical studies. The 'bias adjusted' estimate from the observational studies is then used to specify a prior distribution for the pooled effect from the meta-analysis of the randomised evidence. More formally,

$$Y_i^{RCT} \sim \text{Normal}\left(\delta_i^{RCT}, V_i^{RCT}\right) \text{ and } \delta_i^{RCT} \sim \text{Normal}\left(d^{RCT}, \tau^{2RCT}\right) \qquad (11.2)$$

where Y_i^{RCT} is the effect size (e.g. ln(OR)) in the ith trial with associated variance V_i^{RCT}, δ_i^{RCT} is the 'shrunken' model estimate of the effect size for the ith trial, d^{RCT} is the pooled effect size, and τ^{2RCT} is the between study variance. This is exactly the same as the generic random effects meta-analysis model described in Section 4.3.

The same model is fitted independently to the observational data:

$$Y_j^{OBS} \sim \text{Normal}\left(\delta_j^{OBS}, V_j^{OBS}\right) \text{ and } \delta_j^{OBS} \sim \text{Normal}\left(d^{OBS}, \tau^{2OBS}\right) \quad (11.3)$$

where j now indexes studies and OBS replaces RCT to indicate the observational studies are now being considered.

The observational study meta-analysis forms a prior distribution for the pooled effect from the RCT meta-analysis, i.e.

$$d^{RCT} \sim d^{OBS}|\underline{Y^{OBS}} \quad (11.4)$$

where $\underline{Y^{OBS}}$ represents all the observational data. Stopping at this point would imply the observational data would be used at face value, but including the possibility of bias, but with a mean of 0 can be achieved by considering:

$$d^{OBS} = d^{*OBS} + \gamma \text{ and } \gamma \sim \text{Normal}\left(0, \sigma^2\right) \quad (11.5)$$

where d^{*OBS} is the effect in the observational studies adjusted for bias, γ is the bias associated with the observational studies, and σ^2 represents *a priori* beliefs regarding the possible extent of the bias. This bias could be expressed as a point estimate with no uncertainty, or a (prior) distribution could be specified for σ^2, potentially based on the empirical data mentioned previously. The code for the latter approach is described in detail in Box 11.2.

```
model {

# (a) Meta-analysis of the 19 HRT RCTs

    for(j in 1 : Nstud) {
        rc[j] ~ dbin(pc[j], nc[j])
        rt[j] ~ dbin(pt[j], nt[j])
        logit(pc[j]) <- mu[j]
        logit(pt[j]) <- mu[j] + delta[j] + beta*(duration[j]-5)
        mu[j] ~ dnorm(0.0,1.0E-5)
        delta[j] ~ dnorm(d, prec)
    }

    prec <- 1/tau.sq
```

```
        tau.sq <- tau*tau
        tau ~ dunif(0,5)

        beta ~ dnorm(0.0,1.0E-5)
        OR<- exp(d)

# (b) Meta-meta-analysis of 19 meta-analyses comparing RCTs and
# NRCTs (Ioannidis et al 2001 (6))

        for( j in 1 : Nma) {
        logRRΠ [j] ~ dnorm(d.bias, prec.bias)
                }
# Prior distributions

            prec.bias <- 1/tau.sq.bias
            tau.sq.bias <- tau.bias*tau.bias

        d ~ dnorm(0.27, prec.d)
        prec.d <- 1/tau.sq.d
        tau.sq.d <- 0.0037 + tau.sq.bias
        tau.bias ~ dunif(0,5)
        d.bias ~ dnorm(0.0,1.0E-5)


        }
# Data
list(rt = c(0,2,1,0,1,0,0,2,7,6,1,32,2,1,0,1,0,2,5),
nt = c(84,56,116,62,39,31,30,100,701,1128,37,1380,232,150,215,204,
       243,502,337),
rc = c(4,1,1,1,1,1,1,0,1,0,0,25,1,1,1,0,4,5,5),
nc = c(84,259,40,20,36,70,30,51,174,137,37,1383,232,50,106,105,246,
       504,327),
duration=c(10,2,1,2,1,2.92,1,2,3,2,2,4.08,5,2,1,3.17,3,4.58,2.83), Nstud = 19,
Nma=19, logRRR=c(-1.406497068,-0.182721637, 0.299363577,
0.087094707, 0.805135683, 0.017839918, -0.167235919, 0.133656385,
-0.038740828, 0.969262617, 0.083421608, -0.432322562, 0, 0.347129531,
0.038258712, -0.066139803, 0.206200831, 0.1889661, -0.534435489))

# Initial Values
list(d = 0, tau=1, mu = c(0, 0, 0, 0, 0, 0, 0, 0, 0, 0, 0, 0, 0, 0, 0, 0, 0, 0, 0),
        delta = c(0, 0, 0, 0, 0, 0, 0, 0, 0, 0, 0, 0, 0, 0, 0, 0, 0, 0, 0),
        d.bias=0,  tau.bias=1,beta=0)
```

Box 11.2 WinBUGS code for including bias modelling of the observational studies in the HRT and breast cancer example.

Adopting the former approach of specifying a point estimate for σ^2 and following Deeks et al. [11] the bias/discrepancy on a relative scale is assumed to be

$\pm 30\%$, which for the LOR scale translates into an interval from $\log(0.7)$ to $\log(1.3)$. Assuming that this interval represents a 95% interval for the bias/discrepancy means that $\sigma \approx [\log(1.3) - \log(0.7)]/4 \approx 0.155$, which in turn means that $\sigma^2 \approx 0.02$. This estimate can then be used in Equation (11.5).

As for the power prior analysis in Box 11.1, the meta-analysis of the observational studies (adjusted for length of follow-up) is carried out externally to this code, and the pooled LOR of 0.27 with associated variance of 0.0037 are used as data in the subsequent analysis as described below. Part (a) of the code conducts a standard meta-regression of the RCTs adjusting for duration of treatment, as in Box 11.1, note that the prior distribution for d, the pooled ln(OR), is informative and specified in part (b) of the code. Part (b) of the code fits a normal distribution to empirical data obtained from the study by Ioannidis et al. [9] who compared the ratio of the relative risk (RRR) from RCTs and observational studies in 19 meta-analyses in which both types of studies were included (the 19 RRRs are included as data in the code). The variance of this distribution is then added to the variance of the pooled estimate of the observational study meta-analysis, i.e. since we are assuming Normality and that the effect of bias can be in either direction:

tau.sq.d <- 0.0037 + tau.sq.bias

Once transformed to a precision scale, this variance is used in the prior distribution for the pooled estimate from the meta-analysis together with the mean from the observational data meta-analysis, i.e.

d ~ dnorm(0.27, prec.d)

Thus, in this way the prior distribution has been adjusted for bias, and since no direction for the bias has been assumed (i.e. it has mean 0), this is equivalent to downweighting the observational evidence in a similar spirit to the use of the power prior in the previous section.

The results associated with an analysis using the empirically based estimates of bias in the observational studies are presented in Table 11.1. Also included in this table, for comparison, are the results of treating the observational evidence at 'face value' (i.e. assuming it is totally unbiased), giving an OR = 1.14 (1.07 to 1.20), or totally discounting it (i.e. infinitely biased), giving an OR = 0.87 (0.30 to 1.60),

Table 11.1   Results of allowing for bias in the observational HRT studies.

Belief/Source	Bias (%)	σ^2	OR	95% CrI	P(OR>1)
'Face value'	0	0	1.14	1.07 to 1.20	1.00
Total discounting	∞	∞	0.87	0.30 to 1.60	0.31
Sacks et al. [8]	± 30	0.02	1.08	0.85 to 1.37	0.72
Ioannidis et al. [9]	± 50	0.08	1.00	0.68 to 1.45	0.50
MacLehose et al. [10]	± 100	0.24	0.94	0.56 to 1.49	0.40

from either extreme of Figure 11.3. It can be seen that assuming the studies could be up to 50% bias in either direction, as estimated from Ioannidis *et al.* [9], places the point estimate, 1.00 (0.68 to 1.45), close to midway between these two estimates. Also included in Table 11.1 are results of assuming different levels of bias for the observational studies, as suggested by other empirical studies by Sacks *et al.* [8] and MacLehose *et al.* [10], which translates to up to 30 or 100% biases in either direction, respectively. The estimates obtained after using a prior distribution related to these studies results in ORs of 1.08 (0.85 to 1.37) for 30% bias and 0.94 (0.56 to 1.49) for 100% bias, which intuitively places them at either side of the Ioannidis *et al.* based prior and within the range expressed by the 'face value' and total discounting extremes.

Adopting the second approach and modelling directly the data available from those studies that compared RCTs and Non-Randomised Controlled Trials (NRCTs) in Ioannidis *et al.* [9] produces a posterior distribution for σ^2 of 0.29 (95% CrI 0.15 to 0.60), which is then used as a prior distribution for σ^2 in Equation (11.5). The resulting posterior estimate for the OR is 0.90 (95% CrI 0.38 to 1.85). Not surprisingly, given the estimate for σ^2, this is similar to that using the point estimate of 0.24 adopted from MacLehose *et al.* [10]), but the uncertainty in σ^2 leads to a wide 95% CrI for the OR.

Note that the variance components to model the bias in the observational studies were all centred at zero. This is because the empirical data largely suggest the direction of the bias is unpredictable. If there was thought to be a systematic bias in a particular direction, then this could be expressed by changing the mean of the bias distribution to a value other than zero.

As a footnote to this example, after the above analysis was initially considered, in July 2002 further trial evidence became available including the large Women's Health Initiative (WHI) trial [12] which had a total sample size of 16 608 and observed 290 breast cancers and was stopped early due to adverse event concerns and estimated the OR of breast cancer on HRT to be 1.28 (1.01 to 1.62), which, somewhat intriguingly, is close to the estimate obtained from the observational evidence.

In summary, Sections 11.2 and 11.3 present two different but related frameworks for combining two sources of evidence which result in a downweighting of one of the sources; the observational evidence in the example presented. The HRT and breast cancer example presented is not intended to be definitive, but illustrates what is possible. Many refinements would be possible, for example, the estimates of bias used in the latter framework came from estimates of effectiveness, and since breast cancer was an adverse event of treatment, more closely related prior information would be desirable. Further, as indicated in Section 11.1, these approaches make global adjustments to study types, although it is acknowledged that studies within a certain type may be affected to different levels of bias, and thus a refined approach which adjusts evidence at the study level would be desirable. The next section considers a further modelling approach which considers evidence from different sources distinctly.

11.4 Hierarchical models for evidence from different study designs

In this section we consider an extension to the standard Random Effects model for meta-analysis covered in detail in Chapter 4. Here we model an extra level of variation to allow for variability in effect sizes between different sources of evidence (in addition to allowing for variability between study estimates within each study type). The model can be used when there are three or more different study types to include in the synthesis [13].

As an illustrative example, consider (some of) the evidence for the effect of electronic fetal heart rate monitoring (EFM) on perinatal mortality [14]. Although it is agreed that such equipment should assist with timely deliver, hence reducing the chance of a still birth, EFM has not been shown to reduce perinatal mortality in the nine RCTs available at the time of initial analysis (around 2000), although this may be due to low power since perinatal mortality is rare; thus the potential opportunity to consider a wider evidence base. In the evidence considered here, there are the aforementioned RCTs, comparative cohort studies and before and after studies and the data from these studies are described in Table 11.2. The analysis was conducted on the Risk Difference (RD) scale, although detailed consideration of this data set elsewhere may now suggest that the Relative Risk (RR) may have been a better choice due to issues with excessive heterogeneity on the RD scale [15]. If we assume that the studies of each particular type are exchangeable and that the pooled estimates obtained from each different study type are themselves exchangeable, then this can be expressed formally using the following model:

$$Y_{jl} \sim \text{Normal}[\delta_{jl}, V_{jl}] \qquad j = 1, \ldots, J_l \text{ studies and } l = 1, \ldots L$$

$$\text{type e.g. RCT,CC, etc.}$$

$$\delta_{jl} \sim \text{Normal}[\phi_l, \varphi_l^2] \qquad \phi_l \sim \text{Normal}[d, \tau^2]$$

$$\varphi_l^2 \sim [-, -] \qquad d \sim [-, -] \qquad \tau^2 \sim [-, -]$$

(11.6)

where Y_{jl} and V_{jl} are the effect size and variance in the jth study of type l. In the context of the EFM example, the effect sizes are RDs, and $l = 1, 2, 3$ which relate to RCTs, comparative cohort studies and before and after studies, respectively. d is the overall pooled effect over all sources of evidence, and τ^2 is the between study type variance. ϕ_l is the pooled effect within study type l, and φ_l^2 is the between study variance within study type l. δ_{jl} is the true underlying effect estimated by the observed Y_{jl} with variance V_{jl}. When fitted in WinBUGS, φ_l^2, d and τ^2 require prior distributions with the notation indicating these are to be specified by the user. The schematic of the hierarchical data structure this model imposes in Figure 11.4 may help to conceptualise this model.

The WinBUGS code used to implement this model for the EFM data is presented in Box 11.3. This code can be thought of as split into four sections. The first three sections consider the RCTs, cohort studies and before after studies,

Table 11.2 Data from 9 RCTs, 7 comparative cohort studies and 10 before and after studies examining the effect of EFM on perinatal mortality.

Study ID	Year of publication	Number of subjects given EFM	Number of subjects not given EFM	Number of perinatal deaths in treatment arm	Number of perinatal deaths in control arm	Risk Difference per 1000 births	Standard error of Risk Difference	95% CI for Risk Difference
Randomised Controlled Trials								
R1	1976	175	175	1	1	0.00	8.06	(−15.79 to 15.79)
R2	1976	242	241	2	1	4.12	7.14	(−9.88 to 18.11)
R3	1978	253	251	0	1	−3.98	5.59	(−14.93 to 6.97)
R4	1979	463	232	3	0	6.48	5.03	(−3.38 to 16.34)
R5	1981	445	482	1	0	2.25	3.11	(−3.84 to 8.34)
R6	1985	485	493	0	1	−2.03	2.87	(−7.66 to 3.60)
R7	1985	6530	6554	14	14	0.001	0.81	(−1.58 to 1.59)
R8	1987	122	124	17	18	−5.82	44.54	(−93.11 to 81.48)
R9	1993	746	682	2	9	−10.52	4.76	(−19.85 to −1.18)
Comparative cohort studies								
C1	1973	1162	5427	2	17	−1.41	1.43	(−4.22 to 1.40)
C2	1973	150	6836	0	15	−2.19	4.71	(−11.43 to 7.04)
C3	1975	608	6179	1	37	−4.34	1.91	(−8.10 to −0.59)
C4	1977	4210	2923	1	9	−2.84	1.05	(−4.90 to −0.78)
C5	1978	554	692	1	3	−2.53	3.08	(−8.57 to 3.51)
C6	1979	4978	8634	0	2	−0.23	0.23	(−0.69 to 0.22)
C7	1982	45880	66208	10	45	−0.46	0.12	(−0.70 to −0.22)

(continued overleaf)

Table 11.2 (continued)

Study ID	Year of publication	Number of subjects given EFM	Number of subjects not given EFM	Number of perinatal deaths in treatment arm	Number of perinatal deaths in control arm	Risk Difference per 1000 births	Standard error of Risk Difference	95% CI for Risk Difference
Before and after studies								
B1	1975	991	1024	4	0	−4.04	2.24	(−8.43 to 0.35)
B2	1975	1161	1080	7	9	2.30	3.58	(−4.71 to 9.32)
B3	1975	11599	1950	14	1	−0.69	0.61	(−1.88 to 0.49)
B4	1976	4323	3529	15	1	−3.19	0.94	(−5.03 to −1.35)
B5	1977	4114	3852	53	21	−7.43	2.12	(−11.59 to −3.27)
B6	1978	15357	7312	35	6	−1.46	0.51	(−2.46 to −0.46)
B7	1980	4240	4503	19	2	−4.04	1.07	(−6.14 to −1.93)
B8	1980	6740	8174	15	5	−1.61	0.64	(−2.86 to −0.37)
B9	1984	7582	7911	13	2	−1.46	0.51	(−2.46 to −0.47)
B10	1986	17409	17586	7	5	−0.12	0.20	(−0.51 to 0.27)

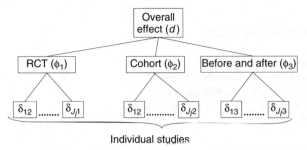

Figure 11.4   Schematic of hierarchical structure of synthesis model. Notation described in Equation (11.6).

respectively and the code is identical in structure for all three. Note that the code does not follow the notational convention of Equation (11.6) and Figure 11.4, as it does not use a double indexing convention. Rather it uses a single index for study within study type and separate code is written for each study design (the reader may want to take on the challenge of rewriting the code using the double index convention). Data are entered as RDs and associated standard errors and combined assuming studies of the same design are exchangeable using a Random Effects model (although the code is a slight reparameterisation of that presented in Section 4.3). For each type of evidence, a different pooled mean (theta[1], theta[2], theta[3]) and between study (within type) standard deviation (sd.theta[1], sd.theta[2], sd.theta[3]) is estimated. In the fourth section of the code, these three pooled estimates are assumed to be themselves exchangeable, with overall mean 'mean' and standard deviation, sd.mean.

```
model {

# Randomised controlled trials

for (i in 1:R) {
    rct.prec[i]  <- 1/(rct.serd[i]*rct.serd[i])
    rct.rd[i]  ~ dnorm(rct.psi[i],rct.prec[i])
    rct.psi[i] <- theta[1] + (rct.z[i]*sd.theta[1])
    rct.z[i] ~dnorm(0,1) }

# Comparative cohort studies model

for (i in 1:C) {
    coh.prec[i]  <- 1/(coh.serd[i]*coh.serd[i])
    coh.rd[i]  ~ dnorm(coh.psi[i],coh.prec[i])
    coh.psi[i] <- theta[2] + (coh.z[i]*sd.theta[2])
    coh.z[i] ~dnorm(0,1)   }
```

```
# Before after studies model

for (i in 1:B) {
    ba.prec[i]  <- 1/(ba.serd[i]*ba.serd[i])
    ba.rd[i]  ~ dnorm(ba.psi[i],ba.prec[i])
    ba.psi[i] <- theta[3] + (ba.z[i]*sd.theta[3])
    ba.z[i] ~dnorm(0,1)   }

# Combining all 3 sources

for(i in 1:T) {
    theta[i] <- mean + (u[i]*sd.mean)
    u[i] ~dnorm(0,1)
    sd.theta[i] ~ dnorm(0,0.1)I(0,)
    var.theta[i] <- sd.theta[i]*sd.theta[i]
    prec.theta[i] <- 1/(sd.theta[i]*sd.theta[i])
                }
    mean  ~ dnorm(0,0.01)
    sd.mean ~ dnorm(0,0.1)I(0,)
    var.mean <- sd.mean*sd.mean
    prec.mean<-1/(sd.mean*sd.mean)
}

Data
list(R=9, C=7, B=10, T=3,
rct.rd=c(-10.51552,-2.028398,4.115085,6.479482,.0078509,0,2.247191,
        -5.817028,-3.984064),
rct.serd=c(4.762193,2.871006,7.142432,5.032322,.8079891,8.058098,
        3.1075,44.53912,5.587013),
ba.rd=c(-4.036327,2.304048,-.6941801,-3.186446,-7.431126,-1.458522,
        -4.036984,-1.613824,-1.461775,-.1177738),
ba.serd=c(2.242277,3.579612,.6056279,.9381518,2.121014,.5100973,
        1.072718,.6358061,.507642,.1981163),
coh.rd=c(-1.41,-2.19,-4.34,-2.84,-2.53,-.23,-.46),
coh.serd=c(1.433,4.71,1.914,1.052,3.081,.232,.123))

Initial values
list(mean=-0.001, sd.mean=0.001, sd.theta=c(0.001,0.001,0.001))
```

Box 11.3 WinBUGS code for three-level hierarchical model allowing for heterogeneity between study types applied to the EFM example.

The results using this code are presented in Figure 11.5 [16] together with standard random effect meta-analysis model estimates included for comparison. It can be seen that the RCT evidence suggests a smaller treatment effect than the observational evidence, although there is considerable uncertainty in that estimate.

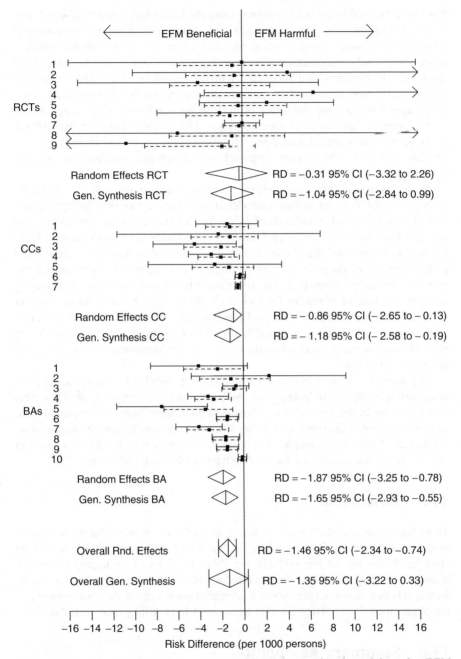

Figure 11.5   Results of applying the three-level hierarchical model to the EFM example with standard meta-analysis results also presented for comparison. RCTs, Randomised Controlled Trials; CCs, Comparative Cohort studies; BAs, Before and After studies. Reproduced from Sutton and Abrams [16].

Note how the study type level estimates from the hierarchical model (labelled Gen. Synthesis estimates) are shrunk towards each other, since there is a borrowing of strength across study designs due to the assumption of exchangeability which is made across study design means. The overall pooled estimate from the hierarchical model is very similar to that obtained if a meta-analysis of all the studies, ignoring study design, were conducted, but the uncertainty around the estimate is considerably larger reflecting the modelling of heterogeneity between study design means in the former. In this way, heterogeneity caused by potential biases in the different study designs has been accounted for. This example is considered in more detail in Section 11.8 where the previous approaches to generalised synthesis of evidence are also applied.

It can be argued that if one evidence type is clearly superior to the others, for example the RCTs in the context considered here, then it may be more appropriate to focus on the shrunken estimate of effect for this specific study type (borrowing strength from the other study type data) compared with the overall mean [17]. In Chapter 4, it was noted that if there are small numbers of studies in a random effect meta-analysis then the prior distribution placed on the heterogeneity parameter can be unintentionally informative. The same issue is relevant here when considering not only the number of studies for each study design type, but also for the number of types of design combined. In the EFM example, there are only three different study types which means it is advisable to conduct sensitivity analyses considering the influence of the prior distribution placed on the heterogeneity between study types (i.e. sd.mean).

A powerful extension to this modelling is the possibility of incorporating prior information on the possible extent of the bias in the different study designs. This could be done in the form of bias adjustment parameters based on empirical data, as was discussed in the previous section. Alternatively, constraints can be placed on the degree of bias. For example, it is possible to impose the prior belief constraint that the RCTs are less biased than either type of observational study [13].

11.5   Discussion

This chapter has presented some relatively simple ways of including observational evidence into a synthesis acknowledging that it may be biased. Whilst there is no 'free lunch' for any of the methods, i.e. they are all based on largely untestable assumptions; they do offer a framework for sensitivity analysis and hence establishing whether decisions are robust to potential beliefs about the shortcomings of the observational data. They are also transparent in how they treat such data.

11.6   Summary key points

- Observational studies could be included along with trials in meta-analyses estimating effectiveness. Such an analysis would ignore the fact that observational studies provide potentially biased estimates of effects. Therefore, there has been a desire to develop methods which include observational evidence but acknowledge this concern.

• Complex methods to adjust individual studies for potential internal and external biases based on empirical data and expert opinion are currently being developed but are not considered further in this chapter.

• What are considered are three different methods of downweighting observational evidence acknowledging it is potentially (more) biased than the randomised evidence. These comprise of a method based on power priors, bias adjusted downweighting based on empirical data and hierarchical models taking between study design variability into account.

• None of the approaches offers a 'free lunch'; they all may be useful as a framework for conducting sensitivity analyses and all are transparent in how they deal with observational data.

11.7   Further reading

In addition to newer methods mentioned in the introduction [2, 3], other approaches to the synthesis of randomised and observational evidence have been considered. Cross-Design Synthesis [18] was an approach started from a concern that results obtained from RCTs may not necessarily generalise to wider patients groups and that RCT and register data should be combined. Methods including covariate adjustment, standardisation and propensity scores could be used to provide adjusted measures of treatment effects from nonrandomised studies.

The Confidence Profile Method (CPM) was the development of a whole system of multi-parameter approaches to synthesis and evaluation [19, 20] (already discussed in Chapter 8). Adjustment for bias was strongly emphasised in this approach, and the CPM literature sets out formulae for adjusting basic or functional parameters for confounding bias, contamination, dilution, errors in measurement, errors in ascertainment, loss to follow-up, patient selection, differences between populations or differences in treatment intensity.

Models for specific situations have been described in the statistics literature. Li and Begg [21] present a model to estimate an overall treatment effect when some comparative studies are to be combined with noncomparative, historically controlled 'single arm' studies. They assume baseline effects are exchangeable in their modelling approach. Larose and Dey [22] describe a grouped Random Effects model which distinguishes between open and closed studies, allowing the degree of between study heterogeneity to be different in each group and thus is similar to the hierarchical model of Section 11.4 although the group means are not assumed to be exchangeable. Finally, a number of authors [23, 24] have investigated the use of hierarchical Bayesian models for interspecies extrapolation of dose-response functions motivated by situations where there was an abundance of precise data available from animals concerning the assessment of cancer risks from environmental agents, but little accurate information on direct effects in humans.

11.8 Exercises

Electronic fetal heart rate monitoring and perinatal mortality

The wide spread use of EFM in the early 1970s in the UK coincided with a fall in the overall perinatal mortality rate. It is plausible that EFM reduces intrapartum and possibly also neonatal deaths since healthy babies sometimes die during labour, and timely Caesarean delivery usually prevents this. They usually exhibit an altered fetal heart rate pattern for some time before hypoxic death and it is difficult to hear and interpret this by intermittent auscultation. Nevertheless evidence-based reviews have concluded that 'EFM... has not been shown to reduce perinatal mortality' [25], that 'intrapartum electronic monitoring significantly increases the chances of Caesarean delivery without any apparent benefits in terms of neonatal outcome' [26], or that 'the only clinically significant benefit ... was in the reduction of neonatal seizures' [27]. However, such reviews ignore the considerable evidence available outside the RCTs.

Randomized evidence

A recent systematic review of the literature yielded nine RCTs which explicitly evaluated EFM compared with control in terms of perinatal mortality. For each trial, the number of expecting mothers and number of perinatal deaths in each arm are reported. From these, an estimate of treatment between the groups, the RD, is calculated (per 1000 births). This is done using the following formula:

$$RD = \left(\frac{r_1}{n_1} - \frac{r_2}{n_2}\right) \times 1000, \qquad (11.7)$$

where r_1 and r_2 are the numbers of deaths in the treatment and control groups, respectively and n_1 and n_2 are the total number of subjects in the treatment and control arms, respectively. For example, for the fifth RCT in *efm RD.xls* the RD calculation is:

$$RD = \left(\frac{1}{445} - \frac{0}{482}\right) \times 1000$$

$$= 2.25 \text{ per 1000 births.}$$

This is interpreted as the difference between the probabilities of an event occurring in the two groups. The variance of this measure is calculated by:

$$\text{var}(RD) = \left(\frac{\frac{r_1}{n_1}\left(1 - \frac{r_1}{n_1}\right)}{n_1} + \frac{\frac{r_2}{n_2}\left(1 - \frac{r_2}{n_2}\right)}{n_2}\right) \times 10^6 \qquad (11.8)$$

For the fifth RCT there are no deaths in the control arm. If Equation (11.8) was used directly the uncertainty in the RD would be underestimated because the variance component due to the control arm would be zero. To get round this problem, a continuity correction is required. Here, 0.5 is added to the number of deaths, and 1 is added to the total number of women in each arm of every study where there are no events in one or both arms. Hence, the calculation of the variance of the RD for the fifth trial is:

$$\text{var}(RD) = \left(\frac{\frac{1.5}{446}\left(1 - \frac{1.5}{446}\right)}{446} + \frac{\frac{0.5}{483}\left(1 - \frac{0.5}{483}\right)}{483} \right) \times 10^6$$

$$= 9.66$$

A 95% confidence interval for the treatment difference can be constructed if the outcome is assumed normally distributed using the following formula: $RD \pm 1.96 \times \sqrt{\text{var}(RD)}$.

Observational evidence

There have also been a number of reports from single units or regions, either before and after the introduction of near universal monitoring (referred to here as before and after studies) or comparing monitored and unmonitored patients in units where monitoring was not universal (referred to here as nonrandomised comparative studies). *efm RD.xls* contains data on 7 nonrandomised comparative studies and 10 before and after studies.

Practical tasks

All the data can be found in the Excel file *efm RD.xls* [16].

11.1 In WinBUGs, use a random effects generic meta-analysis model just for the RCTs to obtain a posterior distribution of the pooled RD/1000 births and calculate the posterior probability that EFM is superior.

11.2 Similarly, considering all the nonrandomised evidence as a whole, in WinBUGS use a random effects generic meta-analysis model to obtain the posterior distribution of the pooled RD/1000 and the posterior probability that EFM is superior.

11.3 Use the posterior distribution of the pooled RD/1000 obtained using all the observational studies to derive a prior distribution for the pooled effect in the RCTs, and calculate the corresponding posterior distribution of the pooled RD/1000 births and the posterior probability that EFM is superior.

11.4 Consider downweighting the prior distribution based on all the observational studies using a power transform prior and obtain the corresponding posterior distributions of the pooled RD/1000 births. (Hint: In WinBUGS you cannot use the same data more than once without it affecting the estimation of model parameters – therefore you need to replicate the data set either in Excel/Stata or WinBUGS the same number of times as you have values of alpha – see *HRT power prior.odc*.)

*11.5 Finally, consider using a three-level hierarchical model to synthesise the RCT, nonrandomised comparative and the before and after studies within a single model. Explore how sensitive this model is to both the prior distributions used for the between study within type precision/variance and also the prior distribution used for the between type precision/variance (see *breast screening.odc*).

References

1. Black N. Why we need observational studies to evaluate the effectiveness of health care. *British Medical Journal* 1996;**312**:1215–1218.

2. Turner R.M., Spiegelhalter D.J., Smith G.C.S., Thompson S.G. Bias modelling in evidence synthesis. *Journal of the Royal Statistical Society, Series A* 2009;**172**:21–48.

3. Welton N.J., Ades A.E., Carlin J., *et al.* Models for potentially biased evidence in meta-analysis using empirically based priors. *Journal of the Royal Statistical Society, Series A* 2009;**172**:119–136.

4. Torgerson D.J., Bell-Syer S.E. Hormone replacement therapy and prevention of vertebral fractures: A meta-analysis of randomised trials. *BMC Musculoskeletal Disorders* 2001;**2**:7.

5. Torgerson D.J., Bell-Syer S.E. Hormone replacement therapy and prevention of nonvertebral fractures: A meta-analysis of randomized trials. *Journal of the American Medical Association* 2001;**285**(22):2891–2897.

6. Collaborative Group on Hormonal Factors in Breast Cancer. Breast cancer and hormone replacement therapy: collaborative reanalysis of data from 51 epidemiological studies of 52,705 women with breast cancer and 108,411 women without breast cancer. *Lancet* 1997;**350**(9084):1047–1059.

7. Ibrahim J.G., Chen M.H. Power prior distributions for regression models. *Statistical Science* 2000;**15**:46–60.

8. Sacks H.S., Chalmers T.C., Smith H. Randomized versus historical controls for clinical trials. *American Journal of Medicine* 1982;**72**:233–240.

9. Ioannidis J.P.A., Haidich A.-B., Pappa M., *et al.* Comparison of evidence of treatment effects in randomised and nonrandomised studies. *Journal of the American Medical Association* 2001;**286**:821–830.

10. MacLehose R.R., Reeves B.C., Harvey I.M., *et al.* A systematic review of comparisons of effect sizes derived from randomised and non-randomised studies. *Health Technology Assessment* 2000;**4**(34):1–154.

11. Deeks J.J., Dinnes J., D'Amico R., *et al.* Evaluating non-randomised intervention studies. *Health Technology Assessment* 2003;**7**(27).

12. Writing Group for the Women's Health Initiative Investigators. Risks and benefits of estrogen plus progestin in healthy postmenopausal women. *Journal of the American Medical Association* 2002;**288**:321–333.

13. Prevost T C., Abrams K.R., Jones D.R. Hierarchical models in generalised synthesis of evidence: an example based on studies of breast cancer screening. *Statistics in Medicine* 2000;**19**:3359–3376.

14. Hornbuckle J., Vail A., Abrams K.R., Thornton J.G. Bayesian interpretation of trials: the example of intrapartum electronic fetal heart rate monitoring. *British Journal of Obstetrics and Gynaecology* 2000;**107**:3–10.

15. Deeks J.J. Issues in the selection of a summary statistic for meta-analysis of clinical trials with binary outcomes. *Statistics in Medicine* 2002;**21**(11):1575–1600.

16. Sutton A.J., Abrams K.R. Bayesian methods in meta-analysis and evidence synthesis. *Statistical Methods in Medical Research* 2001;**10**:277–303.

17. Peters J.L., Rushton L., Sutton A.J., *et al.* Bayesian methods for the cross-design synthesis of epidemiological and toxicological evidence. *Journal of the Royal Statistical Society, Series C* 2005;**54**:159–172.

18. Droitcour J., Silberman G., Chelimsky E. Cross-design synthesis: A new form of meta-analysis for combining results from randomized clinical trials and medical-practice databases. *International Journal of Technology Assessment in Health Care* 1993;**9**:440–449.

19. Eddy D.M. The confidence profile method: A Bayesian method for assessing health technologies. *Operations Research* 1989;**37**:210–228.

20. Eddy D.M., Hasselblad V., Shachter R. *Meta-Analysis by the Confidence Profile Method*. San Diego: Academic Press, 1992.

21. Li Z.H., Begg C.B. Random effects models for combining results from controlled and uncontrolled studies in a metaanalysis. *Journal of the American Statistical Association* 1994;**89**:1523–1527.

22. Larose D.T., Dey D.K. Grouped random effects models for Bayesian meta-analysis. *Statistics in Medicine* 1997;**16**:1817–1829.

23. DuMouchel W.H., Harris J.E. Bayes methods for combining the results of cancer studies in humans and other species (with comment). *Journal of the American Statistical Association* 1983;**78**:293–308.

24. Jones D.R., Peters J., Rushton L., *et al.* Interspecies extrapolation in environmental exposure standard setting: a Bayesian synthesis approach. *Regulatory Toxicology and Pharmacology* 2009;**53**:217–225.

25. Anonymous. Listening to your baby's heartbeat during labour. Midwives Information and Resource Service (MIDIRS) and the NHS Centre for Reviews and Dissemination. Bristol: MIDIRS, 1995.

26. Neilson J. EFM plus scalp sampling vs intermittent auscultation in labour. In: Enkin M.W., Keirse M.J.N.C., Renfrew M.J., Neilson J.P., eds. Cochrane database of systematic reviews: pregnancy and childbirth module. Cochrane updates on disk: Issue 1. Oxford: Update Software, 1994.

27. Thacker S.B., Stroup D.F., Peterson H.B. Continuous electronic fetal heart rate monitoring during labour. In: Neilson J.P., Crowther C.A., Hodnett E.D., Hofmeyer G.J., Keirse M.J.N.C., eds. Cochrane database of systematic reviews: pregnancy and childbirth module. Cochrane updates on disk: Issue 2. Oxford: Update Software, 1997.

12

Expected value of information for research prioritisation and study design

12.1 Introduction

The underlying rationale for performing an evidence synthesis to inform a cost-effectiveness analysis (CEA) is that the resulting decision reflects the body of evidence available, producing joint parameter estimates and corresponding uncertainties. Parameter uncertainty is propagated through the CEA model and manifests itself as decision uncertainty. If we knew the value of the cost-effectiveness model input parameters exactly, then we would know which intervention gives the highest Net Benefit, NB, and there would be no doubt that the best decision would be to recommend this optimal intervention. However, if there is uncertainty in the cost-effectiveness model input parameters, we do not know exactly which parameter values to feed into the Net Benefit function. Instead, we average over the joint distribution that reflects parameter uncertainty to obtain Expected (average) Net Benefit, $E(NB)$. The best decision in the face of parameter uncertainty is to recommend the intervention with the highest $E(NB)$, but we can no longer be sure that this is the best decision, only that *on average* it is the best intervention. There is a probability that the parameters may actually take values that mean our chosen intervention does not have the highest NB, even though it has the highest $E(NB)$. In other words, there is uncertainty as to which is the best decision.

Decision uncertainty is typically measured by the probability that each intervention is the most cost-effective and displayed in a cost-effectiveness acceptability

Evidence Synthesis for Decision Making in Healthcare, First Edition. Nicky J. Welton,
Alexander J. Sutton, Nicola J. Cooper, Keith R. Abrams and A.E. Ades.
© 2012 John Wiley & Sons, Ltd. Published 2012 by John Wiley & Sons, Ltd.

curve (CEAC) as described in Section 3.5. Consider two scenarios – in the first scenario the intervention with highest E(NB) has a probability of being the most cost-effective $p(CE) = 0.9$, whilst in the second scenario it is only $p(CE) = 0.55$. In both scenarios, the intervention would be recommended as the most cost-effective, as it gives the highest E(NB). However, we would be more comfortable with a decision to implement the intervention in the first scenario where $p(CE) = 0.9$ than in the second scenario where $p(CE) = 0.55$, because there is a lower chance that we will get the decision 'wrong'.

If there is a high level of decision uncertainty we may wish to consider commissioning more research to add to the evidence base, and hence reduce decision uncertainty, before deciding to implement the optimal intervention. The value in carrying out further research is therefore dependent on the uncertainty in the decision. However, if the E(NB) lost from choosing a suboptimal intervention is very small, there will be little to gain from reducing uncertainty in the decision. The value in carrying out further research therefore depends on both the uncertainty in the decision, and the E(NB) lost from making the 'wrong' decision. The value of carrying out further research can be quantified with Expected Value of Information (EVI) calculations, which can help prioritise and design new research studies.

Methods for prioritising further research are intrinsically linked to evidence synthesis and CEA. We can think of the research process as a cyclical process (Figure 12.1) of synthesising all available evidence in order to make a decision to either adopt the most cost-effective intervention, reject that intervention, and/or commission further research. If further research is commissioned then a new study needs to be designed. The resulting evidence is then added to the evidence base and the synthesis of the evidence updated to make a new decision, and so on. This process is inherently Bayesian. We begin with priors for our parameters, which are updated by the currently available evidence to give posteriors for the parameters, which feed into the cost-effectiveness model. These posteriors then become the

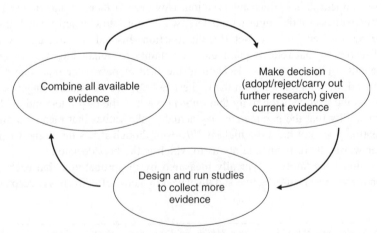

Figure 12.1   Cycle of evidence synthesis, cost-effectiveness analysis, and commissioning and collecting evidence from new research.

priors for the EVI analysis and for a new synthesis that incorporates new evidence collected in a new study. The synthesis produces posteriors for the parameters, which feed into the cost-effectiveness model, and so on.

In this chapter we introduce Expected Value of Perfect Information (EVPI), which measures the value of collecting infinite quantities of evidence on all parameters to eliminate decision uncertainty; Expected Value of Partial Perfect Information (EVPPI), which measures the value of collecting infinite quantities of evidence on just a subset of parameters, whilst retaining uncertainty in the remaining parameters; Expected Value of Sample Information (EVSI), which measures the value of collecting evidence from a given study design to reduce, but not eliminate, decision uncertainty; and Expected Net Benefit of Sampling (ENBS) which measures the net value of running a particular study design minus the costs of such a study, thus providing a basis for determining optimal study design. We illustrate the methods with an expanded multi-parameter evidence synthesis on the epidemiology of HIV in pregnant women that was first introduced in Section 8.3.

Example 12.1   HIV screening in pregnant women [1].

Prevalence model and data sources

We extend the HIV epidemiology evidence synthesis model presented in Section 8.3, to assess the cost-effectiveness of universal screening of all pregnant women as opposed to targeted screening of pregnant women in high risk groups. The model is identical to that presented elsewhere [1]. In Section 8.3, a model for HIV prevalence among pregnant women with five parameters was estimated from six items of data that provided information on various functions of the underlying basic parameters. In the CEA it is important not only to know the prevalence in the different risk groups, but also to distinguish between those who have already been diagnosed, and for whom there is no additional benefit to screening. Figure 12.2 shows the extended model, and Table 12.1 shows the 12 items of data that provide information on functions of the eight model parameters. Parameters a, b and $(1 - a - b)$ represent the proportion of pregnant women in each risk group, parameters c, d and e, the prevalence of HIV in each risk group, and parameters f, g and h the proportion of those HIV positives that have been diagnosed. Note that although data item 12 provides information on the model parameters a, b, d and e, it also depends on the proportion of serotype B in infected women in Sub-Saharan Africa (SSA), w. Data item 12 can only be incorporated in the synthesis model if there is also information on parameter w, which is provided by data item 11. Furthermore, it relies on the assumptions that 100% of infected injecting drug users (IDUs) are serotype B, and that the proportion of serotype B is the same in infected SSA and infected non-SSA. In total then we have 12 items of data providing information on 9 parameters.

The decision problem

The decision problem is to determine the most cost-effective of two screening strategies: targeted testing where only pregnant women in the high risk groups

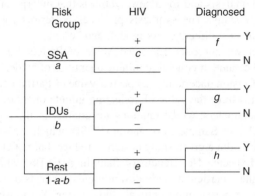

Figure 12.2   HIV epidemiology probability tree, showing for each risk group, the prevalence of HIV, and of those that are HIV positive, the proportion already diagnosed [1].

Table 12.1   Data sources and the parameters that they inform in the HIV epidemiology example [1]. Each data point is a Binomial observation.

Description of data	Function of parameters
1. Proportion of SSA	a
2. Proportion of IDUs	b
3. HIV prevalence in SSA	c
4. HIV prevalence in IDUs	d
5. HIV prevalence in non-SSA	$(db + e(1 - a - b))/(1 - a)$
6. Overall HIV prevalence	$(ca + db + e(1 - a - b))$
7. Proportion of diagnosed HIV+ that are SSA	$fca/(fca + gdb + he(1 - a - b))$
8. Proportion of non-SSA diagnosed HIV+ that are IDUs	$gdb/(gdb + he(1 - a - b))$
9. Overall proportion diagnosed HIV+	$\dfrac{(fca + gdb + he(1 - a - b))}{(ca + db + e(1 - a - b))}$
10. Proportion of IDUs HIV+ that are diagnosed	g
11. Proportion of serotype B in SSA HIV+	w
12. Proportion of serotype B in non-SSA HIV+	$(db + we(1 - a - b))/(db + e(1 - a - b))$

(SSA and IDUs) are tested, or universal testing where all pregnant women are tested. Costs and benefits for the high-risk (SSA and IDUs) risk groups are the same under both strategies. The differences between the strategies are for the low-risk (Rest) risk group. Figure 12.3 shows the decision tree for the Rest risk group, showing incremental costs and benefits of universal testing relative to targeted testing, where T is the cost of the screening test and M is the net maternal benefit of an early diagnosis. The incremental net benefit function for a population with N pregnancies per year is the product along the decision tree of incremental benefits minus incremental costs multiplies by the probability of each branch of the tree:

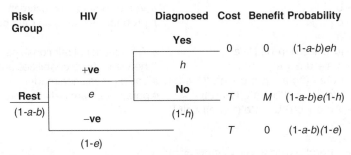

Figure 12.3   HIV screening decision tree [1]. Incremental cost and benefit is shown for universal relative to targeted testing in the low-risk (Rest) risk group.

$$NB(\theta, k) = \begin{cases} 0 & k = 1, \text{Targeted} \\ N(1 - a - b)(Me(1 - h) - T(1 - eh)) & k = 2, \text{Universal} \end{cases}$$
(12.1)

The parameters in the Net Benefit function can be classified into two groups, parameters from the epidemiology prevalence model, and parameters from the economic model:

$$\theta = \begin{cases} N, M, T & \text{Economic parmeters} \\ a, b, e, h & \text{Epidemiology parameters} \end{cases}$$
(12.2)

Following Ades and Cliffe [1], we set the number of pregnancies per year at $N = 105\,000$, the unit cost of an HIV test at $T = £3$, and the net benefit of an early maternal diagnosis M, comes from a previous model:

$$M = 600\,012 - 54\,296 * Y;$$

$$Y \sim \text{Gamma}(0.56, 3) \quad \text{censored to the interval}(0, 2) \tag{12.3}$$

The WinBUGS code for this model is:

```
model{   for(i in 1: 12) {r[i] ~ dbin(p[i],n[i])}   #Likelihood for 12 data points
    a ~ dbeta( 1,2)                        # SET PRIORS
```

```
z ~ dbeta (1,1)                                    # Priors for a, b, and 1-a-b must
b <- z * (1-a)                                     # sum to 1. Code equivalent to a
c ~ dbeta (1,1)                                    # Dirichlet prior.
d ~ dbeta (1,1)
e ~ dbeta (1,1)                                    # Prevalence parameters all
f ~ dbeta (1,1)                                    # given flat Beta priors
g ~ dbeta (1,1)
h ~ dbeta(1,1)
w ~ dbeta(1,1)


p[1] <- a
p[2] <- b                                          # Vector p holds the estimated
p[3] <- c                                          # probabilities for each data point
p[4] <- d
p[5] <- (d*b + e*(1-a-b))/(1- a)                   # The functional relationships
p[6] <- c*a + d*b + e*(1-a-b)                      # between the probabilities and
p[7] <- f*c*a / (f*c*a + g*d*b + h*e*(1-a-b))      # basic prevalence model
p[8] <- g*d*b / (g*d*b + h*e*(1-a-b))              # parameters are defined here
p[9] <- (f*c*a + g*d*b + h*e*(1-a-b)) / p[6]
p[10] <- g
p[11] <- w
p[12] <- d*b/(d*b+e*(1-a-b)) + w*e*(1-a-b)/
(d*b + e*(1-a-b))


M <-  60012 - 54296*Y                              # Distribution for net benefit of
Y ~ dgamma( 0.56,3)I(, 2)                          # maternal diagnosis


nb[1]<-0                                           #  Incremental NB relative to
nb[2] <-  105000*(1-a-b) * (M * e * (1-h) -        # Targeted Testing. k=1, Targeted,
3.0*(1-e*h))                                       # k=2 Universal
```

The posterior mean for node nb[2] gives an E(NB) of universal relative to targeted testing of £1 022 482. This is positive, indicating that the optimal strategy based on current information is universal testing, $k^{current} = 2$.

12.2   Expected value of perfect information

The EVPI measures the average gain in NB from knowing perfectly (exactly) what values the parameters take. In other words, EVPI is the gain from eliminating decision uncertainty altogether. You can think of this as the value of running an infinitely sized study, designed to jointly measure all of the parameters that input into the CEA. Whilst it is unlikely in practise that we could run such a study (although population census studies come close), EVPI is still a useful calculation, first because it is straightforward to calculate, and secondly because it provides an upper bound for the value of running a study of any given design. So, if there is little value in running an infinitely sized study that learns about all of the relevant parameters, there certainly will not be any value in running a smaller trial that only measures some of the model parameter inputs.

Let $NB(\theta, k)$ be the Net Benefit function for intervention, k, given values for the input parameters, θ. Then EVPI is given by:

$$
EVPI = \mathop{\mathrm{E}}_{\theta} \left[\underbrace{\max_{k} \{NB(\theta, k)\}}_{\text{NB based on perfect information}} \right] - \underbrace{\max_{k} \left\{ \mathop{\mathrm{E}}_{\theta} [NB(\theta, k)] \right\}}_{\text{NB based on current information}} \tag{12.4}
$$

Equation (12.4) is made up of two terms:

1. The first measures the Expected Net Benefit obtained if the parameters are known perfectly. For each realisation of the parameters, θ, from their joint distribution, intervention $k^*(\theta)$ is chosen to maximise the Net Benefit. The expectation is then made over the joint distribution of the parameters, to find the average Net Benefit gained from knowing exactly the values that θ take. If EVPI is to be evaluated using simulation, then the maximisation step in the first term is performed at each iteration of the simulation. The resulting simulated maximums are then averaged to get the Expected Net Benefit under perfect information.

2. The second term in Equation (12.4) is the Expected Net Benefit gained using current information, i.e. using the intervention $k^{current}$ which maximises $E(NB)$, where the expectation is over the joint distribution of the parameters. Note that here the maximisation is performed *after* the expectation is formed, and so comes outside the expectation. If EVPI is to be evaluated using simulation, then NB is calculated at each iteration of the simulation, and then averaged to form $E(NB)$ for each intervention. The Expected Net Benefit using current information is simply the maximum $E(NB)$ over all interventions, and $k^{current}$ is the intervention that achieves that maximum.

EVPI is the Expected Net Benefit gained from perfect information minus that gained based on current information (Equation (12.4)).

Equation (12.4) can be rewritten equivalently as a single expectation as shown in Equation (12.5), where $k^{current}$ is the optimal intervention based on current information:

$$
EVPI = \mathop{\mathrm{E}}_{\theta} \left[\underbrace{ \underbrace{\max_{k} \{NB(\theta, k)\}}_{\text{NB based on perfect information}} - \underbrace{NB(\theta, k^{current})}_{\text{NB based on current information}} }_{\text{Gain in NB from perfect information}} \right] \tag{12.5}
$$

Equation (12.5) shows clearly that EVPI is the expected gain in Net Benefit from using perfect rather than current information. This form is particularly useful in the calculation of EVPI from simulation, leading to generic WinBUGS code. Equation (12.5) also highlights one of the computational issues associated with EVI calculations. On simulations where the optimal decision is unchanged (i.e. where $k^*(\theta) = k^{current}$), the terms inside the expectation in Equation (12.5) cancel out to give a gain in NB of zero. The simulated gains in NB are therefore a sequence of zeros (when the decision does not change) and positive values (when the decision does change). This means that long simulated chains are required for the average of these simulated gains to provide precise estimates of EVPI, and this is especially the case when the optimal decision from using perfect compared with current information does not change very often.

Suppose that Net Benefit for intervention k is calculated from a Markov Chain Monte Carlo (MCMC) simulation in WinBUGS in node nb[k]. Two identical runs of the MCMC simulation (with the same random number sequence) are required to calculate EVPI. In the first, posterior summaries are obtained for nodes nb[k], and the optimal intervention based on current information determined as the intervention, $k^{current}$, with greatest posterior mean for nb[k]. The optimal intervention is then entered as a data variable k.current in a repeat run of the MCMC simulation. A single additional line of code is required to calculate EVPI (where N.k is the number of interventions):

```
vpi<-   ranked(nb[ ],N.k)-nb[k.current]      #VPI. Posterior mean gives EVPI
```

The function ranked returns the N.kth smallest element of nb (i.e. the greatest value). Therefore ranked *maximises* the NB function on each iteration of the MCMC simulation, giving the first term inside the expectation in Equation (12.5). nb[k.current] picks out the Net Benefit for the optimal intervention based on current information, giving the second term inside the expectation in Equation (12.5). Monitoring node vpi, and calculating its posterior mean forms the outer expectation in Equation (12.5), and hence gives EVPI. This approach and code is generic and can be applied to any CEA. EVPI is always very straightforward to calculate.

Example 12.1 revisited   HIV screening in pregnant women [1].

Expected value of perfect information

We assume a 10-year time horizon for the screening strategy, and so EVPI is multiplied by 10. However, it is common to discount returns in decision models. Using a discount rate of 5% we multiply EVPI by 7.7127 (rather than 10). In this example there are only two strategies, so the WinBUGS code is:

```
vpi<- 7.7127*(ranked(nb[ ],2)-nb[k.current])      # k.current = 2, Universal Testing
```

Based on a burn-in of 50 000 iterations, and an MCMC sample of 1 000 000, the posterior mean for node vpi gives an EVPI of £71 670. This is positive suggesting that there may be some value in carrying out further research to eliminate uncertainty, however, the actual value is fairly moderate, and in practise would be outweighed by the cost of running such a further study. Figure 12.4 shows the posterior density for the Net Benefit of universal relative to targeted screening. The optimal decision is 'wrong' on those simulations where *NB* is negative, and a decision of targeted rather than universal testing should have been made. In this example, the percentage of simulations where *NB* is negative is only 2.9% (Figure 12.4), which partly explains why EVPI is small in this case. Note the very large number of simulation samples required to obtain stable estimates of the posterior mean of node vpi, again due to the small probability that the decision changes.

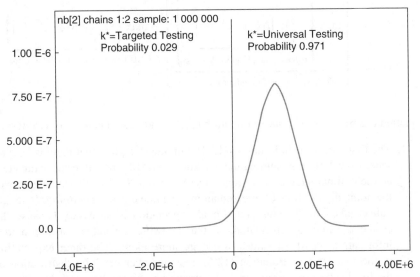

Figure 12.4   Posterior density of Incremental Net Benefit for universal relative to targeted testing for HIV in pregnant women.

12.3   Expected value of partial perfect information

CEA models typically depend on many parameters, which may not all be measurable in the same future study. EVPI assumes that uncertainty is eliminated in *all* of the CEA model parameters. However, we might consider collecting further evidence on only a subset of the CEA model parameters - for example relative treatment effect parameters, natural history parameters describing disease progression, utility parameters or economic parameters. The EVPPI measures the average gain in *NB* from knowing perfectly (exactly) what values a subset of the CEA model parameters take, whilst current uncertainty remains for the other CEA model parameters. In other words, the value of running an infinitely sized study, designed to jointly measure all of the subset of parameters, but no further evidence is collected on other parameters that input into the CEA. As with EVPI, it is unlikely in practise that we could run such an infinitely sized study, however EVPPI is useful to provide an upper bound for the value of running a study on the particular focal subset of parameters, and also as a tool for sensitivity analysis to determine which parameters are the key determinants of decision uncertainty.

Suppose we are interested in the value in eliminating uncertainty in the subset φ of parameters $\theta = \{\varphi, \varphi^C\}$. EVPPI is given by:

$$
EVPPI = \underset{\varphi}{E} \left[\underset{k}{\max} \left\{ \underbrace{\underset{\varphi^C|\varphi}{E} [NB(\varphi, \varphi^C, k)]}_{\text{E(NB) over } \varphi^C \text{ given know } \varphi} \right\} - \underset{k}{\max} \underbrace{\left\{ \underset{\varphi,\varphi^C}{E} \left[NB(\varphi, \varphi^C, k) \right] \right\}}_{\text{NB based on current information}} \right]
$$
$$
\underbrace{\phantom{EVPPI = E\left[\max \left\{ E [NB(\varphi, \varphi^C, k)] \right\} \right.}}_{\text{NB based on perfect information on } \varphi}
$$

(12.6)

Equation (12.6) is very similar to Equation (12.4), and again made up of two terms:

1. The first term is as in Equation (12.4) with the exception that there is now an inner expectation. Assuming that we know perfectly the values of parameters φ, the optimal strategy is to maximise Expected Net Benefit, averaged over the joint distribution of the remaining parameters φ^C *conditional* on the values taken by φ. This conditional expectation is necessary because the φ and φ^C may be correlated, so that knowing the values of φ provides information on which values of φ^C are more likely. The outer expectation in the first term of Equation (12.6) averages over the joint distribution of the focal subset of parameters, φ to obtain the average Expected Net Benefit obtained from eliminating uncertainty in parameters φ.

2. The second term of Equation (12.6) is identical to that in Equation (12.4), and measures the Expected Net Benefit obtained using current information, which is simply the maximum $E(NB)$ over all interventions. $k^{current}$ is the intervention that achieves that maximum.

EVPPI is the Expected Net Benefit obtained from perfect information on subset φ minus that obtained based on current information (Equation (12.6)).

Equation (12.6) can be rewritten equivalently in a more convenient format for computation:

$$EVPPI = \underset{\varphi}{E} \left[\underset{k}{\max} \left\{ \underbrace{\underset{\varphi^C|\varphi}{E} \left[NB \left(\varphi, \varphi^C, k \right) \right]}_{NB \text{ given } \varphi, \text{ based on perfect information}} \right\} - \underbrace{\underset{\varphi^C|\varphi}{E} \left[NB \left(\varphi, \varphi^C, k^{current} \right) \right]}_{NB \text{ given } \varphi, \text{ based on current information}} \right]$$

$$\underbrace{}_{\text{Gain in NB from perfect information conditional on } \varphi}$$

(12.7)

Equation (12.7) shows that EVPPI can be interpreted as the average gain in E(NB) from perfect information on parameters φ.

12.3.1   Computation

Computation of EVPPI is not straightforward because of the inner conditional expectation, and it is often necessary to resort to a nested sequence of simulations. There are, however, some special cases where the inner expectation can readily be calculated within a single simulation [2]:

C1: When Net Benefit is a linear function of parameters φ^C and there are no correlations between φ and φ^C, then the inner conditional expectation can be written:

$$\underset{\varphi^C|\varphi}{E} \left[NB \left(\varphi, \varphi^C, k \right) \right] = NB \left(\varphi, \underset{\varphi^C}{E} \left[\varphi^C \right], k \right)$$ (12.8)

C2: Equation (12.8) also holds if Net Benefit is a multilinear function in parameters φ^C (meaning that it can be written as a sum of products of the parameters φ^C) and there are no correlations between φ and φ^C, *and* there are no correlations between the parameters φ^C.

When either of conditions C1 or C2 holds then Equation (12.7) can be evaluated by two identical runs (with the same random number sequence) of the MCMC simulation. In the first, posterior summaries are obtained for nodes nb[k] and parameters φ^C, phi.C. The optimal intervention based on current information is determined as the intervention, $k^{current}$, with greatest posterior mean for nb[k]. The optimal intervention and posterior means of the φ^C parameters are then entered as data variables k.current and E.phi.C, respectively, in a repeat run of the MCMC simulation. The following additional lines of code are required to calculate EVPPI (where N.k is the number of interventions):

```
nb.phi[k]<- NB formula replacing
phi.C with E.phi.C                          #NB plugging in means for phi.C
vppi.phi<- ranked(nb.phi[ ],N.k)-nb.phi[k.current]  #VPPI. Posterior mean gives EVPPI
```

Example 12.1 revisited   HIV screening in pregnant women [1].

EVPPI for epidemiology parameters a, b, e, h

Let the focal subset of parameters for further research be the HIV epidemiology parameters so that $\varphi = \{a, b, e, h\}$ and the remaining parameter, the net maternal benefit of an early diagnosis, $\varphi^C = \{M\}$. Equation (12.1) shows that Net Benefit is a linear function of $\varphi^C = \{M\}$. Furthermore, the parameter M is estimated from independent data sources to the evidence that informs the epidemiology parameters, so it is assumed that there are no correlations between $\varphi = \{a, b, e, h\}$ and $\varphi^C = \{M\}$. Condition C1 is therefore met, and we can calculate EVPPI in a single MCMC simulation.

A first run of the WinBUGS model gives a posterior mean for M of E.M = 49940.29, and as previously found the optimal strategy based on current information is universal testing, $k^{current} = 2$. The following code allows the calculation of EVPPI for the epidemiology parameters as the posterior mean of node vppi.epi:

```
nb.epi[1]<- 0                                        #E(NB) conditional on
nb.epi[2]<- 105000*(1-a-b) * (E.M * e * (1-h) - 3.0*(1-e*h))   #epi parameters. Plug in
                                                     #posterior mean for
                                                     #M, E.M

vppi.epi<-7.7217*(ranked(nb.epi[ ],2) - nb[k.current])    # Posterior mean gives
                                                     #EVPPI
#DATA                                                #Enter in optimal
list(k.current=2, E.M=49940.29)                      #strategy, and posterior
                                                     #mean for M as data
```

The posterior mean of node vppi.epi gives a value of £2736 for the EVPPI for epidemiology parameters. This suggests that there is very little value in carrying our further research to reduce uncertainty in the epidemiology parameters.

EVPPI for economic parameter, M

Now let the focal parameter for further research be the 'economic' parameter $\varphi = \{M\}$, the net maternal benefit of an early diagnosis, and the remaining parameters on which no further evidence will be obtained be the HIV epidemiology parameters $\varphi^C = \{a, b, e, h\}$. Equation (12.1) shows that Net Benefit is a multi-linear function of $\varphi^C = \{a, b, e, h\}$ because these parameters appear as products in Equation (12.1). However, condition C2 is not directly met because although $\varphi = \{M\}$ is not correlated with $\varphi^C = \{a, b, e, h\}$, there are correlations between the epidemiology parameters $\varphi^C = \{a, b, e, h\}$. This can be seen in Figure 12.5, in particular the negative correlations between e and h. This arises because the majority of the evidence on e and h is on their product eh, inducing a negative posterior correlation between them (on simulations where e is high, h is correspondingly low and vice versa to give a product that is consistent with the evidence).

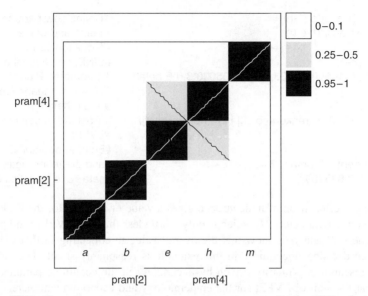

Figure 12.5 Posterior correlations between parameters in the CEA of universal vs targeted testing for HIV in pregnant women. The direction of the line in each cell shows the direction of association (i.e. negative correlation between parameters e and h). The shading indicates the strength of a linear relationship.

We therefore cannot directly exploit conditions C1 or C2. However, by re-parameterisation, we will show that we can apply condition C1 in this case. If we let:

$$\beta_1 = (1 - a - b)e(1 - h)$$

$$\beta_2 = (1 - a - b)(1 - eh) \qquad (12.9)$$

Then the Net Benefit function can be written:

$$NB(\varphi, \varphi^C, k) = \begin{cases} 0 & \text{Targeted, } k = 1 \\ NM\beta_1 - NT\beta_2 & \text{Universal, } k = 2 \end{cases} \qquad (12.10)$$

where $\varphi = \{M\}$ and $\varphi^C = \{\beta_1, \beta_2\}$. Now, Net Benefit is linear in φ^C, and there are no correlations between φ and φ^C, so condition C1 applies, and we can calculate EVPPI in a single MCMC simulation.

Code needs to be added to obtain posterior summaries for $\varphi^C = \{\beta_1, \beta_2\}$. A first run of the WinBUGS model gives posterior means for $\varphi^C = \{\beta_1, \beta_2\}$ of E.beta1= 2.481787E - 4 and E.beta2 = 0.8851898, and as previously found the optimal strategy based on current information is universal testing, $k^{current} = 2$. The following code allows the calculation of EVPPI for the economic parameter M as the posterior mean of node vppi.ec:

```
beta1<- (1-a-b)*e*(1-h)                          #Define new parameters
beta2<-(1-a-b)*(1-e*h)                           #beta1 and beta2
                                                 #(equation 12.9)
nb.ec[1]<-0                                      #E(NB) conditional on ec
nb.ec[2]<- 105000*M*E.beta1 - 105000*3.0*E.beta2  #parameter. Plug in
                                                 #posterior means E.beta1
                                                 #and E.beta2
vppi.ec<-7.7217*(ranked(nb.ec[ ],2) - nb[k.current]))  # Posterior mean gives
                                                 #EVPPI
#DATA                                            #Enter in optimal strategy,
list(k.current.2,E.beta1=2.481787E-4,            #and posterior mean for
E.beta2=0.8851898)                               #beta1 and beta2 as data
```

The posterior mean of node vppi.ec gives a value of £67 743 for the EVPPI for the economic parameter, M, which is only a little less than the EVPI for all parameters. The EVI analyses show that the overall value in collecting further evidence to reduce decision uncertainty in this example is reasonably small. The value of further research is primarily driven by uncertainty in the economic parameter M. Note that the sum of EVPPI for the epidemiology and economic parameters is not equal to EVPI.

12.3.2   Notes on EVPPI

Note that the sum of EVPPI over all sets of parameters will not necessarily equal EVPI. This is because EVPI is not a linear function of the CEA model input parameters. Note also that there can be value in collecting further evidence on parameters that are not directly in the CEA model, due to correlations with parameters that are in the CEA model induced by evidence informing complex functions of parameters (Table 12.1).

12.4   Expected value of sample information

EVPI and EVPPI both assume that uncertainty is eliminated, and therefore provide an upper bound for the value of running further research. In practise, a study with finite sample size can only reduce, not eliminate, uncertainty in the parameters that it is designed to inform. The EVSI measures the average gain in NB from running a study with a specific design and size to inform the subset of parameters φ. It is useful to think of the joint distribution for parameters $\theta = \{\varphi, \varphi^C\}$ based on current information as the prior, and the updated joint distribution for $\theta = \{\varphi, \varphi^C\}$ as the posterior having observed data D generated from the proposed new study.

EVSI is given by:

$$
EVSI = \underset{\varphi,\varphi^C}{E} \left[\underbrace{ \underset{D|\varphi,\varphi^C}{E} \left[\max_k \left\{ \underbrace{ \underset{\varphi,\varphi^C|D}{E} \left[NB\left(\varphi, \varphi^C, k\right) \right] }_{\text{E(NB) over } \varphi \text{ and } \varphi^C \text{ given data D}} \right\} \right] }_{\substack{ \text{NB based on \textbf{sample} information D on } \varphi }} \right]
$$

$$
\underbrace{\text{Average over possible data sets D, given current prior}}
$$

$$
- \underbrace{ \max_k \left\{ \underset{\varphi,\varphi^C}{E} \left[NB(\varphi, \varphi^C, k) \right] \right\} }_{\text{NB based on \textbf{current} information}} \right\} \tag{12.11}
$$

Equation (12.11) is again made up of two terms:

1. The first term measures the average gain in *NB* from running a study of specific design which generates data *D*. The inner expectation finds the E(*NB*) based on the *posterior* for parameters $\theta = \{\varphi, \varphi^C\}$ given observed data *D*. The optimal strategy given new data *D* is to maximise the posterior E(*NB*). The outer two expectations average over all possible data sets *D* given the proposed study design and based on the *prior* for parameters $\theta = \{\varphi, \varphi^C\}$.

2. The second term of Equation (12.11) is identical to that in Equation (12.4), and measures the Expected Net Benefit obtained using current information, which is simply the maximum E(*NB*) over all interventions.

EVSI is the Expected Net Benefit obtained from sample information on subset φ minus that obtained based on current information [Equation (12.11)].

12.4.1   Computation

Computation of EVSI is challenging, and except in cases where the joint prior distribution is *conjugate* with the likelihood for the generated future data (this means that the distribution of the posterior is the same as that for the prior, e.g. both multi-variate Normal), then it is necessary to resort to a nested sequence of simulations to calculate EVSI. Methodology for the evaluation of EVSI is a topic of active research (see Section 12.7), and is beyond the scope of this book.

Example 12.1 revisited   HIV screening in pregnant women [1].

Expected value of sample information

The EVPI and EVPPI calculations have indicated that there is little value in carrying out further research. It is therefore not necessary to perform EVSI calculations in this example.

12.5   Expected net benefit of sampling

EVSI can be calculated and compared for various different research designs to find the research design that is likely to produce the greatest expected gain in NB. For example, we could calculate EVSI for different proposed sample sizes. EVSI will inevitably increase with increasing sample size, however the larger the new study the more expensive it will be to carry out. The ENBS measures the difference between the E(NB) gain for a population (Population EVSI) from the proposed new study and its cost. The cost of the trial should not only include costs of carrying out the study, but also the lost-opportunity costs (in terms of E(NB)) for those patients allocated to interventions that are not, under current information, the intervention with highest E(NB).

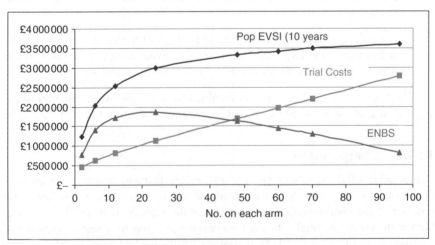

Figure 12.6   Population EVSI (Pop EVSI, discounted over a 10-year time horizon), trial costs and ENBS plotted against the number of clusters per arm in a balanced cluster randomised trial.

Figure 12.6 illustrates how ENBS can be used to determine optimal study design. This example was for a cluster randomised trial, so the number per arm on the x-axis represents the number of *clusters* per arm. EVSI for the population (discounting a 10-year time horizon) increases with the number of clusters on each arm, but at a diminishing rate. The trial costs increase in a near linear relationship with the number of clusters on each arm. The difference between Population EVSI and trial cost is shown by the ENBS which first increases then decreases with the number of clusters on each arm as the additional benefits of increasing the sample size are outweighed by the additional costs. The optimal sample size is at roughly 20 clusters on each arm. Note that this approach to sample size determination differs from a conventional power calculation in that it takes into consideration the CEA model and the impact of increasing sample size on the E(*NB*) gain from reducing decision uncertainty. It is not always feasible to recruit large numbers of clusters/individuals to a trial. An ENBS approach allows us to assess whether there is value in running trials with a suboptimal design. For example, in Figure 12.6, although the optimal number of clusters is around 20 per arm, there is still value in running a trial with only 6 clusters per arm because the ENBS is still positive i.e. the E(*NB*) gains outweigh the trial costs.

12.6   Summary key points

- EVPI measures the expected gain in Net Benefit from running an infinitely sized trial to learn parameter values exactly, over current information.

- EVPI is always straightforward to calculate, although may need very long simulations to obtain precise estimates.

- EVPPI measures the average gain in Net Benefit from knowing perfectly (exactly) what values a subset of the CEA model parameters take, whilst current uncertainty remains for the other CEA model parameters.

- EVPPI can be calculated in a single MCMC simulation under special conditions, otherwise a nested sequence of simulations is required.

- EVSI measures the average gain in Net Benefit from running a study with a specific design and size to inform a subset of parameters.

- EVSI is usually complex to calculate, and this is an area of active research.

- ENBS measures the difference between the Expected Net Benefit gain for a population from a proposed new study of given design, and the cost of such a study.

- ENBS provides a measure on which to determine the optimal design of a future study.

12.7 Further reading

For a good introduction to EVI calculations see Pratt *et al.* [3] and Raiffa and Schlaiffer [4]. The number of examples of applications of EVI analyses is growing in the literature [5–13]. The study of methods for the computation of EVI calculations is an active area of research [2, 14–19].

12.8 Exercises

See Section 7.6 for details of the decision model to compare the prophylactic use of neuraminidase inhibitors (NIs) with standard care for influenza. Use the final CEA model (Exercise 7.3) with uncertainty in d, the Log Odds Ratio of influenza under NI use, and also uncertainty in $p1$, the baseline probability of influenza in the absence of NI use.

12.1 Calculate EVPI, and plot it against willingness to pay per unit of effect.

12.2 Are either of conditions C1 or C2 met for:
(a) EVPPI on Log Odds Ratio, d?

(b) EVPPI on baseline probability of influenza, $p1$?

References

1. Ades A.E., Cliffe S. Markov Chain Monte Carlo estimation of a multi-parameter decision model: consistency of evidence and the accurate assessment of uncertainty. *Medical Decision Making* 2002;**22**:359–371.

2. Ades A., Lu G., Claxton K. Expected value of sample information calculations in medical decision modeling. *Medical Decision Making* 2004;**24**:207–227.

3. Pratt J.W., Raiffa H., Schlaiffer R. *Statistical Decision Theory*. Cambridge, MA: Massachusetts Institute of Technology, 2001.

4. Raiffa H., Schlaiffer R. *Applied Statistical Decision Theory*. New York: Wiley Interscience, 1967.

5. Claxton K., Ades A.E. Efficient research design: an application of value of information analysis to an economic model of zanamivir. In: *Proceedings of the 24th Meeting of the Society for Medical Decision Making*. Baltimore: 2002.

6. Brennan A., Kharroubi S.A. Expected Value of Sample Information for Weibull survival data. *Health Economics* 2007;**16**:1205–1225.

7. Claxton K., Neumann P.J., Araki S., Weinstein M.C. Bayesian value-of-information analysis: An application to a policy model of Alzheimer's disease. *International Journal of Technology Assessment in Health Care* 2001;**17**:38–55.

8. Thompson K.M., Evans J.S. The value of improved national exposure information for perchloroethylene (Perc): a case study for dry cleaners. *Risk Analysis* 1997;**17**:253–271.

9. Claxton K.P., Sculpher M.J. Using value of information analysis to prioritise health research: some lessons from recent UK experience. *Pharmacoeconomics* 2006;**24**:1055–1068.

10. Colbourn T., Asseburg C., Bojke L., *et al*. Prenatal screening and treatment strategies to prevent Group B Streptococcal and other bacterial infections in early infancy: cost-effectiveness and expected value of information analysis. *Health Technology Assessment* 2007;**11**:1–226.

11. Colbourn T.E., Asseburg C., Bojke L., *et al*. Preventive strategies for group B streptococcal and other bacterial infections in early infancy: cost effectiveness and value of information analyses. *British Medical Journal* 2007;**335**:655–661.

12. Yokota F., Thompson K.M. Value of information analysis in environmental health risk management decisions: past, present and future. *Risk Analysis* 2004;**24**:635–650.

13. Yokota F., Thompson K.M. Value of information literature analysis: A review of applications in health risk management. *Medical Decision Making* 2004;**24**:287–298.

14. Brennan A., Kharroubi S.A. Efficient computation of partial expected value of sample information using Bayesian approximation. *Health Economics* 2007;**26**:122–148.

15. Eckermann S., Willan A.R. Expected value of information and decision making in HTA. *Health Economics* 2007;**16**:195–209.

16. Felli J.C., Hazen G.B. Sensitivity analysis and the expected value of perfect information. *Medical Decision Making* 1998;**18**:95–109.

17. Felli J.C., Hazen G. A Bayesian approach to sensitivity analysis. *Health Economics* 1999;**8**:263–268.

18. Tappenden P., Chilcott J.B., Eggington S., *et al*. Methods for expected value of information analysis in complex health economic models: developments on the health economics of interferon-β and glatiramer acetate for multiple sclerosis. *Health Technology Assessment* 2004;**8**(27).

19. Welton N.J., Ades A.E., Caldwell D.M., Peters T.J. Research prioritisation based on Expected Value of Partial Perfect Information: A case study on interventions to increase uptake of breast cancer screening. *Journal of the Royal Statistical Society, Series A* 2008;**171**:807–841.

Appendix 1

Abbreviations

AIC	Akaike's Information Criterion
AIDS	Acquired Immune Deficiency Syndrome
CADTH	Canadian Agency for Drugs and Technology in Health
CE	Cost Effective
CEA	Cost-Effectiveness Analysis
CEAC	Cost-Effectiveness Acceptability Curve
CPM	Confidence Profile Method
DAG	Directed Acyclic Graph
DALYs	Disability Adjusted Life Years
DIC	Deviance Information Criterion
EBM	Evidence-Based Medicine
EFM	Electronic Fetal Heart Rate Monitoring
ENBS	Expected Net Benefit of Sampling
EOGBS	Early Onset Group B Streptococcus
EVI	Expected Value of Information
EVPI	Expected Value of Perfect Information
EVPPI	Expected Value of Partial Perfect Information
EVSI	Expected Value of Sample Information
FDA	Food and Drug Administration
GBS	Group B Streptococcus
Hex	Hospital treated exacerbation
HIV	Human Immunodeficiency Virus
HRT	Hormone Replacement Therapy
ICER	Incremental Cost-Effectiveness Ratio
IDU	Injecting Drug User

Evidence Synthesis for Decision Making in Healthcare, First Edition. Nicky J. Welton,
Alexander J. Sutton, Nicola J. Cooper, Keith R. Abrams and A.E. Ades.
© 2012 John Wiley & Sons, Ltd. Published 2012 by John Wiley & Sons, Ltd.

INB	Incremental Net Benefit
IPD	Individual Patient Data
log	Logarithm (always means log to the base e)
LOR	Log Odds Ratio
MC	Monte Carlo
MCMC	Monte Carlo Markov Chain
MD	Mean Difference
MI	Myocardial Infarction
MLE	Maximum Likelihood Estimate
MPES	Multi-Parameter Evidence Synthesis
MR	Mental Retardation
MSUD	Maple Syrup Urine Disease
NB	Net Benefit
NHS	National Health Service
NICE	National Institute of Health and Clinical Excellence
OR	Odds Ratio
pD	Effective number of parameters
Pex	Primary care treated exacerbation
QALYs	Quality Adjusted Life Years
RCT	Randomised Controlled Trial
RD	Risk Difference
RR	Relative Risk
RSS	Residual Sum of Squares
SSA	Sub-Saharan Africa
STW	Successfully Treated Week
TB	Tuberculosis
TF	Treatment Failure
UTW	Unsuccessfully Treated Week
WHI	Women's Health Initiative

Appendix 2

Common distributions

A2.1 The Normal distribution

Use: Commonly used for both likelihood and priors for continuous variables/ parameters. Note that it covers values from $-\infty$ to $+\infty$.

Notation: Normal(μ, σ^2), mean $= \mu$, variance $= \sigma^2$, precision $= 1/\text{variance}$.

WinBUGS syntax: dnorm(mean,precision).

Flat prior: Set the precision to be small (variance large), e.g. precision $= 0.0001$, dnorm(0,0.0001) or using scientific form dnorm(0,1.0E-4). To restrict prior to positive values (for example for the standard deviation), use the half-normal prior in WinBUGS dnorm(0,1.0E-4)I(0,).

Evidence Synthesis for Decision Making in Healthcare, First Edition. Nicky J. Welton, Alexander J. Sutton, Nicola J. Cooper, Keith R. Abrams and A.E. Ades.
© 2012 John Wiley & Sons, Ltd. Published 2012 by John Wiley & Sons, Ltd.

Probability density for a range of parameter values:

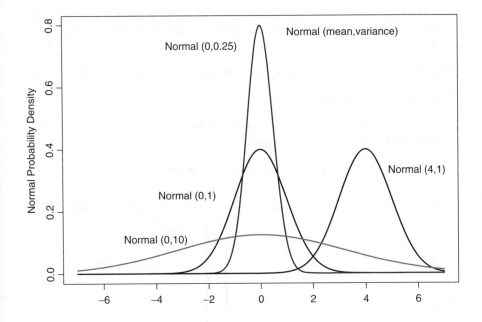

A2.2 The Binomial distribution

Use: Likelihood for number of events out of a given denominator, n.

Notation: Binomial(p, n) where p is the probability/proportion experiencing the event and n is the observed number at risk.

WinBUGS syntax: dbin(p,n).

Flat prior: The Binomial distribution is not used as a prior.

A2.3 The Multinomial distribution

Use: Likelihood for the number of competing events that occur.

Notation: Multinomial($p_1, \ldots, p_k$). Note interpretation p_i is the probability of outcome i. The probabilities $p_1, \ldots, p_k$ must sum to 1.

WinBUGS syntax: dmulti(p[],n), where p[] is the vector ($p_1, \ldots, p_k$).

Flat prior: The Multinomial distribution is not used as a prior.

A2.4 The Uniform distribution

Use: Prior for parameters that can only take values on a specific interval (a, b). Often used for the standard deviation, and for proportion parameters [on interval $(0,1)$].

Notation: Uniform(a, b) or Unif(a, b), mean $= (a + b)/2$, variance $= (b - a)^2/12$.

WinBUGS syntax: dunif(a,b).

Flat prior: Set the range of the Uniform to be large e.g. dunif(-100,100) or dunif(0,100) for positive parameters.

Probability density for a range of parameter values:

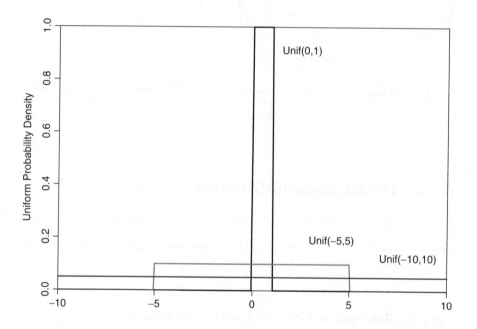

A2.5 The Exponential distribution

Use: Likelihood for positive continuous variables, especially time to events. Often used as a prior for Beta parameters.

Notation: Exponential(λ) or Exp(λ), mean $= 1/\lambda$, variance $= 1/\lambda^2$.

WinBUGS syntax: dexp(lambda).

Flat prior: Set lambda to be small, e.g. dexp(0.01).

Probability density for a range of parameter values:

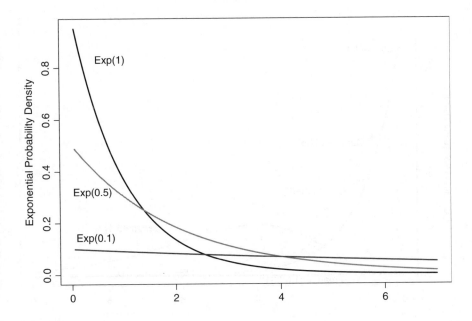

A2.6 The Gamma distribution

Use: Likelihood for positive continuous variables, especially time to events. Often used as a prior for a Normal precision parameter, and prior for Beta parameters.

Notation: Gamma(α,β), mean $= \alpha/\beta$, variance $= \alpha/\beta^2$, shape parameter α, scale parameter β. Setting $\alpha = 1$ gives the Exponential(β) distribution.

WinBUGS syntax: dgamma(alpha, beta).

Flat prior: Set alpha and beta to be small, e.g. dgamma(0.01,0.01).

Probability density for a range of parameter values:

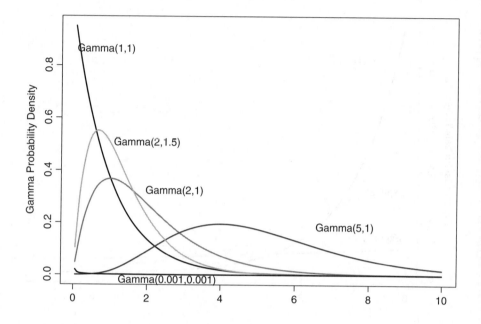

A2.7 The Beta distribution

Use: Prior for proportions/probabilities (takes values between 0 and 1).

Notation: Beta(α, β), mean $= \alpha/(\alpha + \beta)$. Note interpretation α is the prior number of successes, β is the prior number of failures for the Binomial probability parameter.

WinBUGS syntax: dbeta(alpha, beta).

Flat prior: Set alpha and beta equal to 1, dbeta(1,1).

Probability density for a range of parameter values:

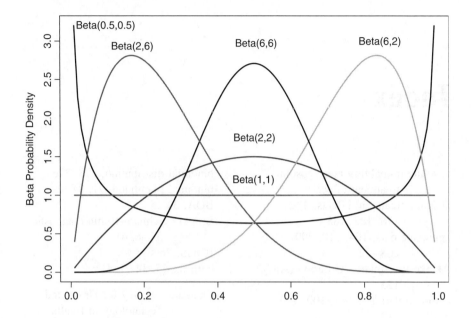

A2.8　The Dirichlet distribution

Use: Prior for multinomial proportions/probabilities (takes values between 0 and 1). This is the extension of the Beta distribution for several probability parameters that must sum to 1.

Notation: Dirichlet($\alpha_1, \ldots, \alpha_k$). Note interpretation α_i is the prior number of outcomes of type i.

WinBUGS syntax: ddirch(alpha[]), where alpha is the vector $(\alpha_1, \ldots, \alpha_k)$.

Flat prior: Set alpha as a vector of 1's: in WinBUGS syntax alpha<-c(1, 1, ..., 1).

Index

Evidence Synthesis for Decision Making in Healthcare, First Edition. Nicky J. Welton,
Alexander J. Sutton, Nicola J. Cooper, Keith R. Abrams and A.E. Ades.
© 2012 John Wiley & Sons, Ltd. Published 2012 by John Wiley & Sons, Ltd.